OBSTETRICS AND GYNECOLOGY ADVANCES

# HANDBOOK ON OVARIAN CANCER

## RISK FACTORS, THERAPIES AND PROGNOSIS

# OBSTETRICS AND GYNECOLOGY ADVANCES

Additional books in this series can be found on Nova's website
under the Series tab.

Additional e-books in this series can be found on Nova's website
under the e-book tab.

OBSTETRICS AND GYNECOLOGY ADVANCES

# HANDBOOK ON OVARIAN CANCER

## RISK FACTORS, THERAPIES AND PROGNOSIS

BETHANY R. COLLIER
EDITOR

*New York*

**Library of Congress Cataloging-in-Publication Data**

Library of Congress Control Number: 2015952555

ISBN: 978-1-63483-874-0

*Published by Nova Science Publishers, Inc. † New York*

# CONTENTS

# PREFACE

Ovarian cancer is the third most diagnosed gynecologic cancer and the first leading cause of death from all of gynecological malignancies. High mortality of the patients is usually associated with the progression of the disease. Most patients are diagnosed within the advanced stages due to lacking relevant diagnostic and screening markers. This handbook discusses several risk factors of ovarian cancer. It also examines the different therapies provided to ovarian cancer patients, and the prognosis of the cancer.

Chapter 1 - The exact causes of the sporadic cases of the most malignant gynecological cancer, ovarian carcinoma, are still difficult to ascertain. However, they account for the vast majority of ovarian cancer cases (~ 85%). The remaining cases may be attributed to genetic alterations in genome, chromosomes, genes and regulatory factors. Within this group, germline mutations in BRCA1/2 and DNA mismatch repair genes are the best known genetic risk factors. The aim of the epidemiological studies is to find out the risk or protective factors, associated with the ovarian cancer. In this review, the authors focus on a brief survey of these factors, with emphasis put particularly on the genetic alterations, reproductive factors and life style factors along with dietary factors. Unfortunately, there is no factor found to be fully protective. On the other hand, there is also no factor known to result in 100% risk of development of ovarian cancer. Further investigations of factors associated with ovarian cancer are warranted, similarly as the search for novel diagnostic markers and improved treatment options.

Chapter 2 - Ovarian cancer (OC) is the third most diagnosed gynecologic cancer and the first leading cause of death from all of gynecological malignancies. OC presents with the highest mortality rate, largely due to its advanced stage at the time of diagnosis. About 90% of these cases are epithelial ovarian cancer (EOC), and 70% are diagnosed with widespread intra-abdominal or distant metastases. Unfortunately, the frequency of invasive and advanced EOC is mostly due to the lack of a suitable and sufficiently reliable screening tool at the moment of diagnosis. Despite new strategies and improvements in surgical techniques and chemotherapeutic options, a 5-year survival rate for invasive EOC is approximately 46%. The main symptoms reported from OC include abnormal vaginal bleeding, pelvic and abdominal pain, weight loss, back pain, urinary urgency, and fatigue, which contribute to the difficulties of an early diagnosis, thereby resulting in low prognosis and survival rates. The treatment of early stage OC involves surgical resection followed by chemotherapy; clinical trials show an overall survival rate with adjuvant platinum-based chemotherapy, but this treatment in sub-groups of patients may vary according to different prognosis. Many risk factors associated with breast cancer are also related to the risk of other gynecologic cancers, such as OC. They include current age, age at menarche, parity, and first-degree family history with a wide inter-individual genetic variations in the susceptibility of OC. Recent studies regarding genome-wide association have reported several single nucleotide polymorphisms that confer low-penetrance susceptibility to EOC. In addition, mutations in BRCA gene, the gene that produces breast cancer-linked protein, are strongly associated with hereditary forms of OC. Hormone replacement therapy is further associated with increased risks of OC, mainly long duration use of both unopposed estrogens and estrogens plus progestins, regardless of treatment regimen. Independent prognostic factors are often considered including those described by International Federation of Gynecology and Obstetrics (FIGO), such as stage, tumor grade, volume of residual OC, and specific biomarkers for predicting survival in ovarian tumor patients. This chapter will discuss the new therapies, major risk factors in early and advanced ovarian cancer stage, and most prognostic factors as a tool for improving the survival rate outcomes in women.

Chapter 3 - Ovarian cancer is the most deadly gynecological cancer. High mortality of the patients is usually associated with the progression of the disease. Most of the patients are diagnosed within the advanced stages due to lacking relevant diagnostic and screening markers. Achieving the diagnosis in the early stages of disease is a prerequisite of the more successful treatment of ovarian cancer. In this review, the authors focus on the recent progress in research focused on circulating, particularly cell-free microRNAs expression in diagnostically relevant samples such as blood, plasma/serum and urine. More research will be needed to establish circulating and extracellular microRNAs as the novel diagnostic markers for ovarian cancer.

Chapter 4 - Ovarian cancer remains the leading cause of death among gynecological malignancies. Surgery should be performed in adnexal masses suspected of ovarian cancer for diagnosis, staging and treatment. The debulking surgery is still the main surgical approach in advanced primary ovarian cancer. The adjuvant treatment is performed with taxanes and platinum-based chemotherapy. The addition of the bevacizumab, an anti-angiogenic agent, is recommended. Adjuvant treatment in ovarian cancer in advanced stage leads to an improvement in disease-free survival in approximately 10-30% of patients, depending on the stage and residual disease. Retrospective data show better outcomes in patients who underwent complete cytoreduction. Immunotherapy can be insufficient to eliminate all tumor when used alone. However, the use after surgery and chemotherapy can be useful to eliminate remaining tumor cells.

In recent years, there was an increase in the use of immunohistochemical markers in ovarian cancer. Most of the published data refers to the use of antibodies for diagnosis, some markers also has prognostic value.

In general, when immunohistochemistry is utilized for diagnosis markers panels provide better information than the use of a single antibody. Ovarian cancer is a heterogeneous disease; each of the subtypes is associated with different genetic risk factors and molecular events during oncogenesis. Each subtype responds differently to chemotherapy.

The tendency of ovarian cancer treatment is moving toward different therapies for their specific subtypes. It is likely that a panel of tumor markers will be required to detect all subtypes of the disease. The ovarian cancer subtypes should be considered as distinct diseases in biomarker studies and clinical trials, in order to relate the biomarker, diagnosis and prognosis.

The main aim of this chapter is to provide an update of the current treatments in ovarian cancer. The section also demonstrates the potential targets of future therapies, such as immunotherapy and target therapies.

Chapter 5 - The physiological actions of dopamine (DA) are mediated by five receptors (DR) that are divided into two major groups: D1 and D2. The D1-like subtypes (DR1 and DR5) can activate the adenylate cyclase thereby increasing the cAMP level, but the D2-like subtypes (DR2, DR3 and DR4) lead to the opposite effect (i.e., decreasing the cAMP level). The role of DA and DR in cancer therapy remains unclear. Human ovarian cancer cells express all DR except DR3. The DR2-mediated inhibition of the Src activation can reverse the permissive microenvironment for tumor growth attributable to chronic stress. DA favors the uptake of cisplatin via stabilizing tumor blood vessels, which results from DR1-mediated activation of the cAMP–kinase A signaling pathway. An antagonist of DR2 can inhibit tumor growth by targeting the VEGFR-2/PI3K/mTOR pathway. The blockage of D2-family proteins inhibits growth of cancer cells (including cancer stem cells). Therefore, DR2 can be a target for cancer treatments.

Chapter 6 - Malignant ovarian germ cell tumors are a very uncommon disorder. The incidence is estimated in 0.5/100000 women. They represent only a 5 percent of ovarian cancers overall. Mostly, ovarian germ cell neoplasms affect women aged between 10-30 years and they constitute in this collective the most frequent ovarian tumor (around 70%).

These type of neoplasms have their origin on the primordial ovarian cells. There are different hystological subtypes: they can be divided into embryo-like neoplasms (immature teratoma and dysgerminoma) and placenta-like neoplasms (similar than extraembrionic fetal-derived cell population), or a mixture. The main malignant ovarian germ cell are: *immature teratoma, dysgerminoma, endodermalsinus (yolksac) tumors, embryonalcell carcinoma, choriocarcinoma, polyembrioma and mixedgermcelltumors.*

Basically, patients present abdominal pain with abdominal enlargement, abnormal vaginal bleeding and/or precocious puberty.Tumor marker tester can be increased, as AFP, beta-HCG, inhibin, CA 125, LDH.

Malignant ovarian germ cell tumors are staged by the International Federation of Gynecology and Obstetrics (FIGO) into: stage I, confined to the ovarian; stage II extension into other pelvic organs; stage III, disease extended into the abdmen or retroperitoneal lymphnodes; stage IV, metastatic disease beyond the abdomen or affecting the liver. Frequently, the tumor is diagnosed at stage I.

Treatment involves primary surgery, depending on the preferences of the patient to conserve or not her fertility. Fertility-sparing surgery must be done laparoscopically with an intraoperative frozen section evaluation. At advanced stages, chemotherapy can be involved to complete the treatment. Malignant ovarian germ cell tumors have an excellent prognosis: 5-years survival after complete suitable treatment is more than 85%.

In this chapter, treatment and prognosis are going to be explained, according to the official international guidelines.

Chapter 7 - Ovarian cancer is one of the commonest malignancy in women worldwide and has an annual incidence of 239 000. It is the most lethal of all the gynaecological malignancies, the fifth leading cause of cancer death, and claimed 151 917 lives in 2012. Ovarian cancer often presents at an advanced stage, with the involvement of the peritoneal surface either at the initial diagnosis or at recurrence. Despite the advances made in the surgical techniques and chemotherapeutic options regarding agents, schedule, and route of administration, majority of the patients recur and eventually succumb to their disease. The change in the surgical approach, in a bid to attain optimal cytoreduction with no gross residual disease, has seen improvement in the survival, as has the use of intraperitoneal chemotherapy in combination with intravenous agents. Cytoreductive surgery (CRS) and hyperthermic intraperitoneal chemotherapy (HIPEC) provide the combined benefits of surgical eradication and effective chemotherapy, and can be performed with acceptable morbidity and mortality. Further trials are being undertaken to examine its role in the primary, as well as recurrent settings of advanced ovarian cancer and to determine the ideal drug combinations and dosages. The authors aim to discuss these increasing controversies.

Chapter 8 - Ovarian cancer is the second most common gynecologic malignancy among women worldwide after endometrial cancer and the most common cause of death in women with gynecologic malignancies. Because of the increasing life expectancy experienced worldwide it is estimated that the incidence of this aggressive disease will significantly increase in the next few decades. Among all cases diagnosed with ovarian cancer the histopathological subtype consisting of epithelial tumors represents the largest part and has been widely studied. However, there is still an important number of patients who are diagnosed in an advanced stage of the disease, when disseminated bulky tumors are already present. It has been demonstrated that the most frequent patterns of spread are represented by the peritoneal, hematogenous and lymphatic route, all of them being responsible in different proportions for the presence of upper abdominal burden which sometimes is present from the moment of initial diagnosis. In all these cases the therapeutic mainstay remains cytoreductive surgery, followed by taxanes and platinum based adjuvant chemotherapy. When it comes to long term outcomes, among various prognostic factors such as age, stage at diagnosis, histopathological subtype, differentiation grade and residual disease, only residual disease has been widely demonstrated to strongly impact survival; at the same time, the amount of residual tumor burden at the end of debulking surgery is the only parameter which is influenced by the treating physician's experience. The presence of upper abdominal disseminations has been considered for a long period of time to be the sign of a tumor with a more aggressive biology and was considered as a poor prognostic factor. The main invaded organs in the upper abdomen consist of liver and porta hepatis, diaphragm, and less common, the spleen. While in cases presenting hepatic involvement the presence of hematogenous disease has been accepted as a poor prognosis factor and was classified the disease as FIGO stage IV, there was no explicit specification whether parenchimatous splenic involvement should be classified as part of the same FIGO stage. Initially a poorer outcome was reported for patients submitted to splenectomy as part of debulking surgery for advanced stage epithelial ovarian cancer, this fact being related to a more aggressive biological behaviour of the tumor. Other studies have stipulated the fact that the presence of splenic metastases is an independent poor prognosis factor but they could not distinguish whether the poorer outcome is related to the presence of hematogenous involvement of the upper abdominal parenchimatous viscera or to the co-existence of bulky left quadrant upper abdominal tumoral burden.

However, the initial results were strongly influenced by the small number of cases included and by the different characteristics of the included patients. For example patients submitted to splenectomy as part of primary and secondary cytoreduction were included in the same study so the results were also influenced by the moment of performing the surgery.

More recently, a significant difference in terms of survival was reported for hematogenous versus peritoneal splenic metastases and concluded that their presence should be considered as an explicit criterion for FIGO stage IV disease. Although it is a safe and effective surgical procedure, performing a splenectomy as part of cytoreductive surgery for advanced stage or relapsed ovarian cancer might associate a higher rate of postoperative morbidity rather due to the fact that in these cases ovarian cancer becomes a systemic disease with multiple visceral involvements, imposing multiple visceral resections in order to achieve an R0 resection; in all these cases the postoperative outcomes are influenced by a cumulative postoperative risk related to each performed resection in part.

However, since splenectomy can be safely performed with acceptable rates of postoperative complications it should be routinely performed in cases presenting splenic tumoral involvement in order to increase the rate of complete cytoreduction. This chapter focuses on the patterns of spread, prognostic factors of patients with splenic involvement, safety and effectiveness of splenectomy as part of cytoreductive surgery for advanced stage and relapsed epithelial ovarian cancer.

Chapter 9 - Ovarian cancer is one of the most aggressive gynecologic malignancies and represents a major cause of death for women worldwide. This aggressive behavior is especially related to the fact that most patients are diagnosed in an advanced stage of the disease when disseminated tumoral burden is already present. Although the intraperitoneal route seems to be the most common pattern of spread, ovarian cancer can also develop distant metastases by hematogenous route and throughout lymphatic channels, the most commonly affected sites by hematogenous spread including the lungs and liver. Historically, patients with liver involvement have been considered as having a systemic, uncontrollable disease and were considered as candidates for supportive care or palliative chemotherapy.

Although the presence of liver metastases at the moment of diagnosis is usually associated with an altered tumor biology and aggressive disease, there was no convincing evidence that cytoreduction in the presence of liver metastases is less efficacious. Starting from this hypothesis, hepatic resection for ovarian cancer liver metastases has been proposed.

However, at this moment it is estimated that the number of patients submitted to liver resection for hepatic metastases from gynecological cancer represent less than 1% of the total resected liver metastases, the role of surgery in patients with ovarian cancer liver metastases being still in question. The main reason for this paucity of hepatectomies in ovarian cancer liver metastases is related to the fact that usually these kinds of tumors develop liver metastases in the settings of obvious systemic or regional dissemination which is not suitable for a complete macroscopic resection. Patients presenting resectable, isolated and limited to liver metastases are rather an exception than a rule in the setting of ovarian cancer. However this small subgroup of patients with isolated hepatic lesions has been initially considered to suit best to liver resection.

According to this principle, initially the main indication for resection in ovarian cancer liver metastases was the presence of solitary liver lesions with no extrahepatic tumoral burden as the best results in terms of survival had been obtained in such cases. More recently, it has been demonstrated that the presence of extrahepatic tumoral burden does not represent a significant prognostic factor for a poorer outcome in all patients and allowed to identify the subsets of patients with extrahepatic tumor burden who could benefit most from liver resections.

A crucial step in studying the long term outcomes after liver resection for ovarian cancer hepatic metastases was demonstrating the different outcomes between the two distinct patterns of hepatic involvement: peritoneal and hematogenous spread. Metastases originating from peritoneal seeding with parenchimatous invasion of at least 2 cm were classified as peritoneal lesions while lesions entirely surrounded by liver parenchyma were considered to have hematogenous origins. Significant differences in terms of survival between patients with peritoneal versus hematogenous lesions submitted to complete resections were observed. Based on these findings, it has been largely accepted that the presence of peritoneal seeding involving the liver included the case in FIGO stage IIIC while the presence of hematogenous liver involvement should be classified as FIGO stage IV.

When it comes to the role of liver resection as part of secondary or even tertiary cytoreduction, literature data is even scarcer, the presence of liver metastases being considered for long time as an exclusion criterion when establishing whether a patient is a candidate for optimal cytoreduction at the moment of surgery for recurrent disease. In time, improved understating of hepatic anatomy in association with the improvement of surgical techniques and postoperative care transformed hepatic resection in a more frequent associated surgical procedure in serial resections for ovarian cancer relapse. Once liver resection has been successfully associated as part of cytoreduction for relapsed ovarian cancer, attention was focused on determining other potential prognostic factors which might influence survival such as initial FIGO stage, disease free survival or histopatologic subtype of the tumor.

This chapter focuses on the subject of liver resection as part of cytoreductive surgery for advanced stage or relapsed ovarian cancer. The influence of different patterns of spread, the safety and effectiveness of performing anatomical or extended liver resections are also presented.

Chapter 10 - Ovarian cancer is the leading cause of death in the gynaecologic cancers within the UK and US. Presently the standard treatment for ovarian cancer entails the use of chemotherapy drugs paclitaxel and carboplatin after aggressive surgical reduction in order to prolong the patient's life for multiple years. However, prolonged use of platinum-based chemotherapy often leads to drug resistance, which causes the ovarian cancer patient to relapse and potential death. Therefore there is an urgent medical need for breakthrough drugs with an effective therapeutic impact on ovarian cancer. Phytochemicals (plant-derived natural products) have been used for thousands of years as treatment for various diseases, because of their huge chemical diversity and wide range of biological activities.

In this review, the role of phytochemicals as chemo-preventive compounds, potential sources of new drugs for ovarian cancer and the benefits of their adoption as mono-therapeutic agents or as chemosensitizers when used in-conjunction with the conventional anti-cancer drugs is highlighted. The authors will describe the phytochemicals: 1) clinically approved drugs such as paclitaxel and camptothecin including its semi-synthetic derivatives topotecan and irinotecan; 2) currently in clinical trials such as epipodophyllotoxin derivatives etoposide and teniposide, ventfolide, phenoxodiol, and combretastatins; 3) in preclinical trials such as quercetin, baicalein, baicalin, thymoquinone, betulinic acid and tetrandrine; and novel compounds which have high potency ($IC_{50}$ less than 10 μM) and have been discovered recently (last 15 years). In particular, several new compounds including bufatrienolides, ipomoeassin D, 2'-(R)-O-acetylglaucarubinone, and molvizarin have $IC_{50}$s lower than 100 nM in ovarian cancer cells and might have different mechanisms of action from those of platinum derivatives/paclitaxel, therefore providing potential ways to attack multidrug resistance in ovarian cancer without jeopardising the patient's treatment.

Chapter 11 - Introduction. Ovarian cancer has the highest rate of mortality among gynecological malignancies and it is the fifth leading cause of cancer-related death in women of developed countries. It is often diagnosed at late stage, therefore, despite optimal cytoreduction by debulking surgery and adjuvant chemotherapy, recurrence is frequent.

New therapeutic strategies are needed to treat relapses and advanced stage chemoresistant ovarian cancer. Ovarian cancer is characterized by different molecular phenotypes, and it can be classified in five tumor types with different clinical, pathologic and prognostic properties, and with different chemosensitivity.

Objective. This review will focus on molecular alterations involved in ovarian cancer carcinogenesis, which may become new targets for therapy in the future. Biological therapies can impact on the prognosis, especially in advanced chemoresistant ovarian cancer patients.

Discussion. The most important pathways involved in ovarian cancer chemoresistance are PI3K/ AKT/ mTOR, KRAS/ MAPK/ ERK, BRCA1/BRCA2, Notch and Forkhead Box M1 pathways.

The amplification of PI3K is more frequent in high-grade ovarian tumors rather than in low grade ones, together with AKT phosphorylation, contributing to disease progression.

KRAS mutations are frequent in low-grade ovarian tumors, and their expression varies in different histopathological types. Loss of PTEN is frequently present in high-grade serous carcinomas and correlates with a poor prognosis.

Several protein kinases and other signaling molecules, such as KRAS, BRAF, PI3KCA and CTNNB1, have been evaluated and their mutations have been correlated with prognosis. Epigenetic modifications are promising targets for ovarian cancer treatment. Several studies on molecular alterations have been conducted on ovarian cancer tissue, but further studies are needed to tailor every therapy to the specific histotype of ovarian cancer.

Actually, the approved biological therapies currently used in ovarian cancer patients are only three: Bevacizumab (a monoclonal antibodies directed against VEGF, usually utilized in platinum-pretreated patients), Pazopanib (tyrosine) and Olaparib (PARP-inhibitor, utilized in BRCA1/2 mutated patients).

Further studies are needed to better evaluate different chemoresistance related pathways, and to find new targets on which to focus clinical research.

Conclusions. Among the analyzed studies, only molecular alterations of PI3KI seem to have the strongest correlation with prognosis. These mutations could be future targets of therapy for chemoresistant patients, but more studies are required.

Chapter 12 - Worldwide, ovarian cancer is the seventh cancer in frequency and the eighth cause of death from cancer in women. Epithelial ovarian cancer is also the leading cause of death among gynaecologic malignancies. Nowadays, the standard management of epithelial ovarian cancer is the correct surgical staging and optimal tumor cytoreduction followed by platinum plus taxane-based chemotherapy. Standard surgical treatment for early stages consists on peritoneal washings, total hysterectomy and bilateral anexectomy, inspection all organs and peritoneum surface, taking samples of suspicious areas, omentectomy and pelvic and para-aortic lymphadenectomy. Laparoscopic approach allows to do this surgical staging with less morbidity and mortality than a more aggressive laparotomy approach. After this complete surgical staging, the International Federation of Gynaecology and Obstetrics (FIGO) staging system for ovarian cancer ought to be applied to determine the management and prognosis of the patient. In advanced stages complete tumor cytoreduction has demonstrated survival advantage compared to incomplete debulking. The morbidity associated with the debulking surgery does not increase mortality. However, some patients with advanced epithelial ovarian cancer undergo debulking surgery but complete cytoreduction is not achieved, with an increase of the morbidity and no improvement in overall survival. There are some criteria to predict the cytoreduction outcomes, based on serum biomarkers levels, preoperative imaging techniques and laparoscopic based scores. Optimization of patient selection for primary cytoreduction would determine which patients could benefit from a complete cytoreduction or which ones might benefit from neoadjuvant chemotherapy and interval surgery.

Chapter 13 - Chemotherapy is limited by toxicity to noncancerous tissues and the development of chemoresistance. Here the authors discuss the use of low intensity ultrasound to modulate chemotherapy against ovarian cancer. Ultrasound can enhance the action of certain drugs, including circumvention of chemoresistance. Ultrasonic cavitation plays the leading role in sonochemotherapy, which permeabilizes the cell membrane favoring the influx of drugs. Recent trials suggest that ultrasound can modulate chemotherapy via multiple pathways, and synergize the sensitization due to a chemical modulator such as verapamil and cyclosporin A. Ultrasound can be efficiently delivered to the preselected volume within the body thus realizing a targeted therapy. This technique can be specifically developed as a non-drug technique to improve the therapeutic outcome of chemotherapy against ovarian cancer.

Chapter 14 - Introduction. Ovarian cancer, the main cause of death among gynaecological malignancies, affects half of women in postmenopausal age. With the increase in older population, this tumor will be more frequent in elderly women, but not all the elderly patients can undertake standard treatments, due to comorbidities and less functional organ reserves.

New therapeutic approaches are needed to obtain an amendable overall survival and quality of life in this kind of patients.

Objective. The author's aim is to propose the best management of elderly ovarian cancer patients, taking account of biological age over chronologic age, with the aim to assure suitable treatments with a better overall survival.

Discussion. Carboplatin-paclitaxel doublet is the standard treatment in patients with ovarian cancer; elderly patients are less treated with this therapy, due both to comorbidities and to the major toxicity. When the standard schedule every 21 days is administered in elderly patients, dose delay or previous stop for toxicity is frequent.

Furthermore, elderly are not candidate for intraperitoneal chemotherapy and HIPEC (hyperthermic intraperitoneal chemotherapy), due to highest toxicity. Chemotherapy is often the only possible choice for these patients, because a surgical debulking can be too much aggressive and associated with several morbidities.

Elderly have the same chemosensitivity than younger: geriatric assessment is fundamental to screen elderly population fitting for chemotherapy, and new strategies with less toxicity have to be investigated. Older patients with ovarian cancer have been underrepresented in clinical trials, so the few clinical studies with this kind of population must be evaluated.

It's not clear whether doublets or single agents are better in the treatment of elderly ovarian cancer patients. Single agent options for elderly patients include liposomal doxorubicin, topotecan, gemcitabine and vinorelbine. Doublet combinations every 21 days have been largerly investigated, but only small clinical trials have been conducted on weekly schedule. Weekly carboplatin and paclitaxel have demonstrated an optimal compliance among elderly patients.

For what concern targeted therapies, there are no elderly-specific data on PARP inhibitors, but they appear to be well tolerated, on the opposite to antiangiogenic agents, which require more caution in the older population.

Metronomic chemotherapy and weekly schedules are the best solutions for elderly patients, for their efficacy and tolerability, contributing to quality of life.

Conclusions. Metronomic therapy, comprising weekly schedules, can be an optimal option for elderly ovarian cancer patients. Prospective studies are needed to develop further strategies for these women.

In: Handbook on Ovarian Cancer
Editor: Bethany R. Collier

ISBN: 978-1-63483-874-0


*Chapter 1*

# RISK FACTORS IN OVARIAN CANCER: A BRIEF OVERVIEW

***Ludek Zavesky[1,*], Eva Jandakova[2] and Radovan Turyna[3]***
[1]Institute of Biology and Medical Genetics, First Faculty of Medicine, Charles University Prague and General University Hospital in Prague, Prague, The Czech Republic
[2]Institute of Pathology, University Hospital Brno, Brno, The Czech Republic
[3]Institute for the Care of Mother and Child, Prague, The Czech Republic

## ABSTRACT

The exact causes of the sporadic cases of the most malignant gynecological cancer, ovarian carcinoma, are still difficult to ascertain. However, they account for the vast majority of ovarian cancer cases (~ 85%). The remaining cases may be attributed to genetic alterations in genome, chromosomes, genes and regulatory factors. Within this group, germline mutations in BRCA1/2 and DNA mismatch repair genes are the best known genetic risk factors. The aim of the epidemiological studies is to find out the risk or protective factors, associated with the ovarian cancer. In this review, we focus on a brief survey of these factors, with emphasis put particularly on the genetic alterations, reproductive factors and life style factors along with dietary factors. Unfortunately, there is no factor found to be fully protective. On the other hand, there is also no factor known to result in 100% risk of development of ovarian cancer. Further investigations of factors associated with ovarian cancer are warranted, similarly as the search for novel diagnostic markers and improved treatment options.

## INTRODUCTION

Ovarian cancer as the most deadly gynecological cancer is a complex disease showing high histological and molecular heterogeneity. Accumulating evidence revealed several pitfalls needed to be resolved in relation to ovarian carcinogenesis. The first one is to

* Corresponding author: e-mail: ludek.zavesky@gmail.com.

elucidate the exact origin of ovarian cancer with suspected roles of various parts of gynecological tract [1-3]. Within the ovarian carcinogenesis, the role of cancer stem cells and the processes of epithelial to mesenchymal (and vice versa) transition and other important factors should be elucidated, particularly in cancer initiation, progression, chemoresistance and recurrence [4, 5].

Most of ovarian cancer cases are attributed to epithelial ovarian cancer (EOC, ovarian carcinomas) with several histological subtypes; serous (~70% of EOC), endometrioid, mucinous, clear cell, transitional cell subtypes have been traditionally recognized. Recently, it has been shown that ovarian cancer may be distinguished into two types I and II, based on their molecular characteristics. Type I are tumors with rare TP53 mutations, early stages and indolent clinical course. Type II is represented by aggressive tumors, with frequent TP53 mutations and genetic instability [6, 7].

Due to high mortality/incidence index of patients with ovarian carcinomas, finding novel diagnostic and screening markers or techniques with high sensitivity and specificity is warranted [8]. The promising markers may be found particularly in body fluids, with a large interest of researchers for microRNAs. They represent the class of non-coding small RNAs functioning as post-transriptional regulators of gene expression involved in fundamental cellular processes and occurring also in extracellular fractions of body fluids [9-11]. Improving treatment options remains as another necessary goal [12].

Last, but not least, hereditary and non-hereditary risk and prognostic factors should be evaluated. Identification of causal factors in ovarian carcinogenesis thus remains the great challenge of the current biomedical research. Therefore, many potential risk factors have been studied to help prevent development of the disease. These factors may be interrelated and associated also with the abovementioned processes.

In this review, we will focus on the risk factors that have been shown to be or not to be associated with ovarian cancer. Their identification might be useful in determination of risk groups within genetic counseling and other prevention programs.

## Genetic Alterations and Ovarian Cancer Risk

Changes in genetic information may be responsible for the development of ovarian cancer. They may be both hereditary and those found in somatic (tumor) tissues.

### Germline Mutations

Hereditary forms of ovarian cancer are less frequent and comprise about 15% of the cases. The germline mutations of tumor suppressor genes BRCA1/2 are a prominent group known to cause hereditary forms of breast and ovarian cancer in susceptible families (i.e., hereditary breast and ovarian cancer syndrome). The BRCA1 and BRCA2 genes are located on chromosomes 17 and 13, respectively, and function as tumor suppressor genes, particularly in repair of DNA double-strand breaks via homologous recombination (HR). Over 1,800 mutations have been identified in BRCA1 and over 1,500 mutations in BRCA2 genes so far [13]. Their carriers develop ovarian cancer much frequently than non-carriers.

The risk for ovarian cancer ranges from 1.4% in normal population to 40% (36% to 46%) in BRCA1 mutations carriers and to 18% (10% to 27%) in BRCA2 mutation carriers [14, 15].

In addition to BRCA1/2 mutations, germline mutations in DNA mismatch repair genes (MMR) may result in development of ovarian cancer within the hereditary non-polyposis colorectal carcinoma syndrome. Most of the cases are attributed to MSH2 and MLH1 homologs mutations, the remaining mutations mostly occur in MSH6 and PSM2 homologs. It has been suggested that 10% to 15% of the hereditary ovarian cancer cases is caused by the mutations in DNA mismatch repair genes, while the risk for development of ovarian cancer is 8% to 15% in their carriers. MMR deficiency with the defects in MMR genes may result in microsatellite instability and consequently in accumulation of single nucleotide mutations and altered length of microsatellite sequences. Interestingly, most of cases with germline MMR mutations were shown to be endometrioid and clear cell histological subtypes (see [16]).

## Somatic Mutations and Genetic Alterations

Mutations in tumor suppressor gene TP53 occur in almost 100% of high-grade serous cancers. Protein p53 is involved in many key cellular processes including DNA repair, co-ordination of cell cycle arrest, and apoptosis associated with DNA damage. These processes are affected also in ovarian cancers. Brachova et al. [17] have investigated the relationship of oncomorphic TP53 mutations and patient outcomes in advanced serous ovarian cancer patients. They divided mutations as oncomorphic (those conferring oncogenic activity), loss of function (LOF), or unclassified. They found significantly worse progression-free survival (PFS), a 60% higher risk of recurrence (HR = 1.60, 95% confidence intervals (CI) 1.09, 2.33, $p = 0.015$), and higher rates of platinum resistance ($p = 0.0024$) in patients with oncomorphic TP53 mutations in comparison with single nucleotide mutations not categorized as oncomorphic [17].

Genomic instability as the hallmark of cancer may be associated with defects in genes involved in homologous recombination (HR), the processes of the repair of double double-strand breaks, for example in BRCA1/2, Fanconi Anemia genes and RAD50. Zhang et al. [18] consider the chromosomal alteration and the mutator phenotype, which can be quantified by the frequency of copy-number change (CNC) and the frequency of somatic mutation, respectively, as the two forms of genomic instability.

Using TCGA database, the authors [18] determined genomic instability score for each sample by the number of CNC regions (n1) and the number of somatic mutations (n2) within a cancer genome, according to the formula: Score = K x n1 + n2. In their study, K was set to 0.5.

The score appeared to be useful to discriminate patients in regard to their outcomes; in the high-score group the 5-year survival rate was 38%, while in the low-score group, this survival rate was 25% [18].

They found that patients with BRCA1 and BRCA2 mutations in tumors had significantly improved survival than wild-type ovarian cancer patients [18]. The 5-year survival rate of BRCA1 mutation carriers was 46% (95% CI, 32%, 68%) while in BRCA2 58% (95% CI, 41%, 83%), i.e., significantly higher than in wild-type patients exhibiting 25% (95% CI, 18%, 33%) 5-year survival rate [18]. Moreover, tumors with germline and somatic BRCA mutations did not differ in outcomes and in genomic instability. However, BRCA2 mutated tumors revealed higher genomic instability than BRCA1-disrupted tumors. High level of both BRCA mutation and CNC was associated with improved overall survival in BRCA mutation carriers compared with wild-type patients [18].

Identification of BRCA mutations with respect to risk of development of ovarian/breast cancer and for the success of treatment thus remain the main goals of this kind of research. Rebbeck et al. [19] have identified associations of differential breast and ovarian cancer risks and particular mutations cluster regions. Although the BRCA mutation status is unknown in majority of patients, the response to chemotherapy may differ between mutation carriers and non-carriers. From this point of view, the PARP inhibitors attract the main attention due to blockage of base excision repair by Poly-ADP ribose polymerase group of enzymes. As the BRCA1/2 mutated tumor cells are defective in homologous recombination repair processes, this treatment might be highly tumor-specific. Moreover, it has been shown in clinical trials that both patients with germline BRCA mutations and without mutations may benefit from this type of therapy. However, challenges still remain to establish markers for identification of patients without BRCA1/2 mutations, responding to PARP inhibitors [20].

Many large chromosomal rearrangements with deletions and amplifications have been reported for ovarian carcinoma tissues previously. For example, Gorringe et al. [21] have analyzed 398 samples and their genome-wide copy number alterations and found that copy number gains were located particularly on 3q (63% of samples with CN gain) and 8q (62%), 20q (47%) and 12p (39%). On the contrary, regions of chromosomes X, 8p, 22q, 17, 4q, 19p and 16 have revealed frequent CN losses. The authors also identified positive CN associations of 17q12/22q losses and 3q13/19q12 gains with overall survival. These associations, however, were not significant for progression-free survival. The alteration in copy numbers may affect thousands of genes in these regions [21].

The Cancer Genome Atlas Network project has analyzed DNA copy numbers, mRNA and microRNA expression and promoter methylation in 489 high-grade serous ovarian adenocarcinomas (HGS-OvCa) and exome DNA sequencing in 316 HGS-OvCa samples [22]. Mutations in TP53 predominated (in at least 96% of samples), mutations in BRCA1 and BRCA2 were detected in 22% of tumors; however several other mutated genes (RB1, NF1, FAT3, CSMD3, GABRA6 and CDK12) were found only in 2 - 6% of samples [22].

# Reproductive Factors and Ovarian Cancer Risk

## Contraceptive Use

During the long-term usage of modern hormonal contraception methods over last decades, specific health impacts have been recognized. The most important effects of hormonal contraception use were decreased risk of ovarian cancer, while the risk of breast cancer increased. As regards other cancers affected by use of oral contraceptives, Gierish et al. [23] have found in their metaanalyses that incidence of cervical cancer increases with the use of contraceptives in women with human papillomavirus infection. They proved the increased risk for breast cancer and decreased risk for colorectal and endometrial cancers [23].

Going back to ovarian cancer, a large study based on 70,259 women (The Shanghai Women's Health Study (SWHS)) investigated impact of various contraception methods and ovarian cancer risk [24]. Non-significant reduction of ovarian cancer risk was observed in ever users of any contraception, and also in long-term users (> 20 years), while the only significant association of contraceptive use and ovarian cancer risk was observed for **intrauterine devices (IUD)**. Increasing duration of IUD use, particularly longer than 20 years had significantly decreased the risk for ovarian cancer [24]. In this study, **higher number of ovulation years and later age of menopause** were significantly associated with increased risk of ovarian cancer [24], the fact known from many previous investigations. Interestingly, a different pattern of protective effect of IUD has been observed in the study of Ness et al. [25]. The authors found protective effect of short using this type of contraception while the longer duration of use resulted in nonsignificantly greater risk of ovarian cancer. In this study, the authors explored data for nine hundred two cases with incident ovarian/peritoneal/tubal cancer and 1,800 population-based control subjects. The results indicated that protective effects may be found in **oral contraceptives, tubal ligation, IUDs and vasectomy** (respective ORs 0.75, 0.63, 0.75, and 0.77) [25].

Charlton et al. [26] investigated associations of oral contraceptive use and causes of mortality in 121,577 women included in Nurses' Health Study. They found no association between ever use of oral contraceptives and all-cause mortality. Increased rates of violent or accidental death and deaths due to breast cancer were found in oral contraceptive users, while ovarian cancer-attributed deaths were less common among women who used oral contraceptives [26].

However, accumulating evidence suggests that use of oral contraceptives is really associated with increased risk of breast cancer, especially in young women [27]. Therefore, the possibility to use oral contraceptives as the prevention of ovarian cancer may be misleading.

## Tubal Ligation

Association of the origin of ovarian cancer and fallopian tube has been recognized recently for one histological subtype; high-grade serous carcinomas (type 2) have been proposed to originate from the epithelium of the fallopian tube [2, 3].

Tubal ligation (TL) has been suggested as the protective factor reducing the risk of ovarian cancer. This mechanical treatment prevents transport of oocytes and sperm, and simultaneously, stops retrograde transport of "substances which hypothetically might trigger epithelial cell carcinogenesis in the peritoneum and on the ovarian surface epithelium." [28]. However, understanding the underlying mechanisms of tubal ligation effects requires more attention. Cibula et al. [28] reviewed the effects potentially responsible for the observations of reduced ovarian cancer risk. The authors proposed that previously suspected factors such as screening effects and altered hormonal levels may not be the true causes of the risk reduction. The use of talc powder, inconsistently reported to increase the risk for ovarian cancer (see [28]), however, may not be ruled out and partially it may explain the reduced risk after TL preventing the ascent of carcinogenic substances from vagina and perineum. The cells coming from the tissues embryologically derived from the Müllerian ducts are the mainly suspected causes of extraovarian origin of ovarian cancer. Fallopian tube, Müllerian rests, rete ovarii and endometrial cells are the sources of this ascent. This may be prevented by TL, and the risk of ovarian cancer development may be attributed to this factor [28].

A large recent Danish study evaluated tubal ligation and salpingectomy and the risk of epithelial ovarian cancer and borderline ovarian tumors [29]. This study included 13,241 epithelial ovarian cancer cases and 3,605 borderline ovarian tumors. The authors found reduced overall epithelial ovarian cancer risk (odds ratios 0.87; 95% confidence interval 0.78 – 0.98) in patients with tubal ligation, particularly for endometrioid cancer (odds ratios 0.66; 95% confidence interval 0.47 – 0.93) and also for rare ovarian tumors (odds ratios 0.60; 95% confidence interval 0.43 – 0.83). No association was found for tubal ligation and risk of borderline ovarian tumors. Moreover, bilateral salpingectomy reduced epithelial ovarian cancer risk by 42% (odds ratios 0.58; 95% confidence interval 0.36 – 0.95) [29].

## Other Reproductive Factors

In a large epidemiological study on ovarian cancer, Gates et al. [30] investigated associations of ovarian cancer risk and various factors. They found an inverse association of **duration of breastfeeding** associated with all 3 subtypes (serous invasive, endometrioid, mucinous), but the association was strongest for mucinous tumors (RR = 0.43 per year). On the contrary, Tsilidis et al. [31] found no association of the risk of ovarian cancer and breastfeeding; this finding is however exceptional among the studies which mostly prove the protective effect [32]. Breastfeeding was proved to decrease the risk of ovarian cancer also in a recent metanalysis of previous studies OR 0.66 (95% CI: 0.57 - 0.76; $P < 0.001$), which identified the most significant decrease when duration of breastfeeding was 8 to 10 months [33].

**Age at natural menopause** may be inversely associated with the risk of ovarian cancer. For example, Tsilidis et al. [31] found that higher age at menopause was associated with a higher risk of ovarian cancer (>52 *vs* ≤ 45 years: HR, 1.46; 95% CI, 1.06 – 1.99; *P*-trend, 0.02). Again, on the contrary, Schildkraut et al. [34] found no association between ovarian cancer risk and age at natural menopause. However, it should be noted that natural menopause before age 40 may be associated with higher rate mortality both all-cause and cause-specific [35, 36], implicating difficulties in interpretation of data.

**In vitro fertilization (IVF) treatment** involving ovarian stimulation has been suspected as another factor potentially altering the risk for ovarian cancer. For example, Van Leeuwen et al. [37] analyzed 19,146 women undergoing IVF and 6,006 sub-fertile women without IVF. They found that ovarian malignancies, mostly borderline tumors were more likely to develop in the former group. This risk was 2-fold. The risk for invasive ovarian cancer was increased even 15 years after the IVF [37]. While the controversies on the issue have been remaining, Li et al. [38] performed a meta-analysis of ten studies not proving the detrimental impact of IVF on the risk of ovarian cancers.

**Hormone replacement therapy (HRT)** has been relatively widely used as the treatment in peri-menopausal women. However, it has become evident that this therapy may increase the risk for ovarian cancer. Collaborative Group on Epidemiological Studies of Ovarian Cancer performed a metaanalysis of 52 epidemiological studies [39], involving 21,488 postmenopausal women participating in 17 prospective and 35 retrospective studies. They found increased risk for ovarian cancer in ever-users than in never-users of hormone therapy, with relative risk (RR) 1.20 in prospective studies, and RR 1.14 for all studies combined. Current or recent HRT use resulted in an RR of 1.37 (95% CI 1.29 – 1.46; $p<0.0001$). There exist differences among histological subtypes. The risk was definitely increased only in serous (RR 1.53, 95% CI 1.40 – 1.66; $p<0.0001$) and endometrioid subtypes (1.42, 1.20 – 1.67; $p<0.0001$). Little heterogeneity was observed for ovarian cancer risk between estrogen-only and estrogen-progestagen preparations giving the same RR 1.37 in prospective studies, and RR 1.32 and RR 1.25 in all studies, respectively. Risk was also significantly increased in current users giving the greatest relative risk (RR 1.41, 95% CI 1.32 – 1.50; $p<0.0001$). However, the long-term effects of HRT persist in those women who had less than 5 years of hormone therapy use in this group (RR 1.43, 95% CI 1.31 – 1.56; $p<0.0001$). The increased risk was also observed for recent ex-users being within 5 years of last use (RR 1.23, 95% CI 1.09 – 1.37; $p = 0.0006$ in prospective studies). There was still an excess of serous or endometrioid tumors about 10 years after stopping long-duration hormone therapy use (RR 1.25, 95% CI 1.07 – 1.46, $p = 0.005$). The risk of ovarian cancer was found to be largely or wholly causal, giving the women who use hormone therapy for 5 years from around age 50 years one extra ovarian cancer per 1000 users [39].

**Parity** has been shown as the protective factor while **nulliparity** may increase the risk of ovarian cancer. Bodelon et al. [40] have evaluated impact of risk factors by parity status using data from two prospective cohorts, the National Institutes of Health-AARP Diet and Health Study (NIH-AARP) and the Prostate, Lung, Colorectal, and Ovarian Cancer Screening Trial (PLCO) with 623 women diagnosed with invasive epithelial ovarian cancer included in the analyses. The authors have shown that parous women may be at a reduced risk of ovarian cancer in comparison with nulliparous women (HR 0.79, 95% CI: 0.63, 0.98). They have also found stronger reduction of the risk with more births. While the authors have not found differences for other risk factors by parity, they observed associations of risk with some other factors. For example, the use of OC reduced the risk of ovarian cancer, while long duration of use of hormone therapy ($\geq$10 years) increased the ovarian cancer risk. An increased risk was observed also in cases with first degree family history of breast and/or ovarian cancer (HR = 1.37, 95% CI: 0.81, 2.34 in nulliparous women; HR = 1.21, 95% CI: 0.97, 1.51 in parous women). There were differences as regards smoking. Nulliparous women who were current smokers exhibited an increased risk of ovarian cancer (HR = 1.40, 95% CI: 0.78, 2.49) in comparison with never smokers. By contrast, parous women who were current smokers have shown an ovarian cancer risk decrease (HR = 0.76, 95% CI: 0.55, 1.05) [40].

## Lifestyle & Dietary Factors and Ovarian Cancer Risk

Factors associated with lifestyle may affect many diseases including cancer. However, data are often inconclusive and difficult to obtain as reliable as possible.

**Smoking** is clearly associated with the development of lung carcinomas but its associations with other carcinomas are less clear. In ovarian cancer, smoking has been shown as the risk factor for mucinous subtype of ovarian cancer. Gram et al. [41] have shown that the risk of mucinous tumors in current smokers was increased by 85% (HR = 1.85, 95% CI 1.08 – 3.16). By contrast, there was not found any association of smoking with serous ovarian cancer. Within the group of endometrioid subtypes, the risk was even decreased in both current (HR = 0.58, 95% CI 0.29 – 1.15) and former (HR = 0.83, 95% CI 0.48 – 1.45) smokers [41].

Indeed, Calle et al. [42] found similar results in a metaanalysis of previous investigations. Increase in incidence of mucinous (mainly borderline than fully malignant) tumors was found in current smokers (RR 1.79, 95% CI 1.60 – 2.00, p<0.0001). On the contrary, current smokers showed decreased risk for both endometrioid (0.81, 95% CI 0.72 – 0.92, p = 0.001) and clear-cell (0.80, 95% CI 0.65 – 0.97, p = 0.03) ovarian cancer subtypes [42]. However, it is far from meaningfulness and reality to use smoking as the prevention of ovarian cancer, particularly due to its detrimental health effects.

Associations between **obesity, diabetes mellitus** and risk of ovarian cancer have been investigated in several studies. Diabetes mellitus (DM) has been found as the risk factor for progression-free survival (PFS) that was 10.3 months for patients with DM in comparison with 16.3 months in patients without DM [43]. Body mass index (BMI), associated with obesity and overweight may be a risk factor for ovarian cancer independent on menopausal status [44]. Physical activity and exercising may potentially reduce risk for ovarian cancer but data are controversial [45].

**Dietary factors** may possibly affect many diseases and have been investigated in many epidemiological studies involving ovarian cancer. We should point out that many results are often contradictory and inconclusive. **Milk and dairy products** have been thoroughly investigated from this point of view. There has not been found any provable effect of milk and dairy products consumption and ovarian cancer risk [46, 47]. However, higher intake of lactose may be associated with lower risk of endometrioid ovarian cancer in adulthood (HR 0.32, 95% CI 0.16-0.65, p (trend) < 0.001) [46].

**Dietary acrylamide** intake is another risk factor not proved to be associated with ovarian cancer risk [48]. However, when focused on non-smokers, there was an increased risk of borderline significance for ovarian cancer in never smoking women associated with high acrylamide intake (RR = 1.39; 95% CI, 0.97 – 2.00) [49].

Similarly, **alcohol consumption** did not prove to be associated with ovarian cancer risk [50]. High consumption of **sugar and sugary food** as the suspicious factor for ovarian cancer risk has been evaluated in several studies. Although being tentative and inconclusive in some studies, sugar consumption in its various forms has been indeed found as the risk factor. King et al. [51] suggested higher risk associated with sugar beverage consumption. A large recent study investigating sugars in diet and risk of cancer in the NIH-AARP Diet and Health Study showed that high consumption of all investigated sugars was inversely associated with risk of ovarian cancer [52].

Do particular **dietary ingredients and quality of food** have impact on ovarian cancer risk? This tempting question raised inconclusive answers in many epidemiological studies. Scoring diet quality using three dietary indices (Eating Index-2005: HEI-2005, Alternative Healthy Eating Index-2010: AHEI-2010, the Alternate Mediterranean Diet Score: aMDS) have not come with proofs of their associations with ovarian cancer risk [53]. Similarly, Chandran et al. [54] have revealed neither individual food groups usable for a prevention of ovarian cancer or the specific impact of food quality previously. Nevertheless, it may be that food quality may improve the survival in patients with ovarian cancer diagnosis [55].

Total dietary intake of **flavonoids** may be associated with decreased risk of ovarian cancer, however this association was found non-significant [56]. Tea consumption in relation to ovarian cancer risk is questionable. Cassidy et al. [56] have found significant protective effect (HR: 0.69; 95% CI: 0.52; 0.93; P-trend = 0.03), however, tea and coffee consumption have not been associated with ovarian cancer risk in metaanalysis elsewhere [57]. Crane et al. [58] suggested that no specific dietary factors are consistently associated with ovarian cancer risk.

**Dietary fat intake** is another factor not clearly associated with ovarian cancer risk. The highest intake of polyunsaturated fat (HR = 1.22, 95% CI = 1.02 – 1.48, P trend = 0.02) may be associated with an increased risk of invasive EOC [59]. Other factors, such as consumption of total fat, animal or plant fat, saturated fat, cholesterol, monounsaturated fat, or fatty fish revealed no association with ovarian cancer risk [59]. Associations of fat consumption and ovarian cancer risk remain elusive as some studies have found no associations, but the other revealed higher risk for ovarian cancer associated with total, animal, and dairy fat [58].

On the other hand, **fish consumption** was not proved to be associated with risk and prevention of ovarian cancer in a metanalysis of the previous studies [60]. Olive oil has been shown as a possibly protective dietary component in relation to ovarian cancer risk (see [61]). Phytoestrogens, isoflavones and enterolignans have been shown inversely, but insignificantly associated with ovarian cancer risk. On the other hand, lignan compounds **matairesinol** (OR 0.72, 95% CI: 0.54; 0.96; P for trend = 0.02) and **lariciresinol** 0.72 (95% CI 0.55; 0.96; P for trend = 0.03) have reached statistical significance [62].

High **soya and its isoflavones** intake has been shown to decrease the risk for ovarian cancer in southern Chinese women [63]. Even though it is congruent with findings reported in breast cancer [64], the protective effects may be more complicated. For example, impact of phytoestrogens consumption on ovarian cancer risk was not proved in Swedish cohort [65]. The results may be affected by the ethnogeographical reasons and other unknown related factors, as the soya consumption was proved as protective in multiethnic cohort involving Japanese Americans, whites, Latinos, African Americans and Native Hawaiians. Within them, the protective effects in relation to breast cancer risk estimates indicated that higher isoflavone intake may be protective only in Latina, African American and Japanese American women [66].

Ethnogeographical factors and related issues should also be taken into account when considering other studies on dietary associations with ovarian cancer. Southern Chinese women have been shown to benefit from **mushroom consumption**, especially from white button mushroom. Their high consumption (more than 2 g per day) resulted in reduced risk of ovarian cancer with adjusted odds ratios 0.68 (95% CI, 0.52 - 0.89) for these women in comparison with those consuming less than 2 g per day [67]. Southern Chinese women have been also reported with decreased risk of ovarian cancer when consuming more fruit and vegetables [68], but for this issue data are generally disputable [58]. On the contrary, higher consumption of preserved foods may be associated with increased risk of ovarian cancer as shown again in Southern Chinese women [69].

Consumption of **red meat** may possibly increase the risk for various cancers, ovarian cancer being among them. Although two previous studies have failed to find an association [70, 71], a more recent study found that red meat consumption increases the risk for ovarian cancer (OR = 1.29; 95% CI: 1.16 - 1.43), and also of the cancers of oral cavity and pharynx, nasopharynx, esophagus, larynx, colon, rectum, pancreas, breast and endometrium [72].

**Nitrate and nitrite** are commonly used additives in many foods. In epithelial ovarian cancer, they have been suggested to increase the risk in women with highest intake. Highest intake of dietary nitrate increases the risk by 31% (95% CI: 1.01 - 1.68), while highest nitrite intake increases this risk by 34% (95% CI: 1.05 - 1.69) in women in highest intake quintile compared with women within the lowest intake quintile [73].

## Occupational Exposure Factors and Ovarian Cancer Risk

There is a huge number of people (125 million people all around the world) working in environments exposed to **asbestos**. Based on the recent metaanalysis, asbestos exposure increases the risk of ovarian cancer in exposed women. The authors showed the overall pooled standardized mortality ratio (SMR) 1.77 (95% CI, 1.37 – 2.28), with a moderate degree of heterogeneity among the studies ($I^2 = 35.3\%$, $p = 0.061$) [74].

Interestingly, Le et al. [75] have evaluated risk of ovarian cancers in various occupation positions. They found significantly higher risk in **teaching-associated occupations**, teaching and related (category SOC 27, adjusted OR 1.77, 95% CI 1.15 – 2.81) and other teaching and related (category SOC 279, adjusted OR 3.11, 95% CI 1.35 – 8.49). Other categories with significant higher risk were bookkeepers and accounting clerks (category SOC 4131, adjusted OR 2.80, 95% CI 1.30 – 6.80). Category SIC 65 (other retail stores) had adjusted OR 2.19, 95% CI 1.16 – 4.38; SIC 85 (educational service) showed adjusted OR 1.45, 95% CI 1.00 – 2.13; and SIC 863, and non-institutional health services revealed adjusted OR 2.54, 95% CI 1.13 – 6.52) [75].

## Conclusion

Ovarian carcinomas with their heterogeneity and relatively low incidence remain the entity difficult to be evaluated from the epidemiological point of view. In this review, we focused on a brief survey of investigated factors. Their causal role, however, deserves more attention and warrants further investigations to be elucidated properly. Therefore, we omitted here to speculate about the reasons why some factors increase the risk for ovarian cancer, while the other decrease the risk, as the arguments may be highly speculative and have been addressed to elsewhere. Genetic factors, particularly mutations in BRCA1/2 and MMR genes, may be the strong risk factors that should be considered in genetic counseling and prevention programs. Some protective factors such as healthy diet and physical activity are vague, and difficult to interpret as their ovarian cancer-specific basis may be only tentative. Several reproductive factors have the impact on risk of ovarian cancer, but there could be hardly any recommendation made as the prevention based on them. However, infertility treatments (particularly hormonal interventions) and associated risks for mother and child should be seriously considered not only for ovarian cancer risk, because their detrimental effects cannot be ruled out. Similarly, application of HRT in peri-menopausal women should be taken into account as the risk factor for ovarian cancer. Epidemiological factors associated with the risk of ovarian cancer should be further investigated to reveal their causal roles. There remain the goals of current medical research endeavoring to reduce the incidence, maximize the early diagnosis and increase the efficiency of treatment with improved outcomes for patients with ovarian cancer.

## ACKNOWLEDGMENTS

The financial support from the Charles University Prague (project PRVOUK-P27/LF1/1) is appreciated.

## REFERENCES

[1] Dubeau, L. (2008). The cell of origin of ovarian epithelial tumours. *Lancet Oncology*, *9*, 1191-1197.

[2] Auersperg, N. (2011). The Origin of Ovarian Carcinomas: A Unifying Hypothesis. *International Journal of Gynecological Pathology*, *30*, 12-21.

[3] Erickson, B. K., Conner, M. G. & Landen, J. (2013). The role of the fallopian tube in the origin of ovarian cancer. *American Journal of Obstetrics and Gynecology*, *209*, 409-414.

[4] Vergara, D., Merlot, B., Lucot, J. P., et al. (2010). Epithelial-mesenchymal transition in ovarian cancer. *Cancer Letters*, *291*, 59-66.

[5] Zavesky, L., Jancarkova, N. & Kohoutova, M. (2011). Ovarian cancer: Origin and factors involved in carcinogenesis with potential use in diagnosis, treatment and prognosis of the disease. *Neoplasma*, *58*, 457-468.

[6] Kurman, R. J. & Shih, I. M. (2011). Molecular pathogenesis and extraovarian origin of epithelial ovarian cancer-Shifting the paradigm. *Human Pathology*, *42*, 918-931.

[7] Koshiyama, M., Matsumura, N. & Konishi, I. (2014). Recent concepts of ovarian carcinogenesis: Type I and type II. *BioMed Research International*, 201*4*, 934261. doi: 10.1155/2014/934261.

[8] Lutz, A. M., Willmann, J. K., Drescher, C. W., et al. (2011). Early diagnosis of ovarian carcinoma: Is a solution in sight. *Radiology*, *259*, 329-345.

[9] Weber, J. A., Baxter, D. H., Zhang, S. L., et al. (2010). The MicroRNA Spectrum in 12 Body Fluids. *Clinical Chemistry*, *56*, 1733-1741.

[10] Zavesky, L., Jandakova, E., Turyna, R., et al. (2015). Evaluation of Cell-Free Urine microRNAs Expression for the Use in Diagnosis of Ovarian and Endometrial Cancers. A Pilot Study. *Pathology Oncology Research*, In press. DOI: 10.1007/s12253-015-9914-y

[11] Zavesky, L., Jandakova, E., Turyna, R., et al. (2015). New perspectives in diagnosis of gynaecological cancers: Emerging role of circulating microRNAs as novel biomarkers. *Neoplasma, 62*(4), 509-520. doi: 10.4149/neo_2015_062.

[12] Banerjee, S. & Kaye, S. B. (2013). New strategies in the treatment of ovarian cancer: Current clinical perspectives and future potential. *Clinical Cancer Research*, *19*, 961-968.

[13] The Human Gene Mutation Database at the Institute of Medical Genetics in Cardiff (2015). http://www.hgmd.cf.ac.uk/ac/gene.php?gene=BRCA1

[14] Kan, C. W. S., Howell, V. M., Hahn, M. A., et al. (2015). Genomic alterations as mediators of miRNA dysregulation in ovarian cancer. *Genes Chromosomes and Cancer*, *54*, 1-19.

[15] McCann, G. A. & Eisenhauer, E. L. (2015). Hereditary cancer syndromes with high risk of endometrial and ovarian cancer: Surgical options for personalized care. *Journal of Surgical Oncology*, *111*, 118-124.

[16] Xiao, X., Melton, D. W. & Gourley, C. (2014). Mismatch repair deficiency in ovarian cancer - Molecular characteristics and clinical implications. *Gynecologic Oncology*, *132*, 506-512.

[17] Brachova, P., Mueting, S. R., Carlson, M. J., et al. (2015). TP53 oncomorphic mutations predict resistance to platinum- and taxane-based standard chemotherapy in patients diagnosed with advanced serous ovarian carcinoma. *International Journal of Oncology*, *46*, 607-618.

[18] Zhang, S., Yuan, Y. & Hao, D. (2014). A genomic instability score in discriminating nonequivalent outcomes of BRCA1/2 mutations and in predicting outcomes of ovarian cancer treated with platinum-based chemotherapy. *PLoS One*. *9*(12), e113169. doi: 10.1371/ journal.pone.0113169.

[19] Rebbeck, T. R., Mitra, N., Wan, F., et al. (2015). Association of Type and Location of BRCA1 and BRCA2 Mutations With Risk of Breast and Ovarian Cancer. *JAMA*. 2015, *313*(13), 1347-1361. doi:10.1001/jama.2014.5985.

[20] Liu, J. F., Konstantinopoulos, P. A. & Matulonis, U. A. (2014). PARP inhibitors in ovarian cancer: Current status and future promise. *Gynecologic Oncology*, *133*, 362-369.

[21] Gorringe, K. L., George, J., Anglesio, M.S., et al. (2010). Copy number analysis identifies novel interactions between genomic loci in ovarian cancer. *PLoS One*. 2010 Sep 10, *5*(9). pii: e11408. doi: 10.1371/journal.pone.0011408.

[22] Bell, D., Berchuck, A., Birrer, M., et al. (2011). Integrated genomic analyses of ovarian carcinoma. *Nature*, *474*, 609-615.

[23] Gierisch, J. M., Coeytaux, R. R., Urrutia, R. P., et al. (2013). Oral contraceptive use and risk of breast, cervical, colorectal, and endometrial cancers: A systematic review. *Cancer Epidemiology Biomarkers and Prevention*, *22*, 1931-1943.

[24] Huang, Z., Gao, Y., Wen, W., et al. (2015). Contraceptive methods and ovarian cancer risk among Chinese women: A report from the Shanghai Women's Health Study. *International Journal of Cancer*, 137(3), 607-14. doi: 10.1002/ijc.29412.

[25] Ness, R. B., Dodge, R. C., Edwards, R. P., et al. (2011). Contraception Methods, Beyond Oral Contraceptives and Tubal Ligation, and Risk of Ovarian Cancer. *Annals of Epidemiology*, *21*, 188-196.

[26] Charlton, B. M., Rich-Edwards, J. W., Colditz, G. A., et al. (2014). Oral contraceptive use and mortality after 36 years of follow-up in the Nurses' Health Study: Prospective cohort study. *BMJ* (Online), *349*, g6356. doi: 10.1136/bmj.g6356.

[27] Beaber, E. F., Malone, K. E. & Tang, M. T. C. (2014). Oral contraceptives and breast cancer risk overall and by molecular subtype among young women. *Cancer Epidemiology Biomarkers and Prevention*, *23*, 755-764.

[28] Cibula, D., Widschwendter, M., Zikan, M., et al. (2011). Underlying mechanisms of ovarian cancer risk reduction after tubal ligation. *Acta Obstetricia et Gynecologica Scandinavica*, *90*, 559-563.

[29] Madsen, C., Baandrup, L., Dehlendorff, C., et al. (2015). Tubal ligation and salpingectomy and the risk of epithelial ovarian cancer and borderline ovarian tumors:

A nationwide case-control study. *Acta Obstetricia et Gynecologica Scandinavica, 94*, 86-94.

[30] Gates, M. A., Rosner, B. A., Hecht, J. L., et al. (2010). Risk Factors for Epithelial Ovarian Cancer by Histologic Subtype. *American Journal of Epidemiology, 171*, 45-53.

[31] Tsilidis, K. K., Allen, N. E., Key, T. J., et al. (2011). Oral contraceptive use and reproductive factors and risk of ovarian cancer in the European Prospective Investigation into Cancer and Nutrition. *British Journal of Cancer, 105*, 1436-1442.

[32] Schuler, S., Ponnath, M., Engel, J., et al. (2013). Ovarian epithelial tumors and reproductive factors: A systematic review. *Archives of Gynecology and Obstetrics, 287*, 1187-1204.

[33] Feng, L. P., Chen, H. L. & Shen, M. Y. (2014). Breastfeeding and the Risk of Ovarian Cancer: A Meta-Analysis. *Journal of Midwifery and Women's Health, 59*, 428-437.

[34] Schildkraut, J. M., Cooper, G. S., Halabi, S., et al. (2001). Age at natural menopause and the risk of epithelial ovarian cancer. *Obstetrics and Gynecology, 98*, 85-90.

[35] Mondul, A. M., Rodriguez, C., Jacobs, E. J., et al. (2005). Age at natural menopause and cause-specific mortality. *American Journal of Epidemiology, 162*, 1089-1097.

[36] Li, S., Rosenberg, L., Wise, L. A., et al. (2013). Age at natural menopause in relation to all-cause and cause-specific mortality in a follow-up study of US black women. *Maturitas, 75*, 246-252.

[37] Van Leeuwen, F. E., Klip, H., Mooij, T. M., et al. (2011). Risk of borderline and invasive ovarian tumours after ovarian stimulation for in vitro fertilization in a large Dutch cohort. *Human Reproduction, 26*, 3456-3465.

[38] Li Y., Zhao J., Zhang, Q., et al. (2015) Does ovarian stimulation for IVF increase gynaecological cancer risk? A systematic review and meta-analysis. *Reproductive BioMedicine Online*, in press.

[39] Collaborative Group on Epidemiological Studies of Ovarian Cancer. (2015). Menopausal hormone use and ovarian cancer risk: Individual participant meta-analysis of 52 epidemiological studies. *Lancet*, 385(9980), 1835-42. doi: 10.1016/S0140-6736(14)61687-1.

[40] Bodelon C., Wentzensen, N., Schonfeld, S. J., et al. (2013). Hormonal risk factors and invasive epithelial ovarian cancer risk by parity. *British Journal of Cancer, 109*(3), 769-76.

[41] Gram, I. T., Lukanova, A., Brill, I., et al. (2012). Cigarette smoking and risk of histological subtypes of epithelial ovarian cancer in the EPIC cohort study. *International Journal of Cancer, 130*, 2204-2210.

[42] Calle, E. E., Gapstur, S. M., Patel, A. V., et al. (2012). Ovarian cancer and smoking: Individual participant meta-analysis including 28 114 women with ovarian cancer from 51 epidemiological studies. *The Lancet Oncology, 13*, 946-956.

[43] Shah, M. M., Erickson, B. K., Matin, T., et al. (2014). Diabetes mellitus and ovarian cancer: More complex than just increasing risk. *Gynecologic Oncology, 135*, 273-277.

[44] Poorolajal, J., Jenabi, E. & Masoumi, S. Z. (2014). Body mass index effects on risk of Ovarian cancer: A meta-analysis. *Asian Pacific Journal of Cancer Prevention, 15*, 7665-7671.

[45] Moorman, P. G., Jones, L. W., Akushevich, L., et al. (2011). Recreational Physical Activity and Ovarian Cancer Risk and Survival. *Annals of Epidemiology, 21*, 178-187.

[46] Merritt, M. A., Poole, E. M., Hankinson, S. E., et al. (2014). Dairy food and nutrient intake in different life periods in relation to risk of ovarian cancer. *Cancer Causes and Control*, *25*, 795-808.

[47] Liu, J., Tang, W., Sang, L., et al. (2015). Milk, yogurt, and lactose intake and ovarian cancer risk: A meta-analysis. *Nutrition and Cancer*, *67*, 68-72.

[48] Obon-Santacana, M., Peeters, P. H. M., Freisling, H., et al. (2015). Dietary intake of acrylamide and epithelial ovarian cancer risk in the european prospective investigation into cancer and nutrition (EPIC) cohort. *Cancer Epidemiology Biomarkers and Prevention*, *24*, 291-297.

[49] Pelucchi, C., Bosetti, C., Galeone, C., et al. (2014). Dietary acrylamide and cancer risk: An updated meta-analysis. *International Journal of Cancer*, *136*, 2912-2922.

[50] Kelemen, L. E., Bandera, E. V., Terry, K. L., et al. (2013). Recent alcohol consumption and risk of incident ovarian carcinoma: A pooled analysis of 5,342 cases and 10,358 controls from the *Ovarian Cancer Association Consortium. BMC Cancer*, *13*, 28. doi: 0.1186/1471-2407-13-28.

[51] King, M. G., Olson, S. H., Paddock, L., et al. (2013). Sugary food and beverage consumption and epithelial ovarian cancer risk: A population-based case-control study. *BMC Cancer*, *13*, 94. doi: 10.1186/1471-2407-13-94.

[52] Tasevska, N., Jiao, L., Cross, A. J., et al. (2012). Sugars in diet and risk of cancer in the NIH-AARP Diet and Health Study. *International Journal of Cancer*, *130*, 159-169.

[53] Xie, J., Poole, E. M., Terry, K. L., et al. (2015). A prospective cohort study of dietary indices and incidence of epithelial ovarian cancer. *Journal of Ovarian Research.*, *7*, 112. doi: 10.1186/s13048-014-0112-4.

[54] Chandran, U., Bandera, E. V., Williams-King, M. G., et al. (2011). Healthy eating index and ovarian cancer risk. *Cancer Causes and Control*, *22*, 563-571.

[55] Thomson, C. A., Crane, T. E., Wertheim, B. C., et al. (2014). Diet Quality and Survival After Ovarian Cancer: Results From the Women's Health Initiative. *JNCI-Journal of the National Cancer Institute.*, *106*(11). pii: dju314. doi: 10.1093/jnci/dju314

[56] Cassidy, A., Huang, T., Rice, M. S., et al. (2014). Intake of dietary flavonoids and risk of epithelial ovarian cancer. *American Journal of Clinical Nutrition*, *100*, 1344-1351.

[57] Braem, M. G. M., Onland-Moret, N. C., Schouten, L. J., et al. (2012). Coffee and tea consumption and the risk of ovarian cancer: A prospective cohort study and updated meta-analysis. *American Journal of Clinical Nutrition*, *95*, 1172-1181.

[58] Crane, T. E., Khulpateea, B. R., Alberts, D. S., et al. (2014). Dietary intake and ovarian cancer risk: A systematic review. *Cancer Epidemiology Biomarkers and Prevention*, *23*, 255-273.

[59] Merritt, M. A., Riboli, E., Weiderpass, E., et al. (2014). Dietary fat intake and risk of epithelial ovarian cancer in the European Prospective Investigation into Cancer and Nutrition. *Cancer Epidemiology*, 2014 Oct;38(5), 528-37. doi: 10.1016/j.canep. 2014. 07.011.

[60] Jiang, P. Y., Jiang, Z. B., Shen, K. X., et al. (2014). Fish intake and ovarian cancer risk: A meta-analysis of 15 case-control and cohort studies. *PLoS ONE*, *9*(4), e94601. doi: 10.1371/journal.pone.0094601

[61] Psaltopoulou, T., Kosti, R. I., Haidopoulos, D., et al. (2011). Olive oil intake is inversely related to cancer prevalence: A systematic review and a meta-analysis of

13800 patients and 23340 controls in 19 observational studies. *Lipids in Health and Disease, 10*, 127. doi: 10.1186/1476-511X-10-127.

[62] Neill, A. S., Ibiebele, T. I., Lahmann, P. H., et al. (2014). Dietary phyto-oestrogens and the risk of ovarian and endometrial cancers: Findings from two Australian case-control studies. *British Journal of Nutrition, 111*, 1430-1440.

[63] Lee, A. H., Su, D., Pasalich, M., et al. (2014). Soy and isoflavone intake associated with reduced risk of ovarian cancer in southern Chinese women. *Nutrition Research, 34*, 302-307.

[64] Kang, H. B., Zhang, Y. F., Yang, J. D., et al. (2012). Study on soy isoflavone consumption and risk of breast cancer and survival. Asian Pacific *Journal of Cancer Prevention, 13*, 995-998.

[65] Hedelin, M., Lo, M., Andersson, T. M. L., et al. (2011). Dietary phytoestrogens and the risk of ovarian cancer in the women's lifestyle and health cohort study. *Cancer Epidemiology Biomarkers and Prevention, 20*, 308-317.

[66] Morimoto, Y., Maskarinec, G., Park, S. Y., et al. (2014). Dietary isoflavone intake is not statistically significantly associated with breast cancer risk in the Multiethnic Cohort. *British Journal of Nutrition, 112*, 976-983.

[67] Lee, A. H., Pasalich, M., Su, D., et al. (2013). Mushroom intake and risk of epithelial ovarian cancer in Southern Chinese women. *International Journal of Gynecological Cancer, 23*, 1400-1405.

[68] Tang, L., Lee, A. H., Su, D., et al. (2014). Fruit and vegetable consumption associated with reduced risk of epithelial ovarian cancer in southern Chinese women. *Gynecologic Oncology, 132*, 241-247.

[69] Lee, A. H., Su, D., Pasalich, M., et al. (2013). Preserved foods associated with increased risk of ovarian cancer. *Gynecologic Oncology, 129*, 570-573.

[70] Larsson, S. C. & Wolk. A. (2005). No association of meat, fish, and egg consumption with ovarian cancer risk. *Cancer Epidemiology Biomarkers and Prevention, 14*, 1024-1025.

[71] Schulz, M., Nöthlings, U., Allen, N., et al. (2007). No association of consumption of animal foods with risk of ovarian cancer. *Cancer Epidemiology Biomarkers Prevention, 16*(4), 852-5.

[72] Di Maso, M., Talamini, R., Bosetti, C., et al. (2013). Red meat and cancer risk in a network of case-control studies focusing on cooking practices. *Annals of Oncology, 24*, 3107-3112.

[73] Aschebrook-Kilfoy, B., Ward, M. H., Gierach, G. L.et al. (2012). Epithelial ovarian cancer and exposure to dietary nitrate and nitrite in the NIH-AARP Diet and Health Study. *European Journal of Cancer Prevention, 21*, 65-72.

[74] Camargo, M. C., Stayner, L. T., Straif, K., et al. (2011). Occupational exposure to asbestos and ovarian cancer: A meta-analysis. *Environmental Health Perspectives, 119*, 1211-1217.

[75] Le, N. D., Leung, A., Brooks-Wilson, A., et al. (2014). Occupational exposure and ovarian cancer risk. *Cancer Causes and Control, 25*, 829-841.

In: Handbook on Ovarian Cancer
Editor: Bethany R. Collier

ISBN: 978-1-63483-874-0


*Chapter 2*

# OVARIAN CANCER: NEW THERAPIES, POTENTIAL RISK FACTORS AND PROGNOSTIC VALUES FOR IMPROVING SURVIVAL OUTCOMES IN WOMEN

***Luiz Gustavo de Almeida Chuffa*[1,*], *Fábio Rodrigues Ferreira Seiva*[2], *João Paulo de Arruda Amorim*[3] and *Luiz Antonio Lupi Júnior*[1]**

[1]Department of Anatomy - IBB/UNESP,
Institute of Biosciences of Botucatu,
Univ. Estadual Paulista, SP, Brazil

[2]Department of Biology and Technology –
UENP/CLM - Universidade Estadual do Norte do Paraná, PR, Brazil

[3]Department of Anatomy - UNIOESTE/FB –
Universidade Estadual do Oeste do Paraná, PR, Brazil

## ABSTRACT

Ovarian cancer (OC) is the third most diagnosed gynecologic cancer and the first leading cause of death from all of gynecological malignancies. OC presents with the highest mortality rate, largely due to its advanced stage at the time of diagnosis. About 90% of these cases are epithelial ovarian cancer (EOC), and 70% are diagnosed with widespread intra-abdominal or distant metastases. Unfortunately, the frequency of invasive and advanced EOC is mostly due to the lack of a suitable and sufficiently reliable screening tool at the moment of diagnosis. Despite new strategies and improvements in surgical techniques and chemotherapeutic options, a 5-year survival rate for invasive EOC is approximately 46%. The main symptoms reported from OC include abnormal vaginal bleeding, pelvic and abdominal pain, weight loss, back pain, urinary

* Corresponding author: Luiz Gustavo de Almeida Chuffa. E-mail: guchuffa@yahoo.com.br. Department of Anatomy, Institute of Biosciences of Botucatu, Univ. Estadual Paulista, SP. Address: Distrite of Rubião Júnior s/n, Botucatu - São Paulo/SP.

urgency, and fatigue, which contribute to the difficulties of an early diagnosis, thereby resulting in low prognosis and survival rates. The treatment of early stage OC involves surgical resection followed by chemotherapy; clinical trials show an overall survival rate with adjuvant platinum-based chemotherapy, but this treatment in sub-groups of patients may vary according to different prognosis. Many risk factors associated with breast cancer are also related to the risk of other gynecologic cancers, such as OC. They include current age, age at menarche, parity, and first-degree family history with a wide inter-individual genetic variations in the susceptibility of OC. Recent studies regarding genome-wide association have reported several single nucleotide polymorphisms that confer low-penetrance susceptibility to EOC. In addition, mutations in BRCA gene, the gene that produces breast cancer-linked protein, are strongly associated with hereditary forms of OC. Hormone replacement therapy is further associated with increased risks of OC, mainly long duration use of both unopposed estrogens and estrogens plus progestins, regardless of treatment regimen. Independent prognostic factors are often considered including those described by International Federation of Gynecology and Obstetrics (FIGO), such as stage, tumor grade, volume of residual OC, and specific biomarkers for predicting survival in ovarian tumor patients. This chapter will discuss the new therapies, major risk factors in early and advanced ovarian cancer stage, and most prognostic factors as a tool for improving the survival rate outcomes in women.

## A General Overview of the Ovarian Cancer (OC) Subtypes

According to the 2014 World Health Organization (WHO) regarding classification and tumour morphology, primary OC are subdivided into three categories: epithelial (60%), germ cell (30%), and sex-cord stromal tumours (8%) (Kurman et al. 2014). The majority of malignant ovarian tumours (80%-85%) are of epithelial type (carcinomas). In contrast, malignant germ cell and sex-cord stromal tumours account for only 10% of all malignant OC. Ovarian carcinomas of epithelial type comprise a heterogeneous group of malignancies, being the most common subtypes classified as serous, endometrioid, clear cell and mucinous (McCluggage, 2011). The current understanding of the mechanisms underlying pathogenesis and initiating molecular events involving different tumour subtypes has gained attention, and although OC is clinically considered as one disease, their various subtypes exhibit different behaviour and prognosis. Serous adenocarcinoma is the primary ovarian epithelial malignancy, and mucinous carcinoma has been regarded as the second most common subtype followed by clear cell and endometroid subtype (McCluggage, 2008). Unfortunately, most ovarian tumours are observed in advanced stage (i.e., stage III or IV; FIGO) at diagnosis. OC is traditionally graded as numbers 1, 2 or 3 (well, moderately or poorly differentiated), but there are many inconsistencies between different laboratories and pathologists (Silverberg, 2000, Sato et al. 2003). The majority of serous carcinomas form glands with papillary architecture, and many psammoma bodies; however, solid variants occur with little or even no papillary aspect. These solid OC merge with undifferentiated carcinoma overlapping with high-grade endometrioid carcinoma (Cramer et al. 1987). Commonly, poorly differentiated serous OC presents psammoma bodies, slit-like as opposed to round glandular spaces, tumour giant cells with bizarre nuclei, smaller and complex papillae, and degree of cellular budding. Previous studies consistently demonstrated that there are two types of ovarian serous carcinoma (OSC), termed low-grade and high-grade OSC. These represent two distinct tumours types displaying different pathogenesis, molecular aspects, resistance to drug treatments, behaviour and prognosis (Singer et al. 2005, 2003, Russell and McCluggage, 2004). Indeed, high-grade OSC is more common than low-grade, and low-grade is thought to arise from a benign borderline cystadenoma with a micropapillary pattern. Conversely, high-grade OSC seems to arise directly from ovarian surface epithelium (OSE) or the inclusion cysts epithelium with no defined precursor lesion (Feeley and Wells, 2001). There is convincing and growing evidence that high-grade OSC may be derived from pre-existing epithelium located near to distal fimbrial portion of the uterine tube (Lee et al. 2006, Medeiros et al. 2007). In addition, high-grade OSC is an aggressive tumour which, in most cases, respond well initially to platinum-based therapy, but the patient typically develop chemoresistance associated with tumour recurrence. Table 1 shows the most common mutations/molecular aberrations occurring in OC.

**Table 1. Histologic subtypes of epithelial and nonepithelial ovarian carcinomas and the most common mutations/molecular aberrations**

| Epithelial | | | | | Nonepithelial |
|---|---|---|---|---|---|
| High-grade serous OC | Low-grade serous OC | Mucinous OC | Clear cell OC | Endo-metrioid OC | Sex-cord stromal |
| *TP53* | *Braf* | *Kras* | *ARID1A* | *ARID1A* | *FOXL2 Granulosa cell* |
| *BRCA 1 and 2* | *Kras* | *Her2* | *PIK3CA* | *PIK3CA* | *DICER1 Sertoli-Leydig cell* |
| *RB1* | *Nras* | *Amplify-cation* | *PTEN* | *PTEN* | |
| *CDK12* | *ERBB2* | | *CTNNB1* | *PPP2R1α* | |
| *NF1* | | | *PPP2R1α* | *MMR deficiency* | |
| *Homologous recombination repair genes* | | | | | |

## Targeted Therapies in Ovarian Cancer

Promising advances in understanding the history of OC, along with surgical and chemotherapeutic strategies, have significantly improved the short-term course of OC. Figure 1 illustrates the most current categories of medications used in the treatment of OC. Despite these improvements, most patients relapse after first treatment and succumb to disease progression (Coward et al. 2015). In general, the risk for OC increases with age and the main group of patients are at postmenopausal stage, with 80% of cases being diagnosed older than fifty years. Surgical reduction (consisting of hysterectomy and bilateral salpingo-oophoretomy, omentectomy, and pelvic lymph node resection) is fundamental to OC diagnosis, staging, and treatment. The major proposal is to resect all macroscopic tumors (i.e., optimal debulking) within the pelvic cavity and to perform abdomen investigation to detect any subtle peritoneal implant (Chi et al. 2009). Notably, the extent of debulking directly influences OC prognosis.

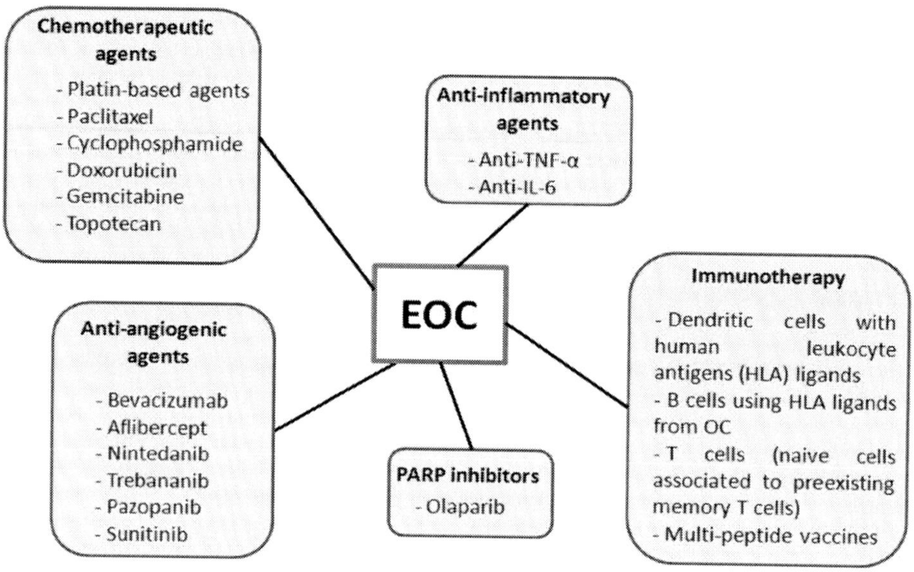


Figure 1. Schematic overview of different categories and drug agents used in the treatment of OC. EOC: epithelial ovarian cancer; TNF-α: tumor necrosis factor α; IL-6: interleukin 6.

Regarding to early-stage OC (i.e., stage Ia and Ib, and II), the patients show good prognosis, and the standard procedure involves cytoreductive surgery followed by observation (first and second look; Sonoda, 2004). For advanced stages of OC, chemotherapy still remains the better choice of adjuvant and neoadjuvant treatment for OC. During the past decades, studies have been conducted to characterize the "gold standard" therapy and to validate the optimal timing, dosage, and route of cytotoxic drug delivery. A pivotal study from gynecologic oncology group in 1996 brought significant initial advance in chemotherapeutic management with the introduction of paclitaxel, in which the combination of cisplatin and paclitaxel conferred a substantial survival rate compared to cisplatin and cyclophosphamide (McGuire et al. 1996). Most lately, the combination of carboplatin and paclitaxel was established as the first-line setting due to a reduced toxicity (Neijt et al. 2000). Other single agents (e.g., gemcitabine, topotecan, doxorubicin) with activity in recurrent disease are used; however, their addition to standard treatment failed to prolong survival.

## Antiangiogenic Therapy

Angiogenesis is thought to trigger the persistence of OC, and therefore, represent a key target in clinical research. Many antiangiogenic agents have been extensively investigated in the treatment of OC, either as single agents or in combination with chemotherapy (Coward et al. 2015). Bevacizumab, a monoclonal antibody that binds to the vascular endothelial growth factor (VEGF)-receptor ligand VEGF-A, has been studied in clinical research. A great benefit of adding bevacizumab was seen in a higher-risk population with advanced stage III-IV disease and residual disease > 1 cm (Burger et al. 2011, Perren et al. 2011). On this basis, the European Society for Medical Oncology suggest bevacizumab in addition to chemotherapy in patients with poor prognosis, such as stage IV or suboptimally debulked OC (Ledermann et al. 2013). Aflibercept, a heterodimeric molecule with domains of VEGFR1 and VEGFR2 conjugated with immunoglobulin, possesses a higher affinity for VEGF isoforms (Aravantinos et al. 2014). Phase II studies were conducted in 46 patients with recurrent OC, and Coleman et al. (2011) found a 54% objective response rate (ORR) after a combination of aflibercept (6 mg/ kg i.v.) and docetaxel (75 mg/m$^2$ i.v.) every 3 weeks. Because the correlation between VEGF signaling and development of ascites, aflibercept has been used for decreasing the frequency of paracentesis. Nintedanib, a triple angiokinase inhibitor, is a drug affecting angiogenesis by targeting VEGF, platelet-derived growth factor (PDGF), and fibroblast growth factor (FGF) (Ledermann et al. 2011). Nintedanib (250 mg twice a day) showed survival rate advantages in a placebo-controlled phase II study, and even a more significant prolonged rate after combined with carboplatin/paclitaxel (Du Bois et al. 2013). Other antiangiogenic compounds (Trebananib, Pazopanib, Sunitinib, etc.) have been consistently combined with different chemotherapies for OC (Coward et al. 2015).

## Poly (Adenosine Diphosphate [ADP]-Ribose) Polymerase(PARPs) Inhibitors

Preclinical data described a role for PARPs in treating tumours with deficient DNA repair by homologous recombination (Bryant et al. 2005, Farmer et al. 2005). These enzymes play a role in DNA repair by regulating base-excision repair pathways, and its inhibition results in an excess of single-strand breaks, which evolves to double-strand breaks during replication (Virág and Szabó, 2002). Such defects are repaired by homologous recombination dependent on intact BRCA proteins. In BRCA1/2 mutation cancers, an efficient sensitivity to PARP inhibition is obtained leading to genomic instability and cell death (Ashworth, 2008). In-human trial of PARP inhibitor (olaparib, 400mg orally twice a day) was conducted in patients with refractory solid tumours, and exhibited antitumor response in the subset of patients with BRCA mutations and no significant toxicity (Fong et al. 2009). Furthermore, platinum-sensitive patients have a more efficient effect of PARP inhibitors than platinum-resistant patients (69% versus 45%, respectively; Fong et al. 2010). In BRCA-mutated recurrent OC, a phase II trial showed a dose-response relationship with a response rate of 13% at 100 mg olaparib compared with 33% at 400 mg olaparib twice a day (Audeh et al. 2010). In a second phase II study, there was an objective response in 41% of patients with recurrent high-grade serous or undifferentiated OC with BRCA 1/2 mutation (Gelmon et al. 2011). As PARP inhibitors are relatively new agents used in the clinical area, all the mechanisms involved in therapeutic resistance are based on preclinical studies.

## Peptides-Based Immunotherapy in OC

Identifying the suitable targets for specific immunotherapy remains a matter of debate. Most peptides used for vaccination in clinical trials exhibit a strong immunological responses but fail in terms of clinical benefit (Peper and Stevanovic, 2015). For immunogenicity testing using human leukocyte antigen (HLA) ligands from OC, there are two in vitro priming methods, either autologous mature dendritic cells (DCs) and B cells or an antigen-presenting cells (APCs) based on streptavidin-coated microspheres loaded with HLA-peptide complexes anti-CD28. Tumor-associated peptides are thought to be immunogenic by in vitro naive T cells from healthy donors and suggest preexisting T cell responses in OC patients. Preexisting memory T cells that recognize a number of vaccine peptides would provide benefit for identifying tumor-associated peptides (Peper and Stevanovic, 2015); however, many T cells failed to counteract and kill the tumor cells, which might be due to the different immune escape in an immunosuppressive tumor microenvironment. Another study reported that strong antigen specific T-cell responses may induce an immunoselection promoting the outgrowth of tumor cells lacking the expression of respective T-cell epitope (Matsushita et al. 2012), implying that previous memory responses may be triggered the loss of epitope. A lack of specific T cells to be activated by the vaccine peptides from OC patients do not mean that these peptides are unsuitable. In OC, most trials relied on NY-ESO-1 and p53 (Diefenbach et al. 2008, Rahma et al. 2012) with no evidence of presentation as HLA ligands. Another challenge was the immunization of patients with peptides to one single antigen only. Importantly, developing multi-peptide vaccines should be fundamental for targeting different antigens in OC immunotherapies.

## Targeting OC-Related Inflammation

Inflammation plays key roles in tumor cell proliferation, migration, angiogenesis, and apoptotic evasion, which together promote an appropriate microenvironment facilitating tumorigenesis. Recent translational studies have showed promising results in targeting proinflammatory cytokines such as tumor necrosis factor α (TNF-α) and IL-6, which both act as principal regulators of these aforementioned tumorigenic processes. Phase II study has been conducted using TNF-α antagonist (etanercept) in 30 patients with advanced OC. Interestingly, six of them showed OC stabilization, and blood cytokine assay revealed a significant decrease in IL-6 (Madhusudan et al. 2005). In another study with advanced OC, 41 patients were treated with infliximab (an anti-TNF antibody) at doses of 5 mg/kg or 10 mg/kg via i.v. every 4 weeks. During the antibody infusion, samples of plasma were analyzed over a 24-96 h period, and IL-6 levels decreased significantly in all patients at 24 and 48 h with both doses (Brown et al. 2008). Coward et al. (2011) investigated the efficacy of anti-IL-6 antibody (siltuximab) in 18 patients with platinum-resistant OC regarding combined evaluation criteria in solid tumors and CA125 criteria. Unfortunately, one from 18 patients had a partial response, and seven others showed periods of disease stabilization after treatment for 6 months. Experimental studies in our laboratory have reported an anti-inflammatory effect of melatonin, an indoleamine secreted by pineal gland at night, upon papillary OC in animals (Chuffa et al. 2015). Importantly, melatonin therapy at doses of 200 μg/100 b.w/day, administered for 60 days, significantly reduced toll-like receptor 4 (TLR4), nuclear factor k-Beta (NFkB), TNF-α and IL-6, besides decreasing OC volume (Chuffa et al. 2013, 2014, 2015).

## RISK FACTORS IN OC: GENETIC MUTATIONS

There are many well-characterized risk factors to OC development, including personal or family history of breast or ovarian cancer, nulliparity or infertility, early menarche and late menopause, and hormone replacement therapy (Lichtenstein et al. 2000; Liang et al. 2010). Growing evidences point to the genetic contribution related to OC (see Figure 2). Some gene mutations are being described to be strongly linked to OC predisposition including BRCA1/BRCA2, hMLH1, hMSH2, hMSH6, PMS1 and PMS2 mutations (Risch et al. 2001; Drek et al. 2003). For instance, female carries of gemline BRCA1 or BRCA2 mutated genes show increased lifetime risk (60% or higher) of developing OC (Lancaster et al. 1997).

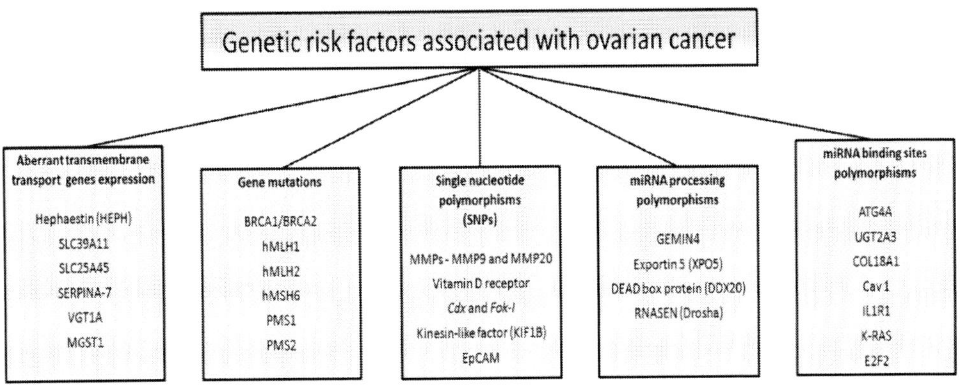


Figure 2. Representative subset of the most common genetic factors related to increased risk of developing OC. miRNA: microRNA.

Genetic polymorphism is now recognized as an important background for several conditions as well as represent valuable tools for screening studies. Single nucleotide polymorphisms (SNPs) have also been implicated to increased risk for OC development. From here will be brought some evidences that associate ovarian cancer risk with gene expression patterns, as well as a brief description of the role of involved proteins.

Matrix metalloproteinases (MMPs) belong to a zinc-dependent enzymes family with more than 20 described isoenzymes (Overall et al. 2006). Up-regulation of MMPs were considered to be found in tumor growth, invasion, and metastasis but new evidences appears to relate MMPs and tissue inhibitors metalloproteinases (TIMPs) with cancer suppressing functions (Egeblad and Werb, 2002). An elegant study performed by Delassus et al. (2010) brought some paradoxical evidences to the role played by signaling pathways involved in cancer development. Evaluating tumor suppressor proteins over several MMPs -1, 2, 7, 13, 14, 16, 19 and 25- expression, authors showed different response patterns to different cancer cell lines, namely PC-3 (human prostate adenocarcinoma), NCI-H460 (lung carcinoma), SNB-19 (brain glioblastoma), and OVSK3 (ovarian adenocarcinoma). This kind of study is relevant in order to elucidate potential targets for more precise and effective cancer therapy. Considering OC cell line, the results have demonstrated that overexpression of E-cadherin, fibulin 1D, p53, PTEN, and RKIP consistently increased MMP2, MMP14/MMP16, MMP16/MMP25, and MMP14 expression, respectively. A large-scale study investigating genetic variants (266 SNP) for 22 MMP and TIMP genes has pointed to two related MMP genes mutations to be associated with overall ovarian cancer risk, MMP9 and MMP20 (Wang et al. 2015). MMP20, identified as "human enamelysin" (Liano et al. 1997), may play a very likely role in the regulation of ovarian cancer. Interestingly, OC risk most significant associated to SNP (doubling the overall risk) was found to be in the intronic region on MMP20 gene, and another MMP20 SNP was found to reduce the risk for OC. These results demonstrate the need for more studies in order to better define and understand the role of genetic alterations in cancer development.

Other gene that seems to be related to OC risk is the kinesin-like factor 1B (KIF1B), a gene which encodes a motor protein involved in organelles, vesicles, protein complexes and RNAs intracellular traffic (Chen et al. 2003; Hirokawa et al. 2009; MacAskill et al. 2010). Aberrant KIF1B expression contributes to tumorigenesis process and downregulation of this gene supports its pro-apoptotic and inhibitory functions (Aulchenko et al. 2008; Yeh et al. 2008; Henrich et al. 2012). Genetic alterations in the intronic region of KIF1B gene reduce the risk for OC. This gene region is predicted to be a transcription binding site modulating gene expression (Shi et al. 2015). These findings may be seem as controversial given that KIF1B has once been identified as tumor suppressor gene, regulating mitochondrial transportation and able to induce cellular apoptosis (Schlisio et al. 2008). In this context, it is worth mentioning that cancer is considered a disease with many complexes and inter-related processes, sometimes leading to data misinterpretation. Another protein involved in OC is the EpCAM, an epithelial cell adhesion molecule (Heubner et al. 2015). The overexpression of EpCAM is a relatively common find in various epithelial neoplasms, including OC (Momburg et al. 1987; Litvinov et al. 2003) in such a way that oncologic therapies seek to target drugs to modulate protein functions (Burges et al. 2007; Simon et al. 2013). Some studies have proposed a putative functional role of EpCAM in tumor progression and carcinogenesis. EpCAM expression is able to upregulate c-myc enhancing proliferation and metabolism (Munz et al. 2004), contributing to cell and tissue differentiation by interaction with E-cadherin (Litvinov et al. 1997; Winter et al. 2003), and more recently, EpCAM has been described as a mitogenic signal transducer (Maetzel et al. 2009).

Vitamin D, a lipid-soluble vitamin, and its interaction with vitamin D receptor (VDR) may be closely associated with increased risk for reproductive cancers, including OC (Anderson et al. 2006; Mun et al. 2015). vitamin D participates in calcium and phosphate transport, regulates cell proliferation, differentiation, and apoptosis (Thomas et al. 1992). After binding to VDR, vitamin D acts in regulating target gene transcription, and involves diverse systems, such as the endocrine system, insulin-like growth factor signaling and estrogen-related pathways (Raimondi et al. 2009; Mun et al. 2015). Anderson et al. (2006) demonstrated VDR polymorphism to be related with increased risk for reproductive cancer, but there is no consensus about the role of polymorphism regardless vitamin D gene expression and OC. Mun et al. (2015) have conducted a meta-analysis study to consider VDR polymorphism and the risk for female reproductive cancer. Although there are many researches looking for polymorphic patterns and OC risk (Lurie et al. 2007; Clendenen et al. 2008; Tworoger et al. 2009; Grant et al. 2013), only two genes have appeared to be most related to OC, the *Cdx-2* and *Fok* I. Other genes, such as BsmI, ApaI and TaqI after data analysis showed no correlation with OC increased risk. It is worth noting that, not all, but most of the studies were performed in Caucasian populations. Further meta-analysis data can be found in Liu et al. (2013) and Li et al. (2014).

In a recent study performed by Chornokur and many others collaborators (2015), SNP in genes encoding cellular transport-related proteins were associated with increased risk for OC. Aberrant expression of transmembrane transport genes has been associated with increased risk of a number of malignancies including breast (Ota et al. 2010; Pinheiro et al. 2011), prostate (Pertega-Gomes et al. 2011), liver (Chen and Chloupkovae, 2009), colorectal and colon (Cross et al. 2011), thyroid (Filetti et al. 1999), neuroblastoma (Ishihara et al. 2011), and ovarian cancer (Chornokur et al. 2015). It has been pointed that six genes have higher association with OC risk, namely HEPH (Hephaestin), SLC39A11, SLC25A45, SERPINA7, UGT1A and MGST1. HEPH gene product is a transmembrane copper-dependent ferroxidase responsible for dietary iron absorption from enterocytes as well as the metal metabolism (Sebastiani and Pantopoulos, 2010; Yeh et al. 2011). Iron homeostasis is crucial in several pathways, being related to cell cycle arrest, apoptosis, DNA synthesis, regulation of potentially carcinogenic kinases and reactive oxygen species generation-induced mutations (Merlot et al. 2013). The solute carrier family 39, member 11, and solute carrier family 25, member 45 (SLC39A11, SLC25A45) are important genes related to membrane protein transporters. The role of the former needs further studies, but it seems to act as zinc-influx transporter (Eide, 2004). SLC24A45 product is an inner mitochondrial membrane protein responsible for transport of long-chain fatty acids and intergenic SNP is strongly correlated with OC, besides that SLC24A45 downregulation is found during OC progression (Palmieri, 2013; Chornokur et al. 2015). SERPINA7 - serpin peptidase inhibitor, clade A (alpha-1 antiproteinase, antitrypsin), member 7 – is a protein that bind T3 and T4 thyroid hormones, both supporting cancer process (Cristofanilli et al. 2005). SNP found in SERPINA7 gene increased risk for some OC subtypes, but not for others (Chornokur et al. 2015). Endometrioid OC was particularly associated with SNP in UDP glucuronosyltransferase 1 family, polypeptide A cluster (UGT1A). This one is a complex locus which encodes nine human UDP-glucuronosyltransferases. These enzymes found in the endoplasmic reticulum membrane are involved in elimination of bilirubin, lipophilic compounds, and several xenobiotics (Tukey and Strassburg, 2000). An important role for UGT1A family genes expression is related with mucosa protection, and Giuliani et al. (2005) discussed the downregulation of UGTA1 as an early event in bladder and colon carcinogenesis. Microsomal glutathione S-transferase 1 (MGST1) gene encodes an antioxidant endoplasmic-reticulum and outer mitochondrial membrane protein related to glutathione metabolism in order to prevent oxidative stress. MGST1 is highly expressed in EOC primary tumors, metastases, and effusions (Morgenstem et al. 2011), and SNP in this gene was associated, in Afro-American descendent women, with OC increased risk (Chornokur et al. 2005).

MicroRNAs (miRNA) are active biomolecules that regulate gene expression patterns. They are associated with several types of human cancer, and furthermore, genetic variants of miRNA are thought to modify the risk for some diseases, including OC (Lu et al. 2005; Lorio et al. 2007; Yang et al. 2008). Previous study evaluating point mutation in 8 miRNA processing genes and 134 genes containing potential miRNA binding sites for OC predisposition have associated SNP in 6 miRNA processing and 7 miRNA binding site genes with OC risk development (Liang et al. 2010). Among these genes, GEMIN4 which encodes a component of a multiprotein complex with multiple role *in vivo*, XPO5 (Exportin 5), DDX20 (DEAD box protein) and RNASEN (Drosha) have shown miRNA processing genes polymorphisms to be strongly associated with ovarian cancer risk. The miRNA binding site genes SNPs that appears to be more related with OC risk were ATG4A (encoding autophagy related protease), UGT2A3 (encoding a detoxifying enzyme), COL18A1 (encoding a type XVIII collagen), Cav1 (multifunctional protein found in cell-surface caveolae), IL1R1 (Interleukin-1 receptor related to inflammatory responses), K-RAS (implicated in various malignancies states) and E2F2 (transcription factor with crucial role in cell cycle regulation).

Taken together, these data point to the importance of a deeper understanding of genetic component as participative in OC development, and furthermore, polymorphic genes are essential elements to design more efficient drugs as well as personalized therapies which could achieve better outcomes.

## Hormone Replacement Therapy

The hormone replacement therapy (HRT) started to be largely used around 1990s as a treatment for the symptoms of menopause in women aged 50 years or older. Declines in postmenopausal hormone use were observed around 2000s, when the Women's Health Initiative published the increased risk of breast cancer, stroke, coronary heart disease and pulmonary embolism in women using the HRT (Rossouw et al. 2002). The current HRT guidelines vary in what they say about the ovarian cancer, but their majority still considers that there is insufficient evidence about the risks for this type of cancer. However, those guidelines were published before the new meta-analysis of postmenopausal women using the HRT from the Collaborative Group on Epidemiological Studies of Ovarian Cancer (CGESOC), which showed the increased risk of developing ovarian cancer in women who received this therapy for menopausal symptoms (CGESOC, 2015). Although some previous studies showed that increased ovarian cancer risk is associated with the HRT, they were too small or limited to a single region, while the CGESOC meta-analysis considered the data from 52 epidemiological studies in different countries of North America and Europe.

There are two different types of HRT: the administration of unopposed estrogens (estrogen therapy - ET) or the administration of estrogens combined with progesterone (estrogen/progesterone therapy - EPT). Previous studies showed the association between the unopposed estrogen therapies and increased ovarian cancer rates (Greiser et al. 2007; Rossing et al. 2007; Santen et al. 2010), but it remains still unclear if the combination estrogen/progesterone is able to reduce the risk as it was observed in patients using both the estrogen therapy and oral contraceptives containing high doses of progesterone (Schildkraut et al. 2002). The hypothesis for the aetiology of epithelial ovarian cancer following HRT is that estrogens may increase and progesterone can reduce ovarian cancer risk through their opposite influences on cell proliferation and apoptosis (Lukanova & Kaaks, 2005), but some recent studies did not support this antagonistic effect of progesterone, as they reported an increased ovarian cancer risk even in patients using the combinatory estrogen/progesterone therapy (Beral et al. 2007; Morch et al. 2009; Trabert et al. 2012).

Recently, the Collaborative Group on Epidemiological Studies of Ovarian Cancer analyzed data from 52 epidemiological studies from 1977 to 2013. The publication reported that ovarian cancer risk was increased in women using the HRT, regardless of treatment duration, even in users with less than five years of HRT usage. The analyses of former users of HRT showed that the risks decreased over the years after the last dose, but even ten years after therapy cessation can be insufficient to completely abolish the risk. Moreover, the study showed that there was no difference between the unopposed estrogen or estrogen/ progesterone therapy, both increasing significantly the risks of developing ovarian cancer. Interestingly, a substantial variation of the tumour type was observed in this study: HRT increased the two most common epithelial tumours (serous and endometrioid tumours), and decreased the other two types (clear-cell and mucinous tumours) (Morch et al. 2012; CGESOC, 2015). The findings about the increased risks of ovarian cancer in women using HRT, even with less than five years of use, are relevant to review the current patterns of HRT use and may be considered for medical advice and worldwide guidelines publications. However, it is very important to note that the HRT is also an effective and well used treatment for vasomotor symptoms during the menopausal period and should be considered being administered in its lowest effective doses (Santen et al. 2010).

## DIET

Ovarian carcinoma is one of the most common types of female cancers, with high incidence rates worldwide, especially in industrialized countries (Ferlay et al. 2010). It has been hypothesized that lifestyle factors, such as diet, may have a broad range of influence over the development of this disease; however, its effective role on the development of ovarian cancer is not clearly understood (Thomson et al. 2014).

A number of different foods have been extensively studied looking for the connections between type of food and cancer development. For example, lactose and its metabolite galactose, has been associated with a potential toxicity to the ovarian germ cells, leading to a subsequent higher gonadotropin secretion related to an increased rate of developing tumors (Larsson et al. 2006; Merritt et al. 2014). The role of dietary fats and cholesterol is controversial since earlier studies reported a positive correlation among ovarian cancer risk and fat intake (Armstrong and Doll, 1975; Prentice and Sheppard, 1990), and recent studies have been reported no association between them (Genkinger et al. 2006; Chang et al. 2007; Gilsing et al. 2011). It is important to observe that there are different types of fat such as total, trans and saturated fat, which have adverse effects for humans. Conversely, long-chain fatty acids, like omega-3 and -6, are strongly associated with antitumorigenic effects (Larsson et al. 2004). Notably, high intake of omega-3 and -6 decreases the risk for developing endometrioid and borderline tumors, respectively, while a greater consumption of trans fat may increase the risk of ovarian cancer (Merritt et al. 2014). Another study reported by Ascherbrook-Kilfoy et al. (2012) found an important association between the consumption of processed meats, a largely consumed type of food in industrialized countries, and a higher risk of ovarian cancer. They suggested that high levels of animal-based nitrites and total nitrates found in these foods may cause influences on ovarian cancer development. Curiously, there was no association between nitrites from plant sources and ovarian cancer risk. The Swedish Mammography Cohort and European Prospective Investigation into Cancer and Nutrition showed an important connection between the total fruit intake and a higher risk of ovarian cancer development (Larsson et al. 2004; Schulz et al. 2005). In addition, both vitamins C and E obtained from food or supplements were marginally associated with an increased risk of developing ovarian cancer, but none showed a significant dose-response relation (Chang et al. 2007).

On the other hand, some foods and drinks including vegetables, tea, citrus fruit, and juice have been implicated in a significant lower risk of developing ovarian cancer. These foods and drinks are the main source of flavonoids, which are categorized in 6 principal classes: flavonols, flavones, flavanones, flavanols, anthocyanidins, and isoflavones. These compounds have been reported to have antiproliferative, antioxidant and antimutagenic effects (Manach et al. 2004). In fact, their anticancer effects and molecular mechanisms are not completely elucidated for ovarian cancer, but a variety of flavonols may interfere in cellular signaling pathways, providing evidences about their possible influences in cancer risk reduction (Lee et al. 2010). This mechanism seems to involve apoptosis induction, activation of autophagy, and inhibition of apoptosis (Gao et al. 2012; De et al. 2013). Also, the estrogenic or antiestrogenic properties of isoflavones, mainly those derived from soybeans such as flavanones, flavanols, and some flavones are linked to a reduced risk of ovarian cancer development (Chen & Anderson, 2001). More recently, Meiyanto et al. (2012) also suggested the effects of flavanones in inhibiting cell growth via cell cycle arrest and apoptosis.

Compiling literature of food-based interventions has reported important evidences involving tea intake and ovarian cancer prevention (Butler and Wu, 2011; Johnson et al. 2012; Trudel et al. 2012). A recent study of Cassidy et al. (2014) showed a strongly inverse association between the black tea intake and ovarian cancer risk. The effects of vegetable consumption are controversial since higher vegetable intake was associated with an increased ovarian cancer risk compared to low intake in the Swedish Mammography Cohort, but no association was demonstrated in two other cohorts (Larsson et al. 2004; Fairfield et al. 2004; Mommers et al. 2005). A recent meta-analysis focusing on cruciferous vegetable such as broccoli, brussels sprouts, and cauliflower showed a positive correlation between high intake and low risk of developing ovarian cancer (Han et al. 2014). In brief, although diet itself may not be the main cause of ovarian cancer development, it is well assumed that a healthy and balanced food consumption can help to reduce the chance of getting cancer.

## Prognostic Factors in OC

The prognosis of OC is generally poor due to the lack of clear and effective diagnostic methods in identifying early stage disease. Most patients are diagnosed with advanced disease, and the five-year survival in OC is about 44% (Siegel et al. 2012). Cytoreductive surgery followed by platinum-based cytotoxic chemotherapy has long been considered to be a suitable treatment, but the mortality rates in advanced ovarian cancer remain considerably high (Hennessy et al. 2009; Morrison et al. 2012).

Prognostic factors are often considered including those described by FIGO, such as tumor stage and grade, amount of residual disease, specific biomarkers, and age for predicting survival in ovarian tumor patients (Benedet et al. 2000; Elattar et al. 2011). Researchers have shown an excellent prognostic in patients after appropriate surgical during stage 1 and grade 1 ovarian tumour (100% disease-free survival rate; Trimbos et al. 1991). In accordance to Ahmed et al. (1996), the 5-year overall survival rates for 194 consecutive patients presenting with FIGO stage I were 93% for stage IA, 92% for stage IB, and 84% for stage IC. In addition, the 5-year disease-free survival rates according to grading were 90% for grade 1, 85% for grade 2, and 45% for grade 3. Grade of differentiation is an important prognostic factor and should be used in the risk classification and for the therapeutic planning. However, the histological classification is hampered by inter-observer differences (Colombo et al. 2006).

In a study of 1,545 patients with invasive epithelial ovarian cancer stage I (FIGO), the grade of differentiation was the most powerful prognosis indicator of disease-free survival in stage I ovarian cancer, in a type 3 level of evidence (Vergote et al. 2001). This was followed by rupture before surgery, rupture during surgery, bilateral distribution of the tumour and age. Patients without tumour rupture had a 5-year disease-free survival of 83% compared with 72% and 70% for patients with tumour rupture before or during surgery. This study confirmed that rupture before surgery is an important independent prognostic factor in the survival rate. More specifically, DNA ploidy, measured using flow cytometry, has been identified as an important prognostic factor in epithelial OC. Vergote et al. (1993) evaluated 219 patients and demonstrated that in stage I the 5-year disease-free survival rates was 90% for patients with diploid tumours and 64% for patients with aneuploid tumours. Taken together, the grade of differentiation, DNA ploidy, and FIGO substage were the only independent prognostic factors (Colombo et al. 2006).

Prognostic in patients with advanced OC is influenced by many factors, but analysts suggest that the most important favorable factors include younger age, good general condition, cell type other than mucinous and clear cell carcinomas, lower stage, absence of ascites and smaller residual tumour following primary cytoreductive surgery (Van Houwelingen et al. 1989; Neijt et al. 1991; Omura et al. 1991; Hoskins et al. 1992; Thigpen et al. 1993). In particular, the amount of residual primary tumour after surgery is an important prognostic factor, on a type 1 level of evidence (Aure et al. 1971; Berek et al. 1999). It has been well accepted from the report of Griffiths and Fuller (1978) that the results of survival (progression-free survival and overall survival) of these patients are directly related to the amount of residual disease left after cytoreductive surgery. On the basis of information from a meta-analysis study, a statistically significant positive correlation is regarded between percent maximal cytoreduction and log median survival time, after controlling all other variables (Bristow et al., 2002). Furthermore, each 10% increase in maximal cytoreduction was associated with a 5.5% increase in median survival time, on a type 1 level of evidence. The definition of an optimal cytoreduction varies from a largest residual tumour mass of 2 cm to no residual tumour. No residual tumor patients had a better survival than those with the largest residual tumour mass of less than 0.5 cm. The latter group had a better prognostic than patients with 0.5–1.5 cm residual tumor (Hacker et al. 1983; Heintz et al. 1986; Redman et al. 1986; Neijt et al. 1987; Heintz et al. 1988; Potter et al. 1991; Hoskins et al. 1992).

Lymphovascular space invasion (LVSI) is defined as the presence of tumor cells within of the capillary lumen of both the lymphatic or microvascular drainage systems inside the primary tumor (Sakuragi et al. 2000). Recently, it has been identified as an important risk factor in the progression of many cancer types (Zaorsky et al. 2012; Bendifallah et al. 2014). The presence of LVSI in tumors is related to increased risk of disease to spread (especially nodal metastases), increased chance of disease recurrence, and reduced survival time. In OC, studies have also suggested the presence of LVSI had linked to worse survival (Matsuo et al. 2012; 2014a; 2014b). Unfortunately, most ovarian cancers progressed fast and has reached advanced stage at the moment of diagnosis (Chen et al. 2015).

Additionally, the VEGF has gained attention as a possible tool because of its association with angiogenesis in many solid tumors, including in OC (Olson et al. 1994). Angiogenesis is essential for cancer growth, progression, and metastasis (Hanahan and Weinberg, 2011). VEGF is a specific mitogen for endothelial cell, involved in cell proliferation, survival and migration. The leaky and permeable vessels induced by VEGF are also barriers to drug penetration (Jain, 2002). Overexpression of VEGF in ovarian tumor cells and malignant cyst fluids has led to investigation of the relationship between their expression and ovarian cancer prognosis (Fujimoto et al. 1998; Hazelton, 1999). Although a large number of works have evaluated the prognostic value of VEGF overexpression in OC survival, there is no clear conclusion yet.

## CONCLUSION

Every year, more than 6,500 women are diagnosed with OC, and around 4,400 die. The survival rate for OC vary greatly according to how early the disease is diagnosed. Although the gold standard of the carboplatin and paclitaxel regimen has remained the "soup of the day" for a long time, small increments in extending OC survival have only been realized with the addition of targeted therapies within the last few years. Current studies on the risks associated with genetic or hormonal replacement treatments either fail to mention OC or conclude that evidence for increased risk is not sufficient to achieve any firm recommendations. Basic research is under way to study biomarkers for detection of OC and both serum and tissue markers for predicting disease progression. Despite emerging and significant contribution has been reached on the OC field in terms of new strategies of treatment, most accurate risk prediction, and OC-related prognostic factors, there is still a main gap in our knowledge to making the effective and precise screening to offer proper treatment of OC at an early stage to improve the ultimate outcomes. Importantly, new insights into the interaction between chemotherapy and genes can maximize the effect of treatment in the future.

## REFERENCES


Ahmed F.Y., Wiltshaw E., A'Hern R.P., Nicol B., Shepherd J., Blake P., Fisher C., Gore M.E. (1996). Natural history and prognosis of untreated stage I epithelial ovarian carcinoma. *Journal of Clinical Oncology*, 14, 2968-2975.

Anderson M.G., Nakane M., Ruan X., Kroeger P.E., Wu-Wong J.R. (2006). Expression ofVDR and CYP24A1 mRNA in human tumors. *Cancer Chemotherapy and Pharmacology*, 57, 234–240.

Aravantinos G., Pectasides D. (2014). Bevacizumab in combination with chemotherapy for the treatment of advanced ovarian cancer: a systematic review. *Jounal of Ovarian Research*, 7, 57.

Armstrong B., Doll R. (1975). Environmental factors and cancer incidence and mortality in different countries with special reference to dietary practices. *International Journal of Cancer*, 15, 617–631.

Aschebrook-Kilfoy B., Ward M.H., Gierach G.L., Schatzkin A., Hollenbeck A.R., Sinha R., Cross A.J. (2012). Epithelial ovarian cancer and exposure to dietary nitrate and nitrite in the NIH-AARP Diet and Health Study. *European Journal of Cancer Prevention,* 21, 65–72.

Ashworth A. (2008). A synthetic lethal therapeutic approach: poly(ADP) ribose polymerase inhibitors for the treatment of cancers deficient in DNA double-strand break repair. *Journal of Clinical Oncology,* 26, 3785–3790.

Audeh M.W., Carmichael J., Penson R.T., Friedlander M., Powell B., Bell-McGuinn K.M., Scott C., Weitzel J.N., Oaknin A., Loman N., Lu K., Schmutzler R.K., Matulonis U., Wickens M., Tutt A. (2010). Oral poly(ADP-ribose) polymerase inhibitor olaparib in patients with BRCA1 or BRCA2 mutations and recurrent ovarian cancer: a proof-of-concept trial. *The Lancet,* 376, 245-251.

Aulchenko Y.S., Hoppenbrouwers I.A., Ramagopalan S.V., Broer L., Jafari N., Hillert J., Link J., Lundström W., Greiner E., Dessa Sadovnick A., Goossens D., Van Broeckhoven C., Del-Favero J., Ebers G.C., Oostra B.A., van Duijn C.M., Hintzen R.Q. (2008). Genetic variation in the KIF1B locus influences susceptibility to multiple sclerosis. *Nature Genetics,* 40, 1402–1403.

Aure J.C., Hoeg K., Kolstad P. (1971). Clinical and histologic studies of ovarian carcinoma. Long-term follow-up of 990 cases. *Obstetrics and Gynecology,* 37, 1-9.

Bendifallah S., Canlorbe G., Raimond E., Hudry D., Coutant C., Graesslin O., Touboul C., Huguet F., Cortez A., Daraï E., Ballester M. (2014). A clue towards improving the European Society of Medical Oncology risk group classification in apparent early stage endometrial cancer? Impact of lymphovascular space invasion. *British Journal of Cancer,* 110, 2640-2646.

Benedet J.L., Bender H., Jones H., Ngan H.Y., Pecorelli S. (2000). FIGO staging classifications and clinical practice guidelines in the management of gynecologic cancers. FIGO Committee on Gynecologic Oncology. *International Journal of Gynaecology and Obstetrics,* 70, 209-262.

Beral V., Bull D., Green J., Reeves G. (2007). Ovarian cancer and hormone replacement therapy in the Million Women Study. *The Lancet,* 369, 1703–1710.

Berek J.S., Trope C., Vergote I. (1999). Surgery during chemotherapy and at relapse of ovarian cancer. *Annals of Oncology,* 1, 3-7.

Bristow R.E., Tomacruz R.S., Armstrong D.K., Trimble E.L., Montz F.J. (2002). Survival effect of maximal cytoreductive surgery for advanced ovarian carcinoma during the platinum era: a meta-analysis. *Journal of Clinical Oncology,* 20, 1248-1259.

Brown E.R., Charles K.A., Hoare S.A., Rye R.L., Jodrell D.I., Aird R.E., Vora R., Prabhakar U., Nakada M., Corringham R.E., DeWitte M., Sturgeon C., Propper D., Balkwill F.R., Smyth J.F. (2008). A clinical study assessing the tolerability and biological effects of infliximab, a TNF-alpha inhibitor, in patients with advanced cancer. *Annals of Oncology,* 19, 1340-1346.

Bryant H.E., Schultz N., Thomas H.D., Parker K.M., Flower D., Lopez E., Kyle S., Meuth M., Curtin N.J., Helleday T. (2005). Specific killing of BRCA2-deficient tumours with inhibitors of poly(ADP-ribose) polymerase. *Nature,* 913-917.

Burger R.A., Brady M.F., Bookman M.A., Fleming G.F., Monk B.J., Huang H., Mannel R.S., Homesley H.D., Fowler J., Greer B.E., Boente M., Birrer M.J., Liang S.X., Gynecologic Oncology Group. (2011). Incorporation of bevacizumab in the primary treatment of ovarian cancer. New England *Journal of Medicine,* 365, 2473-2483.

Burges A., Wimberger P., Kumper C., Gorbounova V., Sommer H., Schmalfeldt B., Pfisterer J., Lichinitser M., Makhson A., Moiseyenko V., Lahr A., Schulze E., Jäger M., Ströhlein M.A., Heiss M.M., Gottwald T., Lindhofer H., Kimmig R. (2007). Effective relief of malignant ascites in patients with advanced ovarian cancer by a trifunctional anti-EpCAM 9 anti-CD3 antibody: a phase I/II study. *Clinical Cancer Research,* 13, 3899–3905.

Butler L.M., Wu A.H. (2011). Green and black tea in relation to gynecologic cancers. *Molecular Nutrition & Food Research,* 55, 931–940.

Chang E.T., Lee V.S., Canchola A.J., Clarke C.A., Purdie D.M., Reynolds P., Anton-Culver H., Bernstein L., Deapen D., Peel D., Pinder R., Ross R.K., Stram D.O., West D.W., Wright W., Ziogas A., Horn-Ross P.L. (2007). Diet and risk of ovarian cancer in the California Teachers Study cohort. *American Journal of Epidemiology,* 165, 802–813.

Chen J., Chloupkova M. (2009). Abnormal iron uptake and liver cancer. *Cancer Biology and Therapy,* 8, 1699–1708.

Chen M., Jin Y., Bi Y., Li Y., Shan Y., Pan L. (2015). Prognostic significance oflymphovascular space invasion in epithelial ovarian cancer. *Journal of Cancer,* 6, 412-419.

Chen X., Anderson J.J. (2001). Isoflavones inhibit proliferation of ovarian cancer cells in vitro via an estrogen receptor-dependent pathway. *Nutrition and Cancer,* 41, 165–171.

Chen Y.Y., Takita J., Chen Y.Z., Yang H.W., Hanada R., Yamamoto K., Hayashi Y. (2003). Genomic structure and mutational analysis of the human KIF1Balpha gene located at 1p36.2 in neuroblastoma. *International Journal of Oncology,* 23, 737–744.

Chi D.S., Eisenhauer E.L., Zivanovic O., Sonoda Y., Abu-Rustum N.R., Levine D.A., Guile M.W., Bristow R.E., Aghajanian C., Barakat R.R. (2009). Improved progression-free and overall survival in advanced ovarian cancer as a result of a change in surgical paradigm. *Gynecologic Oncology,* 114, 26-31.

Chornokur G., et al. (2015). Common genetic variation in cellular transport genes and epithelial ovarian cancer (EOC) risk. *Plos One,* 10, e 0128106.

Chuffa L.G., Fioruci-Fontanelli B.A., Mendes L.O., Fávaro W.J., Pinheiro P.F., Martinez M., Martinez F.E. (2013). Characterization of chemically induced ovarian carcinomas in an ethanol-preferring rat model: influence of long-term melatonin treatment. *PLoS One,* 8: e81676.

Chuffa L.G., Seiva F.R., Fávaro W.J., Amorim J.P., Teixeira G.R., Mendes L.O., Fioruci-Fontanelli B.A., Pinheiro P.F., Martinez M., Martinez F.E. (2013). Melatonin and ethanol intake exert opposite effects on circulating estradiol and progesterone and differentially regulate sex steroid receptors in the ovaries, oviducts, and uteri of adult rats. *Reproductive Toxicology,* 39, 40-49.

Chuffa L.G., Fioruci-Fontanelli B.A., Mendes L.O., Ferreira Seiva F.R., Martinez M., Fávaro W.J., Domeniconi R.F., Pinheiro P.F., Delazari Dos Santos L., Martinez F.E. (2015). Melatonin attenuates the TLR4-mediated inflammatory response through MyD88- and TRIF-dependent signaling pathways in an in vivo model of ovarian cancer. *BMC Cancer,* 6, 15-34.

Clendenen T.V., Arslan A.A., Koenig K.L., Enquist K., Wirgin I., Agren A., Lukanova A., Sjodin H., Zeleniuch-Jacquotte A., Shore R.E., Hallmans G., Toniolo P., Lundin E. (2008). Vitamin D receptor polymorphismsand risk of epithelial ovarian cancer. *Cancer Letters*, 260, 209–215.

Coleman R.L., Duska L.R., Ramirez P.T., Heymach J.V., Kamat A.A., Modesitt S.C., Schmeler K.M., Iyer R.B., Garcia M.E., Miller D.L., Jackson E.F., Ng C.S., Kundra V., Jaffe R., Sood A.K. (2011). Phase 1-2 study of docetaxel plus aflibercept in patients with recurrent ovarian, primary peritoneal, or fallopian tube cancer. *The Lancet Oncology,* 12, 1109-1117.

Collaborative Group On Epidemiological Studies Of Ovarian Cancer, Beral V., Gaitskell K., Hermon C., Moser K., Reeves G., Peto R. (2015). Menopausal hormone use and ovarian cancer risk: individual participant meta-analysis of 52 epidemiological studies. *The Lancet,* 385, 1835-1842.

Colombo N., Van Gorp T., Parma G., Amant F., Gatta G., Sessa C., Vergote I. (2006). Ovarian cancer. *Critical Reviews in Oncology/Hematology,* 60, 59-79.

Coward J., Kulbe H., Chakravarty P., Leader D., Vassileva V., Leinster D.A., Thompson R., Schioppa T., Nemeth J., Vermeulen J., Singh N., Avril N., Cummings J., Rexhepaj E., Jirström K., Gallagher W.M., Brennan D.J., McNeish I.A., Balkwill F.R. (2011). Interleukin-6 as a therapeutic target in human ovarian cancer. *Clinical Cancer Research,* 17, 6083-6096.

Coward J.I., Middleton K., Murphy F. (2015). New perspectives on targeted therapy in ovarian cancer. *International Journal of Women's Health,* 7, 189-203.

Cristofanilli M., Yamamura Y., Kau S.W., Bevers T., Strom S., Patangan M., Hsu L., Krishnamurthy S., Theriault R.L., Hortobagyi G.N. (2005). Thyroid hormone and breast carcinoma. Primary hypothyroidism is associated with a reduced incidence of primary breast carcinoma. *Cancer,* 103, 1122–1128.

Cross A.J., Sinha R., Wood R.J., Xue X., Huang W.Y., Yeager M., Hayes R.B., Gunter M.J. (2011). Iron homeostasis and distal colorectal adenoma risk in the prostate, lung, colorectal, and ovarian cancer screening trial. *Cancer Prevention Research (Phila),* 4, 1465–1475.

De A., Papasian C., Hentges S., Banerjee S., Haque I., Banerjee S.K. (2013). Emblica officinalis extract induces autophagy and inhibits human ovarian cancer cell proliferation, angiogenesis, growth of mouse xenograft tumors. *PLoS ONE,* 8 :e72748.

Delassus G.S., Cho H., Hoang S., Eliceiri G.L. (2010). Many new down- and up-regulatory signaling pathways, from known cancer progression suppressors to matrix metalloproteinases, differ widely in cells of various cancers. *Journal of Cellular Physiology,* 224, 549-558.

Diefenbach C.S., Gnjatic S., Sabbatini P., Aghajanian C., Hensley M.L., Spriggs D.R., Iasonos A., Lee H., Dupont B., Pezzulli S., Jungbluth A.A., Old L.J., Dupont J. (2008). Safety and immunogenicity study of NY-ESO-1b peptide and montanide ISA-51 vaccination of patients with epithelial ovarian cancer in high-risk first remission. *Clinical Cancer Research,* 14, 2740–2748.

Drake A.C., Campbell H., Porteous M.E.M., Dunlop M.G. (2003). The contribution of DNA mismatch repair gene defects to the burden of gynecological cancer. *International Journal of Gynecologic Cancer,* 13, 262–277.

Du Bois A., Kristensen G., Ray-Coquard I., Reub A., Pignata S., Colombo N., Denison U., Vergote I., del Campo J.M., Ottevanger P., Merger M., Harter P. (2013). AGO-OVAR 12: a randomized placebo-controlled GCIG/ENGOT-Intergroup phase III trial of standard frontline chemotherapy/−nintedanib for advanced ovarian cancer [abstract]. *International Journal of Gynecological Cancer,* 23(suppl 1):LBA1.

Egeblad M., Werb Z. (2002). New functions for the matrix metalloproteinases in cancer progression. *Nature Reviews Cancer,* 2, 161–174.

Eide D.J. (2004). The SLC39 family of metal ion transporters. *Pflugers Archiv,* 447, 796–800.

Elattar A., Bryant A., Winter-Roach B.A., Hatem M., Naik R. (2011). Optimal primary surgical treatment for advanced epithelial ovarian cancer. *The Cochrane Database of Systematic Reviews,* 10, CD007565.

Fairfield K.M., Hunter D.J., Colditz G.A., Fuchs C.S., Cramer D.W., Speizer F.E., Willett W.C., Hankinson S.E. (2004). A prospective study of dietary lactose and ovarian cancer. *International Journal of Cancer,* 110, 271–277.

Farmer H., McCabe N., Lord C.J., Tutt A.N., Johnson D.A., Richardson T.B., Santarosa M., Dillon K.J., Hickson I., Knights C., Martin N.M., Jackson S.P., Smith G.C., Ashworth A. (2005). Targeting the DNA repair defect in BRCA mutant cells as a therapeutic strategy. *Nature,* 434, 917-921.

Feeley K.M., Wells M. (2001). Precursor lesions of ovarian epithelial malignancy. *Histopathology,* 32, 87-95.

Ferlay J., Shin H.R., Bray F., Forman D., Mathers C., Parkin D.M. (2010). Estimates of worldwide burden of cancer in 2008: GLOBOCAN 2008. *Journal of the National Cancer Institute,* 127, 2893–2917.

Ferreira G.M., Martinez M., Camargo I.C., Domeniconi R.F., Martinez F.E., Chuffa L.G. (2014). Melatonin Attenuates Her-2, p38 MAPK, p-AKT, and mTOR Levels in Ovarian Carcinoma of Ethanol-Preferring Rats. *Journal of Cancer,* 5, 728-735.

Filetti S., Bidart J.M., Arturi F., Caillou B., Russo D., Schlumberger M. (1999). Sodium/iodide symporter: a key transport system in thyroid cancer cell metabolism. *European Journal of Endocrinology,* 141, 443–457.

Folkman J. (1971). Tumor angiogenesis: therapeutic implications. *The New England Journal of Medicine,* 285, 1182-1186.

Fong P.C., Boss D.S., Yap T.A., Tutt A., Wu P., Mergui-Roelvink M., Mortimer P., Swaisland H., Lau A., O'Connor M.J., Ashworth A., Carmichael J., Kaye S.B., Schellens J.H., de Bono J.S. (2009). Inhibition of poly(ADP-ribose) polymerase in tumors from BRCA mutation carriers. *New England Journal of Medicine,* 361, 123-134.

Fong P.C., Yap T.A., Boss D.S., Carden C.P., Mergui-Roelvink M., Gourley C., De Greve J., Lubinski J., Shanley S., Messiou C., A'Hern R., Tutt A., Ashworth A., Stone J., Carmichael J., Schellens J.H., de Bono J.S., Kaye S.B. (2010). Poly(ADP)-ribose polymerase inhibition: frequent durable responses in BRCA carrier ovarian cancer correlating with platinum-free interval. *Journal of Clinical Oncology,* 28, 2512-2519.

Fujimoto J., Sakaguchi H., Hirose R., Ichigo S., Tamaya T. (1998). Biologic implications of the expression of vascular endothelial growth factor subtypes in ovarian carcinoma. *Cancer,* 83, 2528-2533.

Gao X., Wang B., Wei X., Men K., Zheng F., Zhou Y., Zheng Y., Gou M., Huang M. Guo G., Huang N., Qian Z., Wei Y. (2012). Anticancer effect and mechanism of polymer micelle-encapsulated quercetin on ovarian cancer. *Nanoscale,* 4, 7021–7030.

Gelmon K.A., Tischkowitz M., Mackay H., Swenerton K., Robidoux A., Tonkin K., Hirte H., Huntsman D., Clemons M., Gilks B., Yerushalmi R., Macpherson E., Carmichael J., Oza A. (2011). Olaparib in patients with recurrent high-grade serous or poorly differentiated ovarian carcinoma or triple-negative breast cancer: a phase 2, multicentre, open-label, non-randomised study. *The Lancet Oncology,* 12, 852-861.

Genkinger J.M., Hunter D.J., Spiegelman D., Anderson K.E., Beeson W.L., Buring J.E., Colditz G.A., Fraser G.E., Freudenheim J.L., Goldbohm R.A., Hankinson S.E., Koenig K.L., Larsson S.C., Leitzmann M., McCullough M.L., Miller A.B., Rodriguez C., Rohan T.E,. Ross J.A., Schatzkin A., Schouten L.J., Smit E., Willett W.C., Wolk A., Zeleniuch-Jacquotte A., Zhang S.M., Smith-Warner S.A. (2006). A pooled analysis of 12 cohort studies of dietary fat, cholesterol and egg intake and ovarian cancer. *Cancer Causes Control,* 17, 273–285.

Gilsing A.M., Weijenberg M.P., Goldbohm R.A., van den Brandt P.A., Schouten L.J. (2011). Consumption of dietary fat and meat and risk of ovarian cancer in the Netherlands Cohort Study. *The American Journal of Clinical Nutrition,* 93, 118–126.

Giuliani L., Ciotti M., Stoppacciaro A., Pasquini A., Silvestri I., De Matteis A., Frati L., Aglianò A.M. (2005). UDP-glucuronosyltransferases 1A expression in human urinary bladder and colon cancer by immunohistochemistry. *Oncology Reports,* 13, 185–191.

Grant D.J., Hoyo C., Akushevich L., Iversen E.S., Whitaker R., Marks J., Berchuck A., Schildkraut J.M. (2013). Vitamin D receptor (VDR) polymorphismsand risk of ovarian cancer in Caucasian and African American women. *Gynecologic Oncology,* 129, 173–178.

Greiser C.M., Greiser E.M., Doren M. (2007). Menopausal hormone therapy and risk of ovarian cancer: systematic review and meta-analysis. *Human Reproduction Update,* 13, 453–463.

Griffiths C.T., Fuller A.F. (1978). Intensive surgical and chemotherapeutic management of advanced ovarian cancer. *The Surgical Clinics of North America,* 58, 131-142.

Hacker N.F., Berek J.S., Lagasse L.D., Nieberg R.K., Elashoff R.M. (1983). Primary cytoreductive surgery for epithelial ovarian cancer. *Obstetrics and Gynecology,* 61, 413-420.

Han B., Li X., Yu T. (2014). Cruciferous vegetables consumption and the risk of ovarian cancer: a meta-analysis of observational studies. *Diagnostic Pathology,* 9, 1-7.

Hanahan D., Weinberg R.A. (2011). Hallmarks of cancer: the next generation. *Cell,* 144, 646-674.

Hazelton D., Nicosia R.F., Nicosia S.V. (1999). Vascular endothelial growth factor levels in ovarian cyst fluid correlate with malignancy. *Clinical Cancer Research,* 5, 823-829.

Heintz A.P., Hacker N.F., Berek J.S., Rose T.P., Munoz A.K., Lagasse L.D. (1986). Cytoreductive surgery in ovarian carcinoma: feasibility and morbidity. *Obstetrics and Gynecology,* 67, 783-788.

Heintz A.P., Van Oosterom A.T., Trimbos J.B., Schaberg A., Van der Velde E.A., Nooy M. (1988). The treatment of advanced ovarian carcinoma (I): clinical variables associated with prognosis. *Gynecologic Oncology,* 30, 347-358.

Hennessy B.T., Coleman R.L., Markman M. (2009). Ovarian cancer. *Lancet,* 374, 1371-1382.

Henrich K.O., Schwab M., Westermann F. (2012). 1p36 tumor suppression— a matter of dosage? *Cancer Research,* 72, 6079–6088.

Heubner M., Wimberger P., Kasimir-Bauer S., Singer B.B., Ruf P., Kimmig R., Siffert W. (2015). Single nucleotide polymorphisms of the EpCAM-coding gene TACSTD1 in patients with ovarian cancer and their potential translational aspects. *Archives of Gynecology and Obstetrics* (In Press).

Hirokawa N., Noda Y., Tanaka Y., Niwa S. (2009). Kinesin superfamily motor proteins and intracellular transport. *Nature Reviews Molecular Cell Biology*, 10, 682–696.

Hoskins W.J., Bundy B.N., Thigpen J.T., Omura G.A. (1992). The influence of cytoreductive surgery on recurrence-free interval and survival in small-volume stage III epithelial ovarian cancer: a Gynecologic Oncology Group study. *Gynecologic Oncology,* 47, 159-166.

Iorio M.V., Visone R., Di Leva G., Donati V., Petrocca F., Casalini P., Taccioli C., Volinia S., Liu C.G., Alder H., Calin G.A., Ménard S., Croce C.M. (2007). MicroRNA signatures in human ovarian cancer. *Cancer Research,* 67, 8699–8707.

Ishihara T., Inoue J., Kozaki K., Imoto I., Inazawa J. (2011). HECT-type ubiquitin ligase ITCH targets lysosomal-associated protein multispanning transmembrane 5 (LAPTM5) and prevents LAPTM5-mediated cell death. *The Journal of Biological Chemistry,* 286, 44086–44094.

Jain R.K. (2002). Tumor angiogenesis and accessibility: role of vascular endothelial growth factor. *Seminars in Oncology,* 29, 3-9.

Johnson R., Bryant S., Huntley A.L. (2012). Green tea and green tea catechin extracts: an overview of the clinical evidence. *Maturitas,* 73, 280–287.

Kurman R.J., Carcangiu M.L., Herrington C.S., Young R.H. (2014). WHO classification of tumours of the female reproductive organs. *WHO classification of tumours.* IARC press, Lyon.

Lancaster J.M., Carney M.E., Futreal P.A. (1997). BRCA 1 and 2- A Genetic Link to Familial Breast and Ovarian Cancer. *Medscape Women's Health,* 2, 7.

Larsson S.C., Kumlin M., Ingelman-Sundberg M., Wolk A. (2004). Dietary long-chain n_3 fatty acids for the prevention of cancer: a review of potential mechanisms. *The American Journal of Clinical Nutrition,* 79, 935–945.

Larsson S.C., Holmberg L., Wolk A. (2004). Fruit and vegetable consumption in relation to ovarian cancer incidence: the Swedish Mammography Cohort. *British Journal of Cancer,* 90, 2167–2170.

Larsson S.C., Orsini N., Wolk A. (2006). Milk, milk products and lactose intake and ovarian cancer risk: a meta-analysis of epidemiological studies. *International Journal of Cancer,* 118, 431–441.

Ledermann J.A., Hackshaw A., Kaye S., Jayson G., Gabra H., McNeish I., Earl H., Perren T., Gore M., Persic M., Adams M., James L., Temple G., Merger M., Rustin G. (2011). Randomized phase II placebo-controlled trial of maintenance therapy using the oral triple angiokinase inhibitor BIBF 1120 after chemotherapy for relapsed ovarian cancer. *Journal of Clinical Oncology,* 29, 3798-3804.

Ledermann J.A., Raja F.A., Fotopoulou C., Gonzalez-Martin A., Colombo N., Sessa C., ESMO Guidelines Working Group. (2013). *Newly diagnosed and relapsed epithelial ovarian carcinoma: ESMO Clinical Practice Guidelines for diagnosis, treatment and follow-up. Annals of Oncology,* Suppl 6:vi24-32. doi: 10.1093/annonc/mdt333.

Lee Y., Medeiros F., Kindelberger D., Callahan M.J., Muto M.G., Crum C.P. (2006). Advances in the recognition of tubal intraepithelial carcinoma: applications to cancer screening and the pathogenesis of ovarian cancer. *Advances in Anatomic Pathology*, 13, 1-7.

Lee K.M., Lee D.E., Seo S.K., Hwang M.K., Heo Y.S., Lee K.W., Lcc II.J. (2010). Phosphatidylinositol 3-kinase, a novel target molecule for the inhibitory effects of kaempferol on neoplastic cell transformation. *Carcinogenesis,* 31, 1338–1343.

Li S., Xu H., Li S.C., Qi X.Q., Sun W.J. (2014). Vitamin D receptor rs2228570 polymorphism and susceptibly to ovarian cancer: a meta-analysis. *Tumour Biology,* 35, 1319–1322.

Liang D., Meyer L., Chang D.W., Lin J., Pu X., Ye Y., Gu J., Wu X., Lu K. (2010). Genetic Variants in MicroRNA Biosynthesis Pathways and Binding Sites Modify Ovarian Cancer Risk, Survival, and Treatment Response. *Cancer Research,* 70, 9765-9776.

Liano E., Pendas A.M., Knauper V, Sorsa T., Salo T., Salido E., Murphy G., Simmer J.P., Bartlet J.D., López-Otin C. (1997). Identification and structural and functional characterization of human enamelysin (MMP-20). *Biochemistry,* 36, 15101–15108.

Lichtenstein P., Holm N.V., Verkasalo P.K., Iliadou A., Kaprio J., Koskenvuo M., Pukkala E., Skytthe A., Hemminki K. (2000). Environmental and heritable factors in the causation of cancer—analyses of cohorts of twins from Sweden, Denmark, and Finland. *The New England Journal of Medicine,* 343, 78–85.

Litvinov S.V., Balzar M., Winter M.J., Bakker H.A., Briaire-de Bruijn I., Prins F., Fleuren G.J., Warnaar S.O. (1997). Epithelial cell adhesion molecule (Ep-CAM) modulates cell-cell interactions mediated by classic cadherins. *The Journal of Cell Biology,* 139, 1337–1348.

Litvinov S.V., Velders M.P., Bakker H.A., Fleuren G.J., Warnaar S.O. (1994). Ep-CAM: a human epithelial antigen is a homophilic cell-cell adhesion molecule. *The Journal of Cell Biology,* 125, 437–446.

Liu Y., Li C., Chen P., Li X., Li M., Guo H., Li J., Chu R., Wang H. (2013). Polymorphisms in the vitamin D Receptor (VDR) and the risk of ovarian cancer: a meta-analysis. *PLoS ONE,* 8, e:66716.

Lu J., Getz G., Miska E.A., Alvarez-Saavedra E., Lamb J., Peck D., Sweet-Cordero A., Ebert B.L., Mak R.H., Ferrando A.A., Downing J.R., Jacks T., Horvitz H.R., Golub T.R. (2005). MicroRNA expression profiles classify human cancers. *Nature,* 435, 834-838.

Lurie G., Wilkens L.R., Thompson P.J, McDuffie K.E., Carney M.E., Terada K.Y., Goodman M.T. (2007). Vitamin D receptor gene polymor-phisms and epithelial ovarian cancer risk. *Cancer Epidemiology, Biomarkers & Prevention,* 16, 2566–2571.

MacAskill A.F., Kittler J.T. (2010). Control of mitochondrial transport and localization in neurons. *Trends in Cell Biology*, 20, 102–112.

Madhusudan S., Muthuramalingam S.R., Braybrooke J.P., Wilner S., Kaur K., Han C., Hoare S., Balkwill F., Ganesan T.S. (2005). Study of etanercept, a tumor necrosis factor-alpha inhibitor, in recurrent ovarian cancer. *Journal of Clinical Oncology,* 23, 5950-5959.

Maetzel D., Denzel S., Mack B., Canis M., Went P., Benk M., Kieu C., Papior P., Baeuerle P.A., Munz M., Gires O. (2009). Nuclear signaling by tumour-associated antigen *EpCAM. Nature Cell Biology,* 11, 162–171.

Manach C., Scalbert A., Morand C., Remesy C., Jimenez L. (2004). Polyphenols: food sources and bioavailability. *The American Journal of Clinical Nutrition,* 79, 727–747.

Matsuo K., Sheridan T.B., Yoshino K., Miyake T., Hew K.E., Im D.D., Rosenshein N.B., Mabuchi S., Enomoto T., Kimura T., Sood A.K., Roman L.D. (2012). Significance of lymphovascular space invasion in epithelial ovarian cancer. *Cancer Medicine,* 1, 156-164.

Matsuo K., Yoshino K., Hiramatsu K., Banzai C., Hasegawa K., Yasuda M., Nishimura M., Sheridan T.B., Ikeda Y., Shiki Y., Mabuchi S., Enomoto T., Kimura T., Fujiwara K., Roman L.D., Sood A.K. (2014a). Effect of lymphovascular space invasion on survival of stage I epithelial ovarian cancer. *Obstetrics and Gynecology,* 123, 957-965.

Matsuo K., Sheridan T.B., Mabuchi S., Yoshino K., Hasegawa K., Studeman K.D., Im D.D., Rosenshein N.B., Roman L.D., Sood A.K. (2014b). Estrogen receptor expression and increased risk of lymphovascular space invasion in high-grade serous ovarian carcinoma. *Gynecologic Oncology,* 133, 473-479.

Matsushita H., Vesely M.D., Koboldt D.C., Rickert C.G., Uppaluri R., Magrini V.J., Arthur C.D., White J.M., Chen Y.S., Shea L.K., Hundal J., Wendl M.C., Demeter R., Wylie T., Allison J.P., Smyth M.J., Old L.J., Mardis E.R., Schreiber R.D. (2012). Cancer exome analysis reveals a T-cell-dependent mechanism of cancer immunoediting. *Nature,* 482, 400–404.

McCluggage W.G. (2008). My approach to and thoughts on the typing of ovarian carcinomas. Journal of Clinical Pathology, 61, 152-163.

McCluggage W.G. (2011). Morphological subtypes of ovarian carcinoma: a review with emphasis on new developments and pathogenesis. *Pathology,* 43, 420-432.

McGuire W.P., Hoskins W.J., Brady M.F., Kucera P.R., Partridge E.E., Look K.Y., Clarke-Pearson D.L., Davidson M. (1996). Cyclophosphamide and cisplatin compared with paclitaxel and cisplatin in patients with stage III and stage IV ovarian cancer. *The New England Journal of Medicine,* 334, 1–6.

Medeiros F., Muto M.G., Lee Y., Elvin J.A., Callahan M.J., Feltmate C., Garber J.E., Cramer D.W., Crum C.P. (2007). The tubal fimbria is a preferred site for early adenocarcinoma in women with familial ovarian cancer syndrome. *The American Journal of Surgical Pathology,* 30, 230-236.

Meiyanto E., Hermawan A., Anindyajati. (2012). Natural products for cancer targeted therapy: citrus flavonoids as potent chemopreventive agents. *Asian Pacific Journal of Cancer Prevention,* 13, 427–436.

Merlot A.M., Kalinowski D.S., Richardson D.R. (2013). Novel chelators for cancer treatment: where are we now*? Antioxidants & Redox Signaling,* 18, 973–1006.

Merritt M.A., Poole E.M., Hankinson S.E., Willett W.C., Tworoger S.S. (2014). Dairy food and nutrient intake in different life periods in relation to risk of ovarian cancer. *Cancer Causes Control,* 25, 795-808.

Momburg F., Moldenhauer G., Hammerling G.J., Moller P. (1987). Immunohistochemical study of the expression of a Mr 34,000 human epithelium-specific surface glycoprotein in normal and malignant tissues. *Cancer Research,* 47, 2883–2891.

Mommers M., Schouten L.J., Goldbohm R.A., van den Brandt P.A. (2005). Consumption of vegetables and fruits and risk of ovarian carcinoma. *Cancer,* 104, 1512–1519.

Morch L.S., Lokkegaard E., Andreasen A.H., Kruger-Kjaer S., Lidegaard O. (2009). Hormone therapy and ovarian cancer. *The Journal of the American Medical Association,* 302, 298–305.

Morch L.S., Lokkegaard E., Andreasen A.H., Kjaer S.K., Lidegaard O. (2012). Hormone Therapy and Different Ovarian Cancers: a National Cohort Study. *American Journal of Epidemiology,* 175, 1234–1242.

Morgenstern R., Zhang J., Johansson K. (2011). Microsomal glutathione transferase 1: mechanism and functional roles. *Drug Metabolism Reviews,* 43, 300–306.

Morrison J., Haldar K., Kehoe S., Lawric T.A. (2012). Chemotherapy versus surgery for initial treatment in advanced ovarian epithelial cancer. *The Cochrane Database of Systematic Reviews,* 8, CD005343.

Mun M.J., Kimc T.H. Hwangd J.Y., Janga W.C. (2015). Vitamin D receptor gene polymorphisms and the risk for female reproductive cancers: A meta-analysis. *Maturitas,* 81, 256-265.

Munz M., Kieu C., Mack B., Schmitt B., Zeidler R., Gires O. (2004). The carcinoma-associated antigen EpCAM upregulates c-myc and induces cell proliferation. *Oncogene,* 23, 5748–5758.

Neijt J.P., BokkelHuinink W.W., Van der Burg M.E., Van Oosterom A.T., Willemse P.H., Heintz A.P., Van Lent M., Trimbos J.B., Bouma J., Vermorken J.B. (1987). Randomized trial comparing two combination chemotherapy regimens (CHAP-5v CP) in advanced ovarian carcinoma. *Journal of Clinical Oncology, 5,* 1157-1168.

Neijt J.P., BokkelHuinink W.W., Van Der Burg M.E., Van Oosterom A.T., Willemse P.H., Vermorken J.B., Van Lindert A.C., Heintz A.P., Aartsen E., Van Lent M. (1991). Long-term survival in ovarian cancer. Mature data from The Netherlands Joint Study Group for Ovarian Cancer. *European Journal of Cancer,* 27, 1367-1372.

Neijt J.P., Engelholm S.A., Tuxen M.K., Sorensen P.G., Hansen M., Sessa C., de Swart C.A., Hirsch F.R., Lund B., van Houwelingen H.C. (2000). Exploratory phase III study of paclitaxel and cisplatin versus paclitaxel and carboplatin in advanced ovarian cancer. *Journal of Clinical Oncology,* 18, 3084-3092.

Olson T.A., Mohanraj D., Carson L.F., Ramakrishnan S. (1994). Vascular permeability factor gene expression in normal and neoplastic human ovaries. *Cancer Research,* 54, 276.

Omura G.A., Brady M.F., Homesley H.D., Yordan E., Major F.J., Buchsbaum H.J., Park R.C. (1991). Long-term followup and prognostic factor analysis in advanced ovarian carcinoma: the Gynecologic Oncology Group experience. *Journal of Clinical Oncology,* 9, 1138-1150.

Ota I., Sakurai A., Toyoda Y., Morita S., Sasaki T., Chishima T., Yamakado M., Kawai Y., Ishidao T., Lezhava A., Yoshiura K., Togo S., Hayashizaki Y., Ishikawa T., Endo I., Shimada H. (2010). Association between Breast Cancer Risk and the Wild-type Allele of Human ABC Transporter ABCC11. *Anticancer Research,* 30, 5189–5194.

Overall C.M., Kleifeld O. (2006). Tumour microenvironment —Opinion— Validating matrix metalloproteinases as drug targets and anti-targets for cancer therapy. *Nature Reviews Cancer,* 6, 227–239.

Palmieri F. (2013). The mitochondrial transporter family SLC25: identification, properties and physiopathology. *Molecular Aspects of Medicine,* 34, 465–484.

Perren T.J., Swart A.M., Pfisterer J., Ledermann J.A., Pujade-Lauraine E., Kristensen G., Carey M.S., Beale P., Cervantes A., Kurzeder C., du Bois A., Sehouli J., Kimmig R., Stähle A., Collinson F., Essapen S., Gourley C., Lortholary A., Selle F., Mirza M.R., Leminen A., Plante M., Stark D., Qian W., Parmar M.K., Oza A.M., ICON7 Investigators. (2011). A phase 3 trial of bevacizumab in ovarian cancer. *New England Journal of Medicine,* 365, 2484-2496.

Pertega-Gomes N., Vizcaino J.R., Miranda-Goncalves V., Pinheiro C., Silva J., Pereira H., Monteiro P., Henrique R.M., Reis R.M., Lopes C., Baltazar F. (2011). Monocarboxylate transporter 4 (MCT4) and CD147 overexpression is associated with poor prognosis in prostate cancer. *BMC Cancer,* 11, 312.

Pinheiro C., Sousa B., Albergaria A., Paredes J., Dufloth R., Vieira D., Schmitt F., Baltazar F. (2011). GLUT1 and CAIX expression profiles in breast cancer correlate with adverse prognostic factors and MCT1 overexpression. *Histology and Histopathology*, 26, 1279–1286.

Potter M.E., Partridge E.E., Hatch K.D., Soong S.J., Austin J.M., Shingleton H.M. (1991). Primary surgical therapy of ovarian cancer: how much and when. *Gynecologic Oncology*, 40, 195-200.

Prentice R.L., Sheppard L. (1990). Dietary fat and cancer: consistency of the epidemiologic data, and disease prevention that may follow from a practical reduction in fat consumption. *Cancer Causes Control*, 1, 81–97.

Rahma O.E., Ashtar E., Czystowska M., Szajnik M.E., Wieckowski E., Bernstein S., Herrin V.E., Shams M.A., Steinberg S.M., Merino M., Gooding W., Visus C., Deleo A.B., Wolf J.K., Bell J.G., Berzofsky J.A., Whiteside T.L., Khleif S.N. (2012). A gynecologic oncology group phase II trial of two p53 peptide vaccine approaches: subcutaneous injection and intravenous pulsed dendritic cells in high recurrence risk ovarian cancer patients. *Cancer Immunology, Immunotherapy*, 61, 373–384.

Raimondi S., Johansson H., Maisonneuve P., Gandini S. (2009). Review and meta-analysis on vitamin D receptor polymorphisms and cancer risk. *Carcinogenesis*, 30, 1170–1180.

Redman J.R., Petroni G.R., Saigo P.E., Geller N.L., Hakes T.B. (1986). Prognostic factors in advanced ovarian carcinoma. *Journal of Clinical Oncology*, 4, 515-523.

Risch H.A., McLaughlin J.R., Cole D.E., Rosen B., Bradley L., Kwan E., Jack E., Vesprini D.J., Kuperstein G., Abrahamson J.L., Fan I., Wong B., Narod S.A. (2001). Prevalence and penetrance of germline BRCA1 and BRCA2 mutations in a population series of 649 women with ovarian cancer. *The American Journal of Human Genetics*, 68, 700–710.

Rossing M.A., Cushing-Haugen K.L., Wicklund K.G., Doherty J.A., Weiss N.S. (2007). Menopausal hormone therapy and risk of epithelial ovarian cancer. Cancer Epidemiology, *Biomarkers and Prevention*, 16, 2548–2556.

Rossouw J.E., Anderson G.L., Prentice R.L., LaCroix A.Z., Kooperberg C., Stefanick M.L., Jackson R.D., Beresford S.A., Howard B.V., Johnson K.C., Kotchen J.M., Ockene J.; Writing Group for the Women's Health Initiative Investigators. (2002). Risks and benefits of estrogen plus progestin in healthy postmenopausal women: principal results from the women's health initiative randomized controlled trial. *The Journal of the American Medical Association*, 288, 321-333.

Russell H.E., McCluggage W.G. (2004). A multistep model for ovarian tumorigenesis: the value of mutation analysis in the KRAS and BRAF genes. *The Journal of Pathology*, 203, 617-619.

Sakuragi N., Takeda N., Hareyama H., Fujimoto T., Todo Y., Okamoto K., Takeda M., Wada S.I., Yamamoto R., Fujimoto S. (2000). A multivariate analysis of blood vessel and lymph vessel invasion as predictors of ovarian and lymph node metastases in patients with cervical carcinoma. *Cancer*, 88, 2578-2583.

Santen R.J., Allred D.C., Ardoin S.P., Archer D.F., Boyd N., Braunstein G.D., Burger H.G., Colditz G.A., Davis S.R., Gambacciani M., Gower B.A., Henderson V.W., Jarjour W.N., Karas R.H., Kleerekoper M., Lobo R.A., Manson J.E., Marsden J., Martin K.A., Martin L., Pinkerton J.V., Rubinow D.R., Teede H., Thiboutot D.M., Utian W.H. (2010). Postmenopausal hormone therapy: an Endocrine Society scientific statement. *The Journal*

*of Clinical Endocrinology & Metabolism,* 95 (7 Suppl 1): s1-s66. doi: 10.1210/jc.2009-2509.
Sato Y., Shimamoto T., Amada S., Asada Y., Hayashi T. (2003). Prognostic value of histologic grading of ovarian carcinomas. *International Journal of Gynecological Pathology,* 22, 52-56.
Schildkraut J.M., Calingaert B., Marchbanks P.A., Moorman P.G., Rodriguez G.C. (2002). Impact of progestin and estrogen potency in oral contraceptives on ovarian cancer risk. *Journal of the National Cancer Institute,* 94, 32–38.
Schlisio S., Kenchappa R.S., Vredeveld L.C., George R.E., Stewart R., Greulich H., Shahriari K., Nguyen N.V., Pigny P., Dahia P.L., Pomeroy S.L., Maris J.M., Look A.T., Meyerson M., Peeper D.S., Carter B.D., Kaelin W.G. Jr. (2008). The kinesin KIF1Bbeta acts downstream from eglN3 to induce apoptosis and is a potential 1p36 tumor suppressor. *Genes & Development,* 22, 884–893.
Schulz M., Lahmann P.H., Boeing H., Hoffmann K., Allen N., Key T.J., Bingham S., Wirfält E., Berglund G., Lundin E., Hallmans G., Lukanova A., Martínez Garcia C., González C.A., Tormo M.J., Quirós J.R., Ardanaz E., Larrañaga N., Lund E., Gram I.T., Skeie G., Peeters P.H., van Gils C.H., Bueno-de-Mesquita H.B., Büchner F.L., Pasanisi P., Galasso R., Palli D., Tumino R., Vineis P., Trichopoulou A., Kalapothaki V., Trichopoulos D., Chang-Claude J., Linseisen J., Boutron-Ruault M.C., Touillaud M., Clavel-Chapelon F., Olsen A., Tjønneland A., Overvad K., Tetsche M., Jenab M., Norat T., Kaaks R., Riboli E. (2005). Fruit and vegetable consumption and risk of epithelial ovarian cancer: the European Prospective Investigation into Cancer and Nutrition. *Cancer Epidemiology, Biomarkers and Prevention,* 14, 2531–35.
Sebastiani G., Pantopoulos K (2010). Iron Metabolism and Disease. In: Zalups RK, Koropatnick DJ, editors. *Cellular and molecular biology of metals:* CRC Press.
Shi T.Y., Jiang Z., Jiang R., Yin S., Wang M.Y., Yu K.D., Shao Z.M., Sun M.H., Zang R., Wei Q. (2015). Polymorphisms in the kinesin-like factor 1 B gene and risk of epithelial ovarian cancer in Eastern Chinese women. *Tumor Biology* (In press).
Siegel R., Naishadham D., Jemal A. Cancer statistics. (2012). CA: *A Cancer Journal for Clinicians,* 62, 10-29.
Silverberg S.G. (2000). Histopathologic grading of ovarian carcinoma: a review and proposal. *International Journal of Gynecological Pathology,* 19, 7-15.
Simon M., Stefan N., Pluckthun A., Zangemeister-Wittke U. (2013). Epithelial cell adhesion molecule-targeted drug delivery for cancer therapy. *Expert Opinion on Drug Delivery,* 10, 451–468.
Singer G., Shih Ie.M., Truskinovsky A., Umudum H., Kurman R.J. (2003). Mutational analysis of K-ras segregates ovarian serous carcinomas into two types: invasive MPSC (low-grade tumor) and conventional serous carcinoma (high-grade tumor). *International Journal of Gynecological Pathology,* 22, 37-41.
Singer G., Stöhr R., Cope L., Dehari R., Hartmann A., Cao D.F., Wang T.L., Kurman R.J., Shih Ie.M. (2005). Patterns of p53 mutations separate ovarian serous borderline tumors and low and high grade carcinomas and provide support for a new model of ovarian carcinogenesis: a mutational analysis with immunohistochemical correlation. *The American Journal of Surgical Pathology,* 29, 218-224.
Sonoda Y. (2004). Management of early ovarian cancer. *Oncology,* 18, 343–356.

Thigpen T., Brady M.F., Omura G.A., Creasman W.T., McGuire W.P., Hoskins W.J., Williams S. (1993). Age as a prognostic factor in ovarian carcinoma. The Gynecologic Oncology Group experience. *Cancer,* 71, 606-614.

Thomas M.G., Tebbutt S., Williamson R.C. (1992). Vitamin D and its metabolites inhibitcell proliferation in human rectal mucosa and a colon cancer cell line. *Gut,* 33, 1660–1663.

Thomson C.A., Crane T.E., Wertheim B.C., Neuhouser M.L., Li W., Snetselaar L.G., Basen-Engquist K.M., Zhou Y., Irwin M.L. (2014). Diet Quality and Survival After Ovarian Cancer: Results From the Women's Health Initiative. *Journal of the National Cancer Institute,* 106, 1-8.

Trabert B., Wentzensen N., Yang H.P., Sherman M.E., Hollenbeck A., Danforth K.N., Park Y., Brinton L.A. (2012). Ovarian cancer and menopausal hormone therapy in the NIH-AARP diet and health study. *British Journal of Cancer,* 107, 1181–1187.

Trimbos J.B., Schueler J.A., Van der Burg M., Hermans J., Van Lent M., Heintz A.P., Fleuren G.J. (1991). Watch and wait after careful surgical treatment and staging in well-differentiated early ovarian cancer. *Cancer,* 67, 597-602.

Trudel D., Labbe D.P., Bairati I., Fradet V., Bazinet L., Tetu B. (2012). Green tea for ovarian cancer prevention and treatment: a systematic review of the in vitro, in vivo and epidemiological studies. *Gynecologic Oncology,* 126, 491–498.

Tukey R.H., Strassburg C.P. (2000). Human UDP-glucuronosyltransferases: metabolism, expression, and disease. *Annual Review of Pharmacology and Toxicology,* 40, 581–616.

Tworoger S.S., Gates M.A., Lee I.M., Buring J.E., Titus-Ernstoff L., Cramer D., Hankinson S.E. (2009). Polymorphisms in the vitamin D receptorand risk of ovarian cancer in four studies. Cancer Research, 69, 1885–1891.

Urbich C., Dimmeler S. (2004). Endothelial progenitor cells: characterization and role in vascular biology. *Circulation Research*, 95, 343-353.

Van Houwelingen J.C., BokkelHuinink W.W., Van der Burg M.E., Van Oosterom A.T., Neijt J.P. (1989). Predictability of the survival of patients with advanced ovarian cancer. *Journal of Clinical Oncology,* 7, 769-773.

Vergote I., De Brabanter J., Fyles A., Timmerman D., Vandewalle J., Van Gramberen M., Tropé C.G. (2001). Prognostic importance of degree of differentiation and cyst rupture in stage I invasive epithelial ovarian carcinoma. *Lancet,* 357, 176-182.

Vergote I.B., Kaern J., Abeler V.M., Pettersen E.O., De Vos L.N., Tropé C.G. (1993). Analysis of prognostic factors in stage I epithelial ovarian carcinoma: importance of degree of differentiation and deoxyribonucleic acid ploidy in predicting relapse. *American Journal of Obstetrics and Gynecology,* 169, 40-52.

Virág L., Szabó C. (2002). The therapeutic potential of poly(ADP-ribose) polymerase inhibitors. *Pharmacoligal Reviews,* 54, 375–429.

Wang Y., Ye Y., Lin J., Meyer L., Wu X., Lu K., Liang D. (2015). Genetic variants in matrix metalloproteinase genes as disposition factors for ovarian cancer risk, survival, and clinical outcome. *Molecular Carcinogenesis,* 54, 430-439.

Winter M.J., Nagtegaal I.D., van Krieken J.H., Litvinov S.V. (2003). The epithelial cell adhesion molecule (Ep-CAM) as a morphoregulatory molecule is a tool in surgical pathology. *American Journal of Pathology,* 163, 2139–2148.

Yang H., Kong W., He L., Zhao J.J., O'Donnell J.D., Wang J., Wenham R.M., Coppola D., Kruk P.A., Nicosia S.V., Cheng J.Q. (2008). MicroRNA expression profiling in human ovarian cancer: miR-214 induces cell survival and cisplatin resistance by targeting PTEN. *Cancer Research,* 68, 425–433.

Yeh I.T., Lenci R.E., Qin Y., Buddavarapu K., Ligon A.H., Leteurtre E., Do Cao C., Cardot-Bauters C., Pigny P., Dahia P.L. (2008). A germline mutation of the KIF1B beta gene on 1p36 in a family with neural and nonneural tumors. *Human Genetics,* 124, 279–285.

Yeh K.Y., Yeh M., Glass J. (2011). Interactions between ferroportin and hephaestin in rat enterocytes are reduced after iron ingestion. *Gastroenterology,* 141, 292–299.

Zaorsky N.G., Patil N., Freedman G.M., Tuluc M. (2012). Differentiating lymphovascular invasion from retraction artifact on histological specimen of breast carcinoma and their implications on prognosis. *Journal of Breast Cancer,* 15, 478-480.

In: Handbook on Ovarian Cancer
Editor: Bethany R. Collier

ISBN: 978-1-63483-874-0


*Chapter 3*

# MICRORNAS IN DIAGNOSIS OF OVARIAN CANCER. POTENTIAL, CHALLENGES, PITFALLS

***Ludek Zavesky[1,*], Eva Jandakova[2], Lucie Langmeierova[3], Vit Weinberger[4] and Lubos Minar[4]***

[1]Institute of Biology and Medical Genetics, First Faculty of Medicine, Charles University Prague and General University Hospital in Prague, Prague, The Czech Republic

[2]Institute of Pathology, University Hospital Brno, Brno, The Czech Republic

[3]Faculty Transfusion Centre, General University Hospital in Prague, Prague, The Czech Republic

[4]Department of Obstetrics and Gynecology, University Hospital Brno, Brno, The Czech Republic

## ABSTRACT

Ovarian cancer is the most deadly gynecological cancer. High mortality of the patients is usually associated with the progression of the disease. Most of the patients are diagnosed within the advanced stages due to lacking relevant diagnostic and screening markers. Achieving the diagnosis in the early stages of disease is a prerequisite of the more successful treatment of ovarian cancer. In this review, we focus on the recent progress in research focused on circulating, particularly cell-free microRNAs expression in diagnostically relevant samples such as blood, plasma/serum and urine. More research will be needed to establish circulating and extracellular microRNAs as the novel diagnostic markers for ovarian cancer.

## INTRODUCTION

Ovarian carcinomas represent the most fatal gynecological malignancies. Efforts to establish relevant diagnostic and screening markers still have failed due to a relatively low

* Corresponding author: e-mail: ludek.zavesky@gmail.com.

incidence of the disease, often asymptomatic course of the early stages, and compromised sensitivity and specificity of current diagnostic methods [1]. Histological and molecular heterogeneity of the disease with disputed origin and mechanisms of carcinogenesis make the efforts to manage the disease difficult [2-4].

Pelvic examination, assessment of serum CA-125 antigen level (tumor marker) and transvaginal ultrasound (TVU) have been used for decades as the standard diagnostic procedures for ovarian cancer [1]. HE-4 has become another important diagnostic surrogate marker (along with CA-125) for ovarian cancer recently, applied in various combinations or alone, along with other diagnostic procedures. It may result in similar or better performance in terms of sensitivity and specificity in comparison with CA-125 [5-8]. HE-4 may be superior to CA-125 in detection of type II ovarian cancer [9]. Interestingly, there are ongoing attempts to elucidate proper diagnostic and predictive value of HE-4 and CA-125 not only in ovarian cancer, but also in endometrial cancer [10].

Various algorithms to assign patients to a low or a high ovarian cancer risk have also been applied in ovarian cancer diagnostics; the most common are ROMA, Risk of Malignancy Index (RMI), OVA1 and LR2 index [11]. Several other tumor markers have been under investigation in recent years (e.g., OVX1, CA-125 II, CA-72-4, CA15-3, mesothelin, haptoglobin-α, bikunin, C-reactive protein), however, they are not commonly introduced into clinical practice as their sensitivity and specificity for ovarian cancer may be disputed [12]. Other diagnostic approaches may be applied as well [13].

Although the recent progress in search for novel diagnostic approaches appeared as promising, the data on incidence and mortality in ovarian cancer remain unsatisfactory. The success of ovarian cancer treatment is largely associated with the time of diagnosis. The patients diagnosed during stages I and II have been reported with significantly better 5-year survival (stage I: ~86%, stage II: ~69%) than those in the stage III (~40%) and stage IV (19%), with the overall 5-year survival being ~50% previously [14]. De Angelis et al. [15] analyzed data from 107 cancer registries for more than 10 million patients in different European countries in their retrospective observational study (EUROCARE-5). They found the European mean age-standardized 5-year relative survival for ovarian cancer low (37.6%, 95% CI 37.1–38.0), with the worst values observed in the UK and Ireland (31.0%) and the best survival rates in northern Europe (41.1%). For example, this survival rate was 35.5% in Denmark, 36.3% in the Czech Republic, 39.9% in the Netherlands, 40.1% in France, 40.3% in Germany and 44.1% in Sweden [15]. Similarly, in the USA, the diagnosis of localized stages results in the highest survival rate of 92%, while diagnosis in regional stages accounts for a 72% survival and 27% survival rate is reported for women diagnosed in distant stages. On average, a 5-year survival rate of 44% is reported for ovarian cancer patients [16]. Therefore, novel diagnostic and screening markers for ovarian cancer are urgently needed.

In 2013, it has been 20 years since the publication of discovery of the first microRNA [17]. Since then, the microRNAs (miRNAs) have been shown not only to exist in various organisms including humans, but also in various sample types. These small, single-stranded molecules of RNA with the length of ~22 nucleotides are implicated in key cellular processes within the post-transcriptional regulation of gene expression. With the discovery of miRNAs and their regulatory roles, the previous molecular biology paradigms have been largely reconsidered. During the last decades, much research has been focused on the evaluation of miRNA structure, biogenesis, mechanisms of action, potential mRNA targets of particular miRNAs, and their role in carcinogenesis. Accumulating evidence suggested that their targets may involve tens of mRNA. Untangling the intricate net of interactions of thousands of miRNAs identified so far is a great challenge of the current research as their role may be affected by many factors [18].

Meanwhile, apart from their cellular functions, miRNAs have been suggested to participate in intercellular communications and exchange of genetic material between cells (see [19]). MiRNAs may exist in various extracellular forms bound with lipoprotein complexes or encapsulated within different vesicle structures such as exosomes and shedding vesicles [20-22]. The fact that miRNAs may be found in RNase-rich environments such as blood plasma/serum or urine has appeared not as obvious previously as it is currently. Until 2008, this type of investigations was hindered by wrong assumptions while it became evident that miRNAs may be protected against digestion by RNases (see [23]). The focus of hundreds of previous miRNA investigations on tissue and cell lines samples is worth mentioning, as their impact on diagnostic methods is very limited. This may indicate that the initial efforts were to find candidates for targeted therapies rather than to find out novel diagnostic tools. Despite this, several valuable investigations (e.g., [24]) have launched a handful of following research approaches identifying a novel diagnostic potential in various body fluids. Indeed, body fluids either as the source of cells associated with the disease states, or as the carriers of extracellular miRNAs, may harbor a huge diagnostic potential for many diseases [25].

In this review, we focus on the diagnostic potential of miRNAs coming from blood, plasma/serum and urine samples, revealing their so far underestimated potential as perspective and promising diagnostic biomarkers in ovarian cancer, as shown in recent investigations.

## Urinary microRNAs and Ovarian Cancer

Intentionally, we would like to start this review considering urine and its miRNAs. This is to illustrate how the progress in medicine is difficult. Since the discoveries challenging previous assumptions on lack of miRNAs in blood, plasma or serum, a natural shift of researchers came to these samples. However, the promising investigations focused on tissues and cell lines particularly with therapeutic aspirations continued intensively for good reasons.

Studies employing blood-derived samples represent only a minority of investigations even now. The same holds true for urine. Since the discovery of miRNAs presence in various body fluids including urine being published in 2010 [24], intensive efforts considering urine were focused almost exclusively on urogenital tract-related diseases. The studies used various types of urine samples, but the focus has been put particularly on cells and whole urine rather than on the urinary supernatant. Intriguingly, there has not been any relevant and good basis for such an assumption generally, as the urine miRNA research was in its childhood. Around that time, we hypothesized that urinary miRNAs may reflect a more complex picture of miRNAs excretion. Therefore, we have started to evaluate urinary miRNAs expression in ovarian (and endometrial) cancers [26]. This is the first study on urinary microRNA expression published for these cancers.

## Methodological Remarks

The exceptional stability of miRNAs in urine has been revealed a bit more surprisingly than in blood (see later), so that this research is still in the beginning and suffers with a limited number of studies. Urine, likewise as blood, contains abundant nucleases. Thus, it has been previously dismissed by researchers focused on miRNAs, in the same manner as it has happened in blood miRNAs. However, with the onset of novel approaches it has become evident that urinary miRNAs may be isolated, detected, quantified and used as the potential biomarkers as well. Similarly as miRNAs from various sources, also urinary miRNAs have shown a remarkable degree of stability and resistance. The stability of urinary miRNAs due to nuclease resistance has been attributed to smaller nucleic acid size and/or microvesicular containment (e.g., [27]). Indeed, Mall et al. [28] investigated the impact of various storage conditions on urinary miRNAs (miR-16 and miR-21 investigated) and found their remarkable stability. Even after ten freeze–thaw cycles, 23–37% of the initial miRNA amount remained, while over the 5-day period, 42–56% of miRNA remained after storage at 4°C and 35% remained after the storage at room temperature [28]. Moreover, application of trypsin on exosomal fraction of urine has not resulted in any change of concentration, suggesting that stability of urinary miRNA may not be due to its association with exosome-bound structures or macromolecules in urine [28]. Nevertheless, a detailed view of miRNA resistance in urine and other body fluids remains to be further elucidated.

There exist several pitfalls which may affect the results of urinary miRNAs expression assessment. First one is a proper collection of the urine sample ensuring a limited impact of RNases. We suggest according to our methodology to use the second morning urine, as freshly voided urine is advised rather than using large residues stored in the bladder [29]. We recommend using special tubes with antibiotics and stabilization compounds, particularly to stop the RNases activity and eliminate potential bacterial contamination (e.g., Norgen Biotek, Canada). Alternative sampling is also possible, however, these procedures should be as rapid as possible and samples should be stored at - 80°C. RNase-free environment and equipment should be used for urine processing. RNA concentration may be low in urine samples, therefore larger urine volumes may be used, at least 1-2 ml. When using real-time qPCR methods, an optimization of reverse transcription and real-time PCR protocols may be applied, e.g., increasing the input volumes of RNA and cDNA. Efficiency of PCR reactions should be considered in calculations. Normalization procedures should be tested as there are no endogenous control miRNAs (or sn/snoRNAs) generally proved. Carefully selected control patients (e.g., not male samples, the same menopausal status) should be involved where only female patients are investigated.

## Urinary MicroRNAs Expression in Ovarian Cancer

We explored expression of urine microRNAs in urine of patients with ovarian and endometrial cancers [26]. In ovarian cancer (mostly serous adenocarcinomas), we found miR-92a to be up-regulated, and miR-106b and miR-100 down-regulated, in comparison of cancer samples and controls. These miRNAs were consistently deregulated using various normalization procedures. Interestingly, we could not find differences between pre- and post-surgery urine samples in the miRNAs investigated. We could not also find any miRNA as deregulated significantly using exosomal miRNAs [26]. However, we have demonstrated that particular miRNAs may be enriched or diminished in the exosomal fraction of urine in comparison with supernatant fractions, giving differences also between pathological and control samples. This may indicate that diagnostic potential of particular urinary miRNAs may depend on the isolation procedure and possibly on the degree of involvement of exosomes within the analyzed fractions (Záveský et al., in prep.). Although we did not examine exosomes-depleted fractions, it may be suggested that the differences between this type of urine samples and pure exosomes may be the most important ones.

It was far beyond the reach of our study to investigate the exact sources of origin of urinary miRNAs due to lacking methodology at this moment. Extracellular urinary miRNAs may possibly appear in a variety of forms, carried by extracellular vesicles or other vehicles, such as protein complexes and lipoprotein particles (see [29]). Blood plasma filtered in kidneys may serve as their major source in our case. Their concentrations and proportions detected for example by real-time PCR expression analyses may be affected by many means. During the transport through urinary system the other cells may shed their own miRNAs into urine (e.g., in exosomes). On the other hand, the activity of RNases in urine can change its microRNAs content significantly. Storage in the bladder and releasing other cells into urine there and on the way that urine should pass are other factors possibly changing microRNAs expression. It has been demonstrated previously and also in our study that urinary miRNAs may be associated with diseased conditions. As the abovementioned factors are affected by pathological states, miRNAs then appear to be de-regulated. In cancer, studied in our research, factors associated with carcinogenesis and particularly with tumor-released cells may be suspected to play an important role. It can explain up-regulated expression of miRNAs considered as oncogenes (in our study e.g., miR-92a, miR-21). However, down-regulated expression of microRNAs considered as tumor-suppressors (in our study miR-106b, miR-100) requires more attention to be properly elucidated and interpreted.

We included post-surgery samples in addition to pre-surgery samples and found no significant difference between them. It may indicate that the surgery removing tumor masses did not affect the urinary miRNAs extensively. Indeed, when looking at the data, we observed that down-regulated miR-100 and miR-106b remained down-regulated still after the surgery (see S1 experiment, [26]). We demonstrated also the fact that urinary miRNAs expression is fairly influenced by hormonal regulations. Looking at the miRNAs proportions of post-menopausal patients, and pre-menopausal patients either with or without the contraception use, the differences in exosomal miRNAs proportions could be seen (Záveský et al., in prep.).

Recently, another research group provided insight into urinary miRNAs in ovarian cancer. They found urinary miR-30a-5p upregulated while 37 miRNAs were downregulated in patients with ovarian serous adenocarcinoma in comparison with healthy controls [30]. Interestingly, expression of urinary miR-30a-5p was notably reduced following the surgical removal of the tumor, indicating that it was associated with the tumor tissue. This is in a contradiction with our observations in several candidate individual urinary miRNAs revealing no differences between pre- and post-surgery samples [26].

We and the others [26, 30] have evaluated the novel diagnostic potential of urinary miRNAs expression in ovarian cancer as the only studies so far. It is evident that urinary miRNAs expression reflects a complex and intricate net of interactions that should be further investigated in more detail. For example, the origin of urinary miRNAs, the roles of exosomes, differences between various urine fractions (e.g., cellular versus extracellular, exosomal versus other) and the functional aspects of the miRNAs excretion should be further evaluated. This may improve not only diagnostic potential of urinary microRNAs in future, but also can help elucidate biological processes that have been hidden till now. Further investigations on urinary miRNAs should be encouraged to be performed in gynecological cancers and also in many other cancers and diseases to utilize their promising diagnostic potential. Such an effort has been published for breast cancer recently [31]. We expect and hope that the number of such studies will increase somewhat more rapidly.

For details on urinary miRNAs expression in ovarian cancer see Table 1.

## Blood, Plasma and Serum as the Source of MicroRNAs in Ovarian Cancer Diagnostics: Methodological Remarks

### 1. A Complex Nature of MicroRNAs in Blood-Derived Samples

Blood is a complex body fluid composed particularly of blood cells (erythrocytes, leukocytes and thrombocytes) and plasma. As the origin of miRNAs must be sought in cells, miRNAs appearing in plasma and serum samples should be derived from these cells both being with nucleus and anucleate ones (erythrocytes, platelets), and consequently to a particular extent, it mirrors the alterations in these blood components.

In 2008 and following years, many studies have demonstrated that blood plasma/serum miRNAs may reflect disease states. For example, they may be derived from tumor tissues in cancer patients. In many tissues, there could be tissue-specific miRNAs among the others; however, many miRNAs occur generally in the tissues. Therefore, it is very difficult to distinguish the true origin of particular miRNA in blood-derived samples (see [23]).

Indeed, many miRNAs reported as the tumor markers may be found expressed abundantly in the blood plasma. Blood cells have been shown to substantially affect plasma microRNAs expression. Pritchard et al. [32] demonstrated that 58% of the 79 miRNAs reported as cancer biomarkers may be found highly expressed in one or more blood cell types. In more detail, ten miRNAs were then investigated to test the potential correlations of the miRNA expression and blood cell counts. Myeloid-expressed miRNAs (let-7a, miR-223, miR-197, and miR-574-3p) were positively correlated with the myeloid blood cell counts (neutrophils and platelets), and the lymphoid-enriched miR-150 was correlated with lymphocyte counts [32].

Recently, it has been shown that the platelets should be considered as the specific source of circulating miRNAs [33]. The levels of miR-24, miR-197, miR-191, and miR-223 identified to be abundant in platelets were increased in serum in comparison with platelet-poor plasma. Moreover, several miRNAs have been found to be affected and responsive to the anti-platelet therapy [33].

Lymphocytes have attracted attention of miRNA investigations due to their key role in host immune system for many years. As there exist many functional subpopulations of T cells, their miRNA expression diverges between them [34]. Moreover, different miRNAs have been implicated in the differentiation of both T cells and B cells [35]. Interestingly, corresponding miRNA de-regulations may be found in different sample sources including immune cells. For example, in multiple sclerosis there were several miRNAs up-regulated in both peripheral blood mononuclear cells (PBMCs) and brain white matter lesions, and also miRNAs up-regulated in regulatory T cells (Tregs), plasma, blood cells, PBMCs and brain white matter tissues [36].

How to distinguish the tumor-derived miRNAs occurring in plasma? One of the first efforts provided Taylor & Taylor [37], isolating tumor-derived EpCAM positive exosomes in plasma of ovarian cancer patients. They found that miRNAs expressions of the EpCAM positive exosomes circulating in the blood were broadly consistent with the ovarian tumour cells of the same patients. Among 218 detected miRNAs, 175 miRNAs (i.e., ~80%) were not significantly different between the ovarian tumour cells and their corresponding exosomes, 12 were up-regulated in cells, and 31 were found with increased expression in exosomes. The study corroborated that cancer-specific signatures based on miRNA expression are shared both in cellular (tumor) and exosome (plasma) compartments of ovarian cancer patients. However, they failed to find EpCAM-positive exosomes in control samples [37].

Exosomes are vesicles ranging from 30-100 nm, secreted by live cells, exhibiting various functions in inter-cellular communications, and occurring in higher concentrations in the peripheral circulation during pregnancy and cancer. They may contain proteins, DNA, RNA, miRNA and non-coding RNA (see [22]). Leidinger et al. [38] focused on evaluating the differences among CD3, CD14, CD15, CD19, CD56 positive blood cells, and exosomes as well. They found that a decreased number of miRNAs is found in exosomes in comparison with blood cells. They found CD15 positive cells with the most complex miRNome consisting of 328 miRNAs, while only 186 miRNAs were found in CD19 positive cells, and even less, i.e., 128 miRNAs were found in serum exosomes. Interestingly, 16 miRNAs (miR-1299, miR-3124, miR-4290, miR-2278, miR-32*, miR-3149, miR-877*, miR-584, miR-3148, miR-122, miR-718, miR-670, miR-3680*, miR-193b*, miR-3911 and miR-1228) appeared specific only for exosomes and not for other cells investigated [38].

However, in addition to above-mentioned sources, there exist the other carriers where miRNAs may be found in plasma. Evidently, tumor cells themselves are important contributors to the plasma miRNAs pool either as the source of exosomal miRNAs, or extracellular miRNAs may be released as the by-products of cell lysis. Two major theories suggested recently consider extracellular miRNAs as 1) "by-products" of cellular activity and cell death, and/or 2) on-purpose released cell-cell signaling messengers [20]. The possible mechanisms of miRNA secretion include packaging into various forms of apoptotic bodies, shedding microvesicles, exosomes and lipoprotein HDL particles or binding with associated AGO proteins [20]. Interestingly, microvesicle-associated miRNAs appeared as the least represented fraction while AGO-protein-bound form represented 90-95% of cell-debris-free plasma miRNAs [39, 40]. The exact functions and sources of extracellular miRNAs remain to be further elucidated, as they may be also affected by various external factors such as smoking [41] and food [42]. However, there is lacking a convincing evidence for the transfer and function of dietary miRNAs in human body fluids [43].

To distinguish the different origin of particular miRNAs in blood-derived samples remains the great challenge of the current research. As the result, most of the recent miRNAs expression studies focused on miRNA diagnostic potential cannot attribute the results to their exact source. Instead, the "pooled" miRNome of plasma or other samples is usually investigated.

## 2. Stability of MicroRNAs in Blood

Initially, the presence of RNases in blood hindered the investigations assuming that RNA should not be present in the body fluids rich in ribonucleases such as serum, or considered as being a result of cell death and lyses [see 44].

However, the reports on RNA detection in plasma of nasopharyngeal carcinoma patients [45] and serum of malignant melanoma patients [46] showed that RNA may be readily detected in these biological fluids. In 2008, three ground-breaking studies of Lawrie et al. [47], Mitchell et al. [48] and Chen et al. [49] proving the remarkable stability of endogenous extracellular miRNAs and differences between cancer and control patients were published. Moreover, miRNAs in serum were shown to be highly stable in the harsh conditions (extreme temperature and pH) and even more resistant to RNase digestion than tissue or cellular miRNAs [49].

Further investigations proved that miRNAs may be readily isolated and investigated to assess their expression. However, it became evident that the extracellular miRNAs are a heterogeneous entity consisting of various fractions. The stability of circulating miRNAs was then attributed to their carriers, i.e., various kinds of the microvesicles (microparticles, exosomes, and other vesicular structures) providing the protection of trapped miRNAs against digestion by RNases while naked miRNAs appeared to be RNase-sensitive [48]. Meanwhile, the stability of miRNAs has been shown to be associated also with argonaute proteins [50], explaining their stability in non-vesicle-associated forms of their occurrence in blood.

## Whole Blood MicroRNA Expression in Ovarian Cancer

Up to date, there is only one study profiling miRNAs expression in whole blood available for ovarian cancer [51]. This study evaluated whole blood-borne miRNAs expression in microarray profiles from 24 post-menopausal patients with relapsed ovarian cancer (mostly of the serous type) and 15 age- and sex-matched healthy controls of unknown menopausal status. Among 147 significantly deregulated miRNAs, miR-30c1* has been shown significantly up-regulated, and miR-342-3p, miR-181a* and miR-450b-5p were shown significantly down-regulated still after Benjamini–Hochberg adjustment. Within this investigation, miR-30c-1*, miR-191, miR-155, miR-16, miR-106b, miR-146a, miR-29a and miR-383 previously found to be de-regulated in ovarian cancer have been shown up- or down-regulated similarly as in previous investigations [51] (see Table 1).

## Serum/Plasma MicroRNA Expression in Ovarian Cancer

The first pioneer research focused on exosome miRNAs in serum of ovarian cancer patients has been published in 2008 [37]. The study showed a correlation of miRNA expression between tumor tissues and the tumor-released EpCAM-positive exosomes. However, a limited diagnostic potential of the approach resulted from the absence of exosomes and/or exosomal small RNA in control samples.

Resnick et al. [52] analyzed miRNA expression in serum of ovarian cancer patients and found miRNAs-21, 92, 93, 126 and 29a significantly over-expressed. On the contrary, miRNAs-155, 127 and 99b were significantly under-expressed in comparison of sera between cancer and control patients.

Oncogenic miR-21 and its serum levels were investigated elsewhere [53]. Elevated expression were found in sera of ovarian cancer patients, and the increased miR-21 expression was associated also with advanced FIGO stage, high tumor grade, and shortened overall survival. It has been shown recently that miR-92 may be found up-regulated in serum of ovarian cancer patients [54]. Within this study, 50 ovarian cancer patients and 50 controls were enrolled, and miR-16 was used as an endogenous control. Up-regulation of miR-92a was associated with regional lymph node involvement and advanced clinical stages (III–IV) [54]. Interestingly, as we have shown above, miR-92a was the only one miRNA among investigated miRNAs, which we have found up-regulated in urine of ovarian cancer patients [26].

Back to blood-based samples; the large recent study [55] investigated plasma miRNAs from 360 EOC patients and 200 healthy controls. The study revealed higher levels of miR-205 and lower let-7f expression in cancer samples than in controls, the lower expression of let-7f was also associated with a poor prognosis in EOC patients. In the comparison of early and advanced stages, miR-483-5p expression was increased in stages III and IV [55].

Chung et al. [56] have found down-regulated serum microRNA expression in ovarian cancer patients (18 serous cancers, 12 controls) most markedly and significantly in miR-132, miR-26a, let-7b, miR-145, and miR-143.

The patients with endometriosis, endometriosis-associated ovarian cancer (EAOC) and healthy controls may reveal distinct miRNA signatures in plasma samples [57]. Both miRNAs associated with endometriosis and EAOC, respectively, found to be de-regulated significantly in comparison with healthy controls, were shown up-regulated (miR-21, miR-191, miR-16, miR-15b, miR-1977, miR-1979, miR-1973, miR-1974, miR-4284, and miR-195) [57].

A combined approach using the deep sequencing technology (Solexa) and real-time PCR for miRNAs analysis of serum in ovarian cancer has been applied recently [58]. This study involving 31 patients with ovarian carcinomas, 23 patients with benign ovarian tumors, and 8 control samples confirmed the differential expression of four miRNAs. Here, miR-22 and miR-93 were shown to be consistently (> 2-fold) up-regulated and miR-451 up-regulated in sera of ovarian cancer patients.

On the other hand, miR-106b appeared significantly down-regulated in cancer samples [58]. Again to compare with urine, we have observed miR-106b down-regulated in urine of ovarian cancer samples [26].

**Table 1. List of de-regulated microRNAs found in ovarian carcinomas in blood, plasma/serum and urine samples**

| Type of cancer | Detailed specification | Up-regulated microRNAs | Down-regulated microRNAs | Sample source | Methodology | Reference |
|---|---|---|---|---|---|---|
| Ovarian carcinoma | Relapsed ovarian cancer: serous (n = 22), endometrioid (n = 2). Control samples (n = 15). | miR-16, miR-30c-1*, miR-187, miR-191, miR-383, miR-423-3p, miR-499-3p, miR-574-5p, miR-1181, miR-1228, miR-1253, miR-1254, miR-1289, miR-1908, miR-1915 | miR-28-3p, miR-29a, miR-106b, miR-138-2*, miR-146a, miR-155, miR-181a*, miR-181a-2*, miR-192, miR-342-3p, miR-450-5p, miR-616*, miR-628-5p, miR-1287, let-7f-1* | Whole blood | Geniom Biochip miRNA homo sapiens array. | [51] |
| Ovarian carcinoma | Serous carcinomas (n = 50), benign samples (n = 10), control samples (n = 10) | miR-21, miR-141, miR-200a, miR-200b, miR-200c, miR-203, miR-205, miR-214 | | EpCAM-positive tumor exosomes in blood | Ocean Ridge Biosciences microarrays, GenePix 4000A | [37] |
| Ovarian carcinoma | EOC (n = 28), serous (60%), clear cell (21.2%), endometrioid (12%), mucinous (6%). Control samples (n = 15). | miR-21, miR-29a, miR-92, miR-93, miR-126 | miR-99b, miR-127, miR-155 | Blood serum | TaqMan Array Human MicroRNA Panel, single tube TaqMan MicroRNA Assays | [52] |
| Ovarian carcinoma | Serous carcinomas (n = 68), others (n = 26). Control samples (n = 40). | miR-21 | n/a | Blood serum | TaqMan microRNA assay | [53] |
| Ovarian carcinoma | EOC samples (non-specified) (n = 50). Control samples (n = 50). | miR-92 | | Blood serum | SYBR green qRT-PCR | [54] |

| Type of cancer | Detailed specification | Up-regulated microRNAs | Down-regulated microRNAs | Sample source | Methodology | Reference |
|---|---|---|---|---|---|---|
| Ovarian carcinoma | Total EOC cases (n = 360), incl. 179 serous tumors (49.7%), 86 endometrioid tumors (23.9%), 33 mucinous tumors (9.2%), 15 clear cell tumors (4.2%), and 47 adeno-carcinomas, Not Otherwise Specified (NOS) (13.0%). Control samples (n = 200). | miR-205 | let-7f | Blood plasma | TaqMan Array (TLDA) | [55] |
| Ovarian carcinoma | Serous carcinomas (n = 18), control samples (n = 12). | | miR-132, miR-26a, let-7b, miR-145, and miR-143 | Blood serum (filtration through a 0.2μm filter) | Microarray Affymetrix miRNAV2.0. TaqMan qRT-PCR. | [56] |
| Ovarian carcinoma | Ovarian carcinomas (type unspecified) (n = 31), benign samples (n = 23). Control samples (n = 8). | miR-22 and miR-93 | miR-106b | Blood serum | SYBR green qRT-PCR | [58] |
| Ovarian carcinoma | Serous carcinomas (n = 42), benign samples (n = 36). Control samples (n = 23). | miR-1274a, miR-625-3p, and miR-720 | miR-106a, miR-126, miR-146a, miR-150, miR-16, miR-17, miR-19b, miR-20a, miR-223, miR-24, and miR-92a, miR-106b, miR-191, miR-193a-5p, miR-30b, miR-30a-5p, | Blood plasma (ultracentrifugation, plasma without exosomes) | Taqman Open Array MicroRNA | [59] |

**Table 1. (Continued)**

| Type of cancer | Detailed specification | Up-regulated microRNAs | Down-regulated microRNAs | Sample source | Methodology | Reference |
|---|---|---|---|---|---|---|
| | | | miR-30c, miR-320, and miR-328 | | | |
| Ovarian carcinoma | Serous carcinomas (n =28). Control samples (n = 28). | miR-200a, miR-200b and miR-200c | | Blood serum | Exiqon MiRCURY™ Locked Nucleic Acid Arrays | [60] |
| Ovarian carcinoma | Clear cell carcinomas (n = 21) (pre-operative versus post-operative sera) | miR-130a, miR-138, miR-187, miR-202 | | Blood serum | SYBR green/Taqman microRNA real time PCR | [61] |
| Ovarian carcinoma | EOC, serous carcinomas (n = 5), others (n = 4), benign ovarian samples (n = 3). Control samples (n = 13). | miR-92a | miR-106b | Urine | Taqman microRNA real time PCR | [26] |
| Ovarian carcinoma | 39 ovarian serous adenocarcinoma patients, 26 patients with benign gynecological disease and 30 healthy controls. | miR-30a-5p | 37 miRNAs | Urine | miRNA microarray + real time PCR | [30] |

Another study on serum circulating miRNAs has been published recently [59], investigating 42 serous epithelial cancer samples, 36 benign samples and 23 control samples. The down-regulated expression (at least 10-fold) in cancer samples compared to control samples was found in miR-106a, miR-126, miR-146a, miR-150, miR-16, miR-17, miR-19b, miR-20a, miR-223, miR-24, and miR-92a. The down-regulated expression was also observed in miR-106b, miR-191, miR-193a-5p, miR-30b, miR-30a- 5p, miR-30c, miR-320, and miR-328. Three miRNAs, miR-1274a, miR-625-3p, and miR-720 were up-regulated in cancer samples, but they were shown not to be good discriminators between cancer and control samples [59]. In another study, three serum miRNAs (miR-200a, miR-200b and miR-200c) appeared to be up-regulated significantly in serous ovarian carcinomas (n = 28). A multivariate combination of miR-200b + c resulted in AUC = 0.784 within ROC-AUC analysis [60].

The recent study focused on the clear cell ovarian carcinomas enrolled 21 patients with this histological subtype [61]. The authors have not employed normal healthy controls. Instead, they investigated expression of 270 miRNAs in pre-operative and post-operative samples in 4 patients, identifying eighteen miRNAs with >1.25 fold changes between pre- and postoperative sera. Next, the levels of miR-130a, miR-138, miR-187 and miR-202 have been found with increased expression in the pre-operative sera than in the post-operative sera (11 pairs of sera used). The authors further suggested that miR-130a may be a marker for recurrence (four patients with cancer recurrence, six patients without recurrences were included). Increasing trends of miR-130a expression were seen in all four patients with recurrent cancer and decreasing trends in this miRNA expression were found in three (50%) out of six patients without recurrence [61].

Very recently, Langhe et al. [62] identified a panel of four serum miRNAs (let-7i-5p, miR-122, miR-152-5p and miR-25-3p), which were found significantly down-regulated in ovarian cancer patients, comparing 20 serous ovarian carcinomas and 20 benign serous cystadenomas. Interestingly, these miRNAs target WNT signaling, AKT/mTOR and TLR-4/MyD88, involved in ovarian carcinogenesis.

For details on serum/plasma miRNAs expression see Table 1.

## Pitfalls and Challenges of the Current Research

Despite the recent progress in miRNAs diagnostic research achieved also in ovarian cancer, it is evident that many obstacles yet prevent introducing cell-free miRNAs as novel clinical diagnostics. There is only a limited number of studies investigating miRNAs in blood-derived samples, and only two studies focused on urine in ovarian cancer. With respect to the ethnogeographical issues and underestimated biological variation, their results could not be generally applied unless the international validation and large patients' cohorts will provide a more comprehensive and reliable picture on miRNAs de-regulations. As there are over 2,000 individual miRNAs known in human genome and this number is still increasing, large-scale profiling will be necessary. Methodological challenges include sample collection, stabilization, storage, miRNA isolation, detection, normalization, quantitation, statistical processing and interpretations. As the body fluids-based miRNA research is still in its infancy, no generally applicable procedures may be available for various types of samples/diseases (e.g., endogenous controls in normalization), and individual approach and optimizations might be applicable. Appropriate usage of control healthy samples is strongly recommended, although it is clear that some studies do not include them. Clearly described methodology should be included in the papers; however, the reality is often far from the ideal state. More research will be needed to elucidate also the factors affecting the miRNAs expression at the epigenetic and transcriptional control levels known for cellular processes of miRNA functioning.

## Conclusion

MicroRNAs represent not only the key regulatory molecules, but also diagnostically attractive biomarkers. Due to their presence in various body fluids, a huge potential associated with them should now be explored more intensively. Gynecological cancers including ovarian cancer are less investigated cancers; therefore the scarcity of reports limits the application of their results in the clinical practice at this moment. In ovarian cancer, various types of miRNA samples coming from blood, serum, plasma, leukocytes of various subtypes, urine, ascites, or saliva may exhibit diagnostic or prognostic potential worth investigating. Therefore, more research should now focus on these issues, providing the chance for better outcomes of the affected patients.

## Acknowledgments

The financial support from the Charles University Prague (project PRVOUK-P27/LF1/1) and from the Ministry of Health of the Czech Republic (project FNBr 65269705) is appreciated.

## References

[1] Lutz, A. M., Willmann, J. K., Drescher, C. W., et al. (2011). Early diagnosis of ovarian carcinoma: Is a solution in sight. *Radiology*, *259*, 329-345.

[2] Kurman, R. J. & Shih, I. M. (2011). Molecular pathogenesis and extraovarian origin of epithelial ovarian cancer-Shifting the paradigm. *Human Pathology*, *42*, 918-931.

[3] Zavesky, L., Jancarkova, N. & Kohoutova, M. (2011). Ovarian cancer: Origin and factors involved in carcinogenesis with potential use in diagnosis, treatment and prognosis of the disease. *Neoplasma*, *58*, 457-468.

[4] Koshiyama, M., Matsumura, N. & Konishi, I. (2014). Recent concepts of ovarian carcinogenesis: Type I and type II. *BioMed Research International*, 2014, 934261.

[5] Jacob, F., Meier, M., Caduff, R., et al. (2011). No benefit from combining HE4 and CA125 as ovarian tumor markers in a clinical setting. *Gynecologic Oncology*, *121*, 487-491.

[6] Yu, S., Yang, H. J., Xie, S. Q., et al. (2012). Diagnostic value of HE4 for ovarian cancer: A meta-analysis. *Clinical Chemistry and Laboratory Medicine*, *50*, 1439-1446.

[7] Karlan, B., Thorpe, Y., Watabayashi, J., et al. (2014). Use of CA125 and HE4 serum markers to predict ovarian cancer in elevated-risk women. *Cancer Epidemiology Biomarkers and Prevention*, *23*, 1383-1393.

[8] Stiekema, A., Lok, C. A. R., Kenter, G. G., et al. (2014). A predictive model combining human epididymal protein 4 and radiologic features for the diagnosis of ovarian cancer. *Gynecologic Oncology*, *132*, 573-577.

[9] Gasiorowska, E., Michalak, M. Warchol, et al. (2015). Clinical application of HE4 and CA125 in ovarian cancer type I and type II detection and differential diagnosis. *Ginekologia Polska*, *86*, 88-93.

[10] Antonsen, S., Hoqdall, L., Christensen, E., et al. (2013). HE4 and CA125 levels in the preoperative assessment of endometrial cancer patients: A prospective multicenter study (ENDOMET). *Acta Obstetricia et Gynecologica Scandinavica*, *92*, 1313-1322.

[11] Chudecka-Glaz, A. M. (2015). ROMA, an algorithm for ovarian cancer. *Clinica Chimica Acta*, *440*, 143-151.

[12] Husseinzadeh, N. (2011). Status of tumor markers in epithelial ovarian cancer has there been any progress? A review. *Gynecologic Oncology*, *120*, 152-157.

[13] Zhang, F. & Zhang, Z. L. (2015). The Diagnostic Value of Transvaginal Sonograph (TVS), Color Doppler, and Serum Tumor Marker CA125, CEA, and AFP in Ovarian Cancer. Cell Biochemistry and Biophysics Cell Biochemistry and Biophysics, in press.

[14] Heintz, A. P. M., Odicino, F., Maisonneuve, P., et al. (2006). Carcinoma of the ovary. *International Journal of Gynecology & Obstetrics*, *95*, S161-S192.

[15] De Angelis, R., Sant, M., Coleman, M. P., et al. (2014). Cancer survival in Europe 1999-2007 by country and age: Results of EUROCARE-5-a population-based study. *The Lancet Oncology*, *15*, 23-34.

[16] Siegel, R., Ma, J., Zou, Z., et al. (2014). Cancer statistics, 2014. *CA Cancer Journal for Clinicians*, *64*, 9-29.

[17] Lee, R. C., Feinbaum, R. L. & Ambros, V. (1993). The C. elegans heterochronic gene lin-4 encodes small RNAs with antisense complementarity to lin-14. *Cell*, *75*, 843-854.

[18] Iorio, M. V. & Croce, C. M. (2012). MicroRNA dysregulation in cancer: diagnostics, monitoring and therapeutics. A comprehensive review. *Embo Molecular Medicine*, *4*, 143-159.

[19] Turchinovich, A., Samatov, T. R., Tonevitsky, A. G., et al. (2013). Circulating miRNAs: Cell-cell communication function? *Frontiers in Genetics*, *4*, 119. doi: 10.3389/fgene.2013.00119.

[20] Turchinovich, A., Weiz, L. & Burwinkel, B. (2012). Extracellular miRNAs: The mystery of their origin and function. *Trends in Biochemical Sciences*, *37*, 460-465.

[21] Turchinovich, A. & Cho, W. C. (2014). The origin, function and diagnostic potential of extracellular microRNA in human body fluids. *Frontiers in Genetics*, 2014, 5, 30.

[22] Beach, A., Zhang, H. G., Ratajczak, M. Z., et al. (2014). Exosomes: An overview of biogenesis, composition and role in ovarian cancer. *Journal of Ovarian Research*, 2014, 7, 14.

[23] Zavesky, L., Jandakova, E., Turyna, R., et al. (2015). New perspectives in diagnosis of gynaecological cancers: Emerging role of circulating microRNAs as novel biomarkers. *Neoplasma 62*(4), 509-520. doi: 10.4149/neo_2015_062.

[24] Weber, J. A., Baxter, D. H., Zhang, S. L., et al. (2010). The MicroRNA Spectrum in 12 Body Fluids. *Clinical Chemistry*, *56*, 1733-1741.

[25] Kosaka, N., Iguchi, H. & Ochiya, T. (2010). Circulating microRNA in body fluid: A new potential biomarker for cancer diagnosis and prognosis. *Cancer Science, 101*, 2087-2092.

[26] Zavesky, L., Jandakova, E., Turyna, R., et al. (2015). Evaluation of cell-free urine microRNAs expression for the use in diagnosis of ovarian and endometrial cancers. A pilot study. *Pathology Oncology Research*, in press, DOI, 10.1007/s12253-015-9914-y.

[27] Schwarzenbach, H., Hoon, D. S. B. & Pantel, K. (2011). Cell-free nucleic acids as biomarkers in cancer patients. *Nature Reviews Cancer, 11*, 426-437.

[28] Mall, C., Rocke, D. M., Durbin-Johnson, B., et al. (2013). Stability of miRNA in human urine supports its biomarker potential. *Biomarkers in Medicine, 7*, 623-631.

[29] Witwer, K. W, Buzas, E. I., Bemis, L. T., et al. Standardization of sample collection, isolation and analysis methods in extracellular vesicle research. *Journal of Extracellular Vesicles.*, 2013 May 27, 2. doi: 10.3402/jev.v2i0.20360. eCollection 2013.

[30] Zhou, J., Gong, G., Tan, H., et al. (2015). Urinary microRNA-30a-5p is a potential biomarker for ovarian serous adenocarcinoma. *Oncology Reports, 33*, 2915-2923.

[31] Erbes, T., Hirschfeld, M., Rucker, G., et al. (2015). Feasibility of urinary microRNA detection in breast cancer patients and its potential as an innovative non-invasive biomarker. *BMC Cancer, 15*, 193.

[32] Pritchard, C. C., Kroh, E., Wood, B., et al. (2012). Blood cell origin of circulating microRNAs: A cautionary note for cancer biomarker studies. *Cancer Prevention Research, 5*, 492-497.

[33] Willeit, P., Zampetaki, A., Dudek, K., et al. (2013). Circulating MicroRNAs as novel biomarkers for platelet activation. *Circulation Research, 112*, 595-600.

[34] Smigielska-Czepiel, K., Van Den Berg, A., Jellema, P., et al. (2014). Comprehensive analysis of miRNA expression in T-cell subsets of rheumatoid arthritis patients reveals defined signatures of naive and memory Tregs. *Genes and Immunity, 15*, 115-125.

[35] Belver, L., Papavasiliou, F. N. & Ramiro, A. R. (2011). MicroRNA control of lymphocyte differentiation and function. *Current Opinion in Immunology, 23*, 368-373.

[36] Ma, X., Zhou, J., Zhong, Y., et al. (2014). Expression, regulation and function of MicroRNAs in multiple sclerosis. *International Journal of Medical Sciences, 11*, 810-818.

[37] Taylor, D. D. & Gercel-Taylor, C. (2008). MicroRNA signatures of tumor-derived exosomes as diagnostic biomarkers of ovarian cancer. *Gynecologic Oncology, 110*, 13-21.

[38] Leidinger, P., Backes, C., Meder, B., et al. (2014). The human miRNA repertoire of different blood compounds. *BMC Genomics, 15*, 474.

[39] Arroyo, J. D., Chevillet, J. R., Kroh, E. M., et al. (2011). Argonaute2 complexes carry a population of circulating microRNAs independent of vesicles in human plasma. *Proceedings of the National Academy of Sciences of the United States of America, 108*, 5003-5008.

[40] Turchinovich, A., Weiz, L., Langheinz, A., et al. (2011). Characterization of extracellular circulating microRNA. *Nucleic Acids Research, 39*, 7223-7233.

[41] Momi, N., Kaur, S. Rachagani, et al. (2014). Smoking and microRNA dysregulation: A cancerous combination. *Trends in Molecular Medicine, 20*, 36-47.

[42] Tarallo, S., Pardini, B. Mancuso, et al. (2014). MicroRNA expression in relation to different dietary habits: A comparison in stool and plasma samples. *Mutagenesis*, *29*, 385-391.

[43] Witwer, K. W. (2014). Diet-responsive mammalian miRNAs are likely endogenous. *Journal of Nutrition*, *144*, 1880-1881.

[44] Iguchi, H., Kosaka, N. & Ochiya, T. (2010). Secretory microRNAs as a versatile communication tool. *Commun Integr Biol*, 3(5), 478-481.

[45] Lo, K. W., Lo, Y. M. D., Leung, S. F., et al. (1999). Analysis of cell-free Epstein-Barr virus-associated RNA in the plasma of patients with nasopharyngeal carcinoma. *Clinical Chemistry*, *45*, 1292-1294.

[46] Kopreski, M. S., Benko, F. A., Kwak, L. W., et al. (1999). Detection of tumor messenger RNA in the serum of patients with malignant melanoma. *Clinical Cancer Research*, *5*, 1961-1965.

[47] Lawrie, C. H., Gal, S., Dunlop, H. M., et al. (2008). Detection of elevated levels of tumour-associated microRNAs in serum of patients with diffuse large B-cell lymphoma. *British Journal of Haematology*, *141*, 672-675.

[48] Mitchell, P. S., Parkin, R. K., Kroh, E. M., et al. (2008). Circulating microRNAs as stable blood-based markers for cancer detection. *Proceedings of the National Academy of Sciences of the United States of America*, *105*, 10513-10518.

[49] Chen, X., Ba, Y., Ma, L., et al. (2008). Characterization of microRNAs in serum: A novel class of biomarkers for diagnosis of cancer and other diseases. *Cell Research*, *18*, 997-1006.

[50] Winter, J. & Diederichs, S. (2011). Argonaute proteins regulate microRNA stability: Increased microRNA abundance by Argonaute proteins is due to microRNA stabilization. *RNA biology*, *8*, 1149-1157.

[51] Hausler, S. F. M., Keller, A., Chandran, P. A., et al. (2010). Whole blood-derived miRNA profiles as potential new tools for ovarian cancer screening. *British Journal of Cancer*, *103*, 693-700.

[52] Resnick, K. E., Alder, H., Hagan, J. P., et al. (2009). The detection of differentially expressed microRNAs from the serum of ovarian cancer patients using a novel real-time PCR platform. *Gynecologic Oncology*, *112*, 55-59.

[53] Xu, Y. Z., Xi, Q. H., Ge, W. L., et al. (2013). Identification of serum microRNA-21 as a biomarker for early detection and prognosis in human epithelial ovarian cancer. *Asian Pacific Journal of Cancer Prevention*, *14*, 1057-1060.

[54] Guo, F., Tian, J., Lin, Y., et al. (2013). Serum microRNA-92 expression in patients with ovarian epithelial carcinoma. *Journal of International Medical Research*, *41*, 1456-1461.

[55] Zheng, H., Zhang, L., Zhao, Y., et al. (2013). Plasma miRNAs as diagnostic and prognostic biomarkers for ovarian cancer. *PLoS ONE*, *8*, e77853.

[56] Chung, Y. W., Bae, H. S., Song, J. Y., et al. (2013). Detection of microRNA as novel biomarkers of epithelial ovarian cancer from the serum of ovarian cancer patients. *International Journal of Gynecological Cancer*, *23*, 673-679.

[57] Suryawanshi, S., Vlad, A. M., Lin, H. M., et al. (2013). Plasma MicroRNAs as novel biomarkers for endometriosis and endometriosis-associated ovarian cancer. *Clinical Cancer Research*, *19*, 1213-1224.

[58] Ji, T., Zheng, Z. G., Wang, F. M., et al. (2014). Differential microRNA expression by solexa sequencing in the sera of ovarian cancer patients. *Asian Pacific Journal of Cancer Prevention*, *15*, 1739-1743.

[59] Shapira, I., Oswald, M., Lovecchio, J., et al. (2014). Circulating biomarkers for detection of ovarian cancer and predicting cancer outcomes. *British Journal of Cancer*, *110*, 976-983.

[60] Kan, C. W. S., Hahn, M. A., Gard, G. B., et al. (2012). Elevated levels of circulating microRNA-200 family members correlate with serous epithelial ovarian cancer. *Bmc Cancer*, *12*, 627.

[61] Chao, A., Lai, C. H., Chen, H. C., et al. (2014). Serum microRNAs in clear cell carcinoma of the ovary. *Taiwanese Journal of Obstetrics and Gynecology*, *53*, 536-541.

[62] Langhe, R., Norris, L., Saadeh, F. A., et al. (2015). A novel serum microRNA panel to discriminate benign from malignant ovarian disease. *Cancer Letters*, *356*, 628-636.

In: Handbook on Ovarian Cancer
Editor: Bethany R. Collier

ISBN: 978-1-63483-874-0


*Chapter 4*

# IMMUNOTHERAPY AND TARGET THERAPY: NEW APPROACHES IN OVARIAN CANCER

***Rosekeila Simões Nomelini[1*], Millena Prata Jammal[1], Agrimaldo Martins Filho[1] and Eddie Fernando Candido Murta[1]***

[1]Discipline of Gynecology and Obstetrics, Oncological Research Institute (IPON), Federal University of the Triângulo Mineiro, Uberaba, MG, Brazil

## ABSTRACT

Ovarian cancer remains the leading cause of death among gynecological malignancies. Surgery should be performed in adnexal masses suspected of ovarian cancer for diagnosis, staging and treatment. The debulking surgery is still the main surgical approach in advanced primary ovarian cancer. The adjuvant treatment is performed with taxanes and platinum-based chemotherapy. The addition of the bevacizumab, an anti-angiogenic agent, is recommended. Adjuvant treatment in ovarian cancer in advanced stage leads to an improvement in disease-free survival in approximately 10-30% of patients, depending on the stage and residual disease. Retrospective data show better outcomes in patients who underwent complete cytoreduction. Immunotherapy can be insufficient to eliminate all tumor when used alone. However, the use after surgery and chemotherapy can be useful to eliminate remaining tumor cells.

In recent years, there was an increase in the use of immunohistochemical markers in ovarian cancer. Most of the published data refers to the use of antibodies for diagnosis, some markers also has prognostic value.

In general, when immunohistochemistry is utilized for diagnosis markers panels provide better information than the use of a single antibody. Ovarian cancer is a heterogeneous disease; each of the subtypes is associated with different genetic risk

* Corresponding author: Prof. Rosekeila Simões Nomelini, Oncological Research Institute (IPON)/Discipline of Gynecology and Obstetrics, UFTM, Av. Getúlio Guaritá, s/n, Bairro Abadia, 38025-440 Uberaba-MG, Brazil. E-mail: rosekeila@terra.com.br.

factors and molecular events during oncogenesis. Each subtype responds differently to chemotherapy.

The tendency of ovarian cancer treatment is moving toward different therapies for their specific subtypes. It is likely that a panel of tumor markers will be required to detect all subtypes of the disease. The ovarian cancer subtypes should be considered as distinct diseases in biomarker studies and clinical trials, in order to relate the biomarker, diagnosis and prognosis.

The main aim of this chapter is to provide an update of the current treatments in ovarian cancer. The section also demonstrates the potential targets of future therapies, such as immunotherapy and target therapies.

## INTRODUCTION

Ovarian cancer is one of the most lethal types of malignant tumors in women around the world [1, 2]. It is often found in advanced stages due to lack of effective strategies and displays nonspecific symptom in the early stage of the disease. At diagnosis, more than 70% of patients present with advanced or metastatic [3].

The American Cancer Society estimates that 21,290 women will be diagnosed with some type of ovarian cancer in the United States and of these 14,180 will die from the disease in 2015 [4]. The estimated incidence worldwide is approximately 224,000 cases diagnosed each year, while nearly 150,000 women die from this disease annually [5]. Ovarian cancer ranks fifth in cancer deaths among women, accounting for more deaths than any other cancer of the female reproductive system. Most patients are diagnosed in advanced stage of the disease, and this fact is closely correlated with a poor prognosis [6].

Although there have been advances in surgical techniques and conventional chemotherapy, the prognosis of patients with ovarian cancer was not have improved significantly [3]. In most cases, recurrence occurs in two years, and some patients become resistant to chemotherapy and the five-year survival is only 45% [7]. Unlike cancer in other organs, ovarian cancer may spread by direct extension to adjacent organs, and exfoliated tumor cells can be carried throughout the peritoneal cavity [8]. Thus, the elucidation of the mechanism involved in the invasion of ovarian cancer and its progression are crucial for the development of new therapies [9].

Ovulation can increase levels of inflammatory agents that may still lead to mutations in the DNA. Ovulation creates breaks in the ovarian surface, which leads to healing with increased levels of inflammatory mediators and reactive oxygen species [10]. These reactive oxygen species can interact directly with the DNA by oxidizing its structures, increasing exponentially the chances of developing mutations in the DNA chains [10, 11]. An alternative theory proposes that the tumors with a Mullerian phenotype, such as serous, endometrioid and clear cell carcinoma, are derived from mülleriano tissue. This columnar epithelium tissue cysts may originate paratubal and paraovarian cysts. According to this theory, ovarian tumors develop from these ovarian cysts, and not the superficial epithelium. The tumor growth compresses and destroy the ovarian tissue, resulting in ovarian tumor that appears to have arisen in the ovary [12].

## Ovarian Carcinogenesis

Recent studies have proposed an ovarian carcinogenesis model. In this model, epithelial ovarian tumors are divided into two groups, Type I and Type II, according pathological, genetic and molecular characteristics. Type I ovarian tumors are slow-growing tumors that can develop from precursor lesions. They are serous borderline tumors with micropapillary default, low-grade serous and low-grade mucinous carcinomas, endometrioid and clear cell carcinomas. They usually present as large masses, confined to an ovary (stage Ia). They are genetically stable, have a good prognosis and are characterized by mutations in several genes. In contrast, Type II ovarian tumors grow rapidly and are highly aggressive. Most of them are diagnosed in advanced stages. Examples of such tumors are high-grade serous carcinomas, malignant mesodermal mixed tumor (carcinosarcoma) and undifferentiated tumors.

They have TP53 mutation in 50% to 80% of cases and have a high level of genetic instability [13, 14].

## Treatment

Optimal debulking surgery combined with postoperative chemotherapy (paclitaxel and platinum based agents) are the current standard of epithelial ovarian cancer therapy [15]. The addition of bevacizumab can be performed in recurrent disease [16]. Although this treatment is effective for early stage epithelial ovarian cancer, over 60% of women with advanced stage disease will have recurrent disease [17].

There is no well-defined treatment strategy for recurrent ovarian epithelial cancer. The survival rate at 5 years is even below 30% [18]. A new chemotherapy and second debulking surgery are the two major therapeutic strategies for recurrent ovarian epithelial cancer. The recurrence of epithelial ovarian cancer may suggest a poor prognosis and it is often lethal. The general principle for the treatment of recurrent cancer is palliative, and the main objectives are increasing the survival time, relieve symptoms and improve quality of life [19].

The ideal treatment of ovarian cancer has not been satisfactorily established due to poor understanding of its natural history, histopathologic features, tumor immunology, treatment response and prognostic factors [20]. Further clarification of new prognostic factors in ovarian cancer are needed to help further stratification of patients into risk groups and to allow further refinement of adjuvant treatment recommendations.

## Potential Targets of Future Therapies: Immunotherapies and Target Therapies

Immunotherapy is the cancer treatment that promotes the stimulation of the immune system with substances that modify biological response. The purpose is to present tumor-associated antigens in the context of appropriate costimulatory molecules, and achieve blocking the tumor evasion mechanisms that tend to lead to immunological tolerance [21]. New therapies need to be integrated in ovarian cancer treatment strategies to achieve durable clinical outcomes.

Over the past two decades, advances in understanding the immunogenicity of ovarian cancer have shown new immunotherapy approaches in treatment [22]. Antibodies are excellent anti-cancer agents because of their high specificity for antigen, stability and simplicity to be produced by bioengineering. The ideal target for antibodies should be selectively or highly expressed by tumor cells and not by normal cells.

Antibodies can induce apoptosis of tumor cells through several mechanisms, such as blocking receptor or blocking growth factors that are essential to the cell and inducing apoptosis, antibody-dependent cellular cytotoxicity (ADCC) or complement-dependent cytotoxicity (CDC) [23]. Antitumor effects are exerted through two complementary paths. Firstly the specific antibody facilitates cytotoxicity mediated by T cells through location in the tumor tissue. Simultaneously, Natural Killer cells (NK) promote tumor lysis [24].

The antibody therapy has been increasingly used in ovarian cancer. Tumor angiogenesis plays a critical role in tumor growth and progression. In the absence of neovascularization, most solid tumors stop growing and enter an inactive phase [25]. The following sections describe some immunotherapies and targeted therapies studied as potential treatments in ovarian cancer.

## Angiogenesis and Vascular Endothelial Growth Factor Inhibitors

Angiogenesis is an interesting target in ovarian cancer. Longer maintenance therapy may improve efficiency, because the benefit of therapy may be lost when the inhibition of angiogenesis ends [25].

The main pathway involved in tumor angiogenesis is modulated by the VEGF family (vascular endothelial growth factor) and their receptors. VEGF is a key mediator of angiogenesis and it can regulate tumor vasculature. The anti-VEGF antibody therapy has been proven effective in several subtypes of cancer [22].

Ovarian cancer is a promising candidate for therapy with VEGF. In ovarian tumor tissues, the expression of the VEGF gene correlates with a poor prognosis [26]. Recently, attention turned to the role of angiopoietin family. The angiopoietin family consists of four elements. Ang-1 is produced predominantly by vascular mural cells, and it is a pro-angiogenic factor that acts upon the endothelial cells modulating cellular interactions and it promotes cellular differentiation.

Ang-2 is produced by endothelial cells, and it binds to the same receptor Ang-1. Angiopoietin (Ang) 1 and 2 are important selective growth factors of endothelial cells [27]. Ang-4, almost exclusively expressed in lung, is relatively poorly characterized, whereas Ang-3 is ortholog of mouse Ang-4. They act on specific binding and stimulate the tyrosine kinase receptors of endothelial cells Tie 2. Tie 1 and 2 are specific receptors expressed on vascular endothelial cells and lymphatic endothelial cells. Ang1 binds to the Tie2 receptor promoting stability of blood vessels by enhancing the interactions between perivascular cells and endothelium, improves survival of endothelial cells and the vasculature leading to vascular stability with reduction of permeability. Ang2 interferes with vascular normalization mediated by Ang1 resulting in vascular destabilization and increase of vascular permeability [25].

Various types of angiogenesis inhibitors are studied in ovarian cancer, including VEGF monoclonal antibodies (bevacizumab) or VEGFR2 (ramucirumab), VEGF (VEGF Trap, Aflibercept) or inhibitors of tyrosine kinase (TKI) [25].

The anti-angiogenic drug most investigated (non angiopoietin) is bevacizumab, a human monoclonal antibody (Mab) that binds all isoforms of vascular endothelial growth factor (VEGF). The results of research involving bevacizumab show that it leads to increased progression-free survival [28, 29]. The benefits in overall survival and progression free survival were greater among those patients at high risk of disease progression (14.5 months of progression-free survival with standard therapy versus 18.1 months with addition of bevacizumab, and overall survival of 28.8 and 36.6 months, respectively) [29].

The GOG 218 is a phase III randomized study that evaluated the use of bevacizumab at or above 10 months of chemotherapy with paclitaxel and carboplatin. Its utilization can prolong the median progression-free survival of about 4 months in patients with advanced epithelial ovarian cancer, indicating that VEGF promotes the progression of ovarian cancer and that blocking VEGF can inhibit tumor growth, metastasis and ascites formation, thus supporting a synergistic action of anti-VEGF MoAb to conventional chemotherapy [30].

The addition of bevacizumab to chemotherapy with gemcitabine-carboplatin reduces the risk of disease progression by more than half of women with recurrent epithelial ovarian cancer. Therefore, bevacizumab is a therapeutic option for recurrent ovarian cancer. The toxicity of bevacizumab in ovarian cancer and other solid tumors include hypertension, thrombosis, hemoptysis, proteinuria and headache [31].

Besides VEGF, other factors related to angiogenesis also represent promising therapeutic targets in cancer therapy. The Platelet-derived growth factor (PDGF) is essential for pericyte recruitment, which is an important component of the maturation of blood vessels. Preclinical studies have shown that activation of the PDGF receptor increases angiogenesis. More importantly, interactions with VEGF signaling have been described both in the PDGF / VEGF as in the activation of PDGF on the resistance to inhibition of VEGF [32]. This evidence explains the combination of PDGF and VEGF inhibition [33].

Preclinical studies have demonstrated reduction in vascularization and pericytes when the approach was used in tumor models in mice. The association of its expression also demonstrates the importance of PDGF in ovarian cancer prognostic. Similarly the PDGF family, fibroblast growth factor (FGF) has also been implicated in the resistance of the VEGF pathway inhibitors. FGF is a well known activator of angiogenesis and has been found in high levels in ovarian cancer compared to benign tumors [34].

The angiopoietin antagonist "AMG 386" (Trebananib, Amgen®, Thousand Oaks, CA, US) belongs to a new type of formulation mimicking the molecular structure of traditional human immunoglobulin IgG1: peptibody. A peptibody is a fusion of a protein and an Fc-peptide engineered through the chimerization of a functional peptide with a fragment of immunoglobulin that carrier Fc domain (Crystallizable Region Fragment).

The most promising representative of the family is AMG386. This molecule has been produced with the goal of achieving tumor anti-angiogenesis by interference in the activity of angiopoietins (Ang 1/2) and its connection with the Tie2 receptor. Therefore, the AMG 386 hinders the new tumor angiogenesis [35].

In 2012, Karlan et al. reported the results of a phase II, randomized, double-blind, placebo-controlled study which evaluated the effects of AMG 386 (3 or 10 mg / kg iv, weekly) in combination with paclitaxel (80 mg / m2 iv, weekly, 3 weeks and a week without medication) in 161 patients with recurrent advanced ovarian cancer, primary peritoneal cancer or tubal carcinoma. The median disease-free survival was 7.2 months in the group A (AMG 386 10 mg / kg), 5.7 months in the group B (AMG 386 3 mg / kg), and 4.6 months in the group C (placebo). All patients evaluated in Group A had a reduction in serum CA-125 compared to 84% of patients in group B 63% of patients in group C [36]. Current literature demonstrates an adequate safety profile of AMG 386, unlike other anti-angiogenic agents, also suggesting that the combination of AMG 386 with another cytotoxic therapy would probably be safe.

## ANTIBODIES

Catumaxomab (Removab®, Fresenius Biotech GmbH) is a bispecific antibody directed against the epithelial cell adhesion molecule (EpCAM) and the CD3 T cell antigen. Primary and metastatic epithelial ovarian tumors express EpCAM in significantly higher level in comparison with the normal surface epithelium [24].

Cetuximab is a chimeric monoclonal IgG1 antibody that binds to the receptor extracellular portion for the epidermal growth factor (EGFR), which is present on the surface of some cancer cells, preventing its signaling. This binding inhibits phosphorylation of the EGFR and the chain of biochemical events that result in stimulation of cell proliferation. Cetuximab is administered routinely in the treatment of metastatic colorectal and head and neck cancer. Up to 70% of ovarian cancer tumors are EGFR-positive, being a promising therapeutic target for this disease. In vitro, treatment of cell lines of ovarian cancer with cetuximab inhibits cell growth, enhances apoptosis, and impairs tumor metastasis [22].

In response to unique aspects of ovarian cancer, including platinum resistance development and role of primary cells in the tumor miroenvironment, researchers strive to find additional strategies in the treatment of ovarian cancer [37].

The term "platinum resistant" is used to describe patients whose recurrence of the disease occurs within 6 months after the platinum-based therapy. Agents studies used to reverse the in vitro platinum resistance are in progress [38, 39].

A clear difference was found between non-serous and serous carcinomas in relation to expression of folate receptor (FR), in particular the isoform overexpression of FRα on the surface of almost all epithelial ovarian cancers. Thus it could be an excellent "antigen associated with tumor" and it could be utilized the treatment of ovarian cancer resistant to platinum [40]. It has been suggested that FRα can affect cell proliferation through signaling pathways, and it can increase tumor progression. Studies show their association with ovarian cancer of high-grade platinum resistance. For this reason, FRα is an attractive target for immunotherapy based on monoclonal antibodies against the cancer [40, 41].

Some studies have shown the expression of steroid receptors and HER2 (stimulator of epidermal growth receptor - subtype 2) can be associated with prognosis and therapeutic response, but the results are conflicting [42]. The monoclonal antibody trastuzumab (Herceptin) and Pertuzumab (both from Roche) are antibodies against human HER2. Clinical evidence has shown a limited amount of trastuzumab use in recurrent ovarian cancer. However Pertuzumab, which inhibits the dimerization of HER2 with other HER receptors, can be promising platinum resistance diseases in conjunction with other treatments [42].

The HER3 may be associated with poor prognosis in ovarian cancer and resistance to chemotherapy. The ErbB3 monoclonal antibody (MM-121, Merrimack Pharmaceuticals, Cambridge, US) in combination with paclitaxel is under investigation in advanced cancer and platinum-resistant ovarian cancer [43].

## Toll-Like Receptors (TLRs)

Toll-like receptor (TLR) expressed on leukocytes (e.g., macrophages) have an important role in early immune response by activating numerous pro-inflammatory pathways that result in secretion of cytokines and activation of immune cells, including adaptive immune response [44]. The population of leukocytes infiltrating the tumor environment differs between the types of cancer and has been demonstrated that specific leukocyte at the site profile has a profound effect on tumor progression or regression. Activation of Toll-like receptor in immune cells can promote anti-tumor immune response, through the activation of anti-tumor T cells (NK cells, cytotoxics T lymphocytes).

Several clinical trials have been conducted in an attempt to stimulate Toll-like receptor for ovarian cancer therapy including the use of TLR agonists in combination with other immunostimulatory agents such as dendritic cell vaccines. Overall, these studies point to the promising effects of stimulation of TLR in ovarian cancer, especially integrated with conventional treatments or as adjuvants to other immunotherapies [45].

In 2009, Zhou and colleagues described the expression of TLRs in tissue samples of human ovarian, including normal and neoplastic tissue (benign and malignant). TLR2, TLR3, TLR4, TLR5 were found in ovarian epithelial tissue [46]. It has been shown that TLRs expressed in epithelial cells was functional and it was suggested that its activation could be a mechanism by which epithelial cancer cells can lead to inflammatory pathways to stimulate tumor growth. The last decade research on TLRs in tumor cells suggests that TLR activation in cancer cells leads to increased production of angiogenic cells and molecules, facilitating the immune evasion.

The TRL signal can be attributed to more aggressive disease, risk for metastasis and poor prognosis. Thus, specific inhibitors of TRLs (derived from tumor cells) can be operated with potential therapeutic targets in some patients with ovarian cancer, especially those with advanced stage and with few therapeutic options [47].

## Tumor Associated Macrophages (TAMs)

Tumor associated macrophages (TAMs) are a major component of solid tumors and facilitating tumor growth by stimulating the cancer cells proliferated by these cells assist in the avoidance processes of the immune system and promote angiogenesis.

In cancer patients, high levels of TAMs are often correlated with poor prognosis. In this context, most of them have focused on destroying the TAMs. In ovarian tumor microenvironment, they are many TAMs. Thus, these cells are important targets for new cancer therapies [48]. The TAMs are classified into two sub-groups with different profiles of cytokine.

In the class M1 (polarized), macrophages are activated by interferon-γ (IFN-γ) and are characterized by the production of pro-inflammatory cytokines and immune stimulatory (for e.g., IL-6, IL-12). By stimulating the immune system and antigen presentation, M1 macrophages have a tumoricidal effect. In the class M2, macrophages (polarized) are activated by Th2 cytokines (e.g., IL-4, IL-10) and exert anti-inflammatory effects [49].

In ovarian tumors, M2 macrophages contribute to immunosuppressive mechanisms mediated TAMs. Ovarian tumor macrophages secrete CCL22 cytokine that promotes the passage of regulatory T cells (Treg) to the tumor, having anti tumor effect. While anti-CCL22 mAbs and anti-B7-H4 scFvs exert antitumor effects by modulating the interaction between macrophages and T cells, there is stimulating factor-1 receptor (CSF-1R) acting directly on the immunosuppressive TAMs, depleting them [49].

In 2011, an anti-CSF-1R mAb humanized, RG7155 (Roche) entered in clinical trials. The results of the Phase Ia / Ib trial (NCT01494688) indicate that treatment with RG7155 is well tolerated and effective against TAMs, showing a promising therapeutic approach for ovarian cancer [50].

## Cytotoxic T-Lymphocyte-Associated Protein 4 CTLA-4

The cytotoxic T-lymphocyte-associated protein 4 (CTLA-4 or CD152) plays a key role in the regulation of T cell activation [51]. Activation is triggered by antigen recognition by the T cell receptor (TCR), but co-stimulatory or co-inhibitory signal determining the intensity of the response. The cell surface molecule CD28 and its ligand CD80 (B7-1) and CD86 (B7-2) are major sources of co-stimulatory signal. CD80 and CD86 are found predominantly in antigen presenting cells such as monocytes, activated B cells and dendritic cells. By limiting or reversing activation of T cells, CTLA-4 acts as an important immune checkpoint that helps contain immune responses [51].

The immunosuppressive tumor microenvironment, CTLA-4 blockade has the potential of activate CD4 + T cells and CD8 + effector T cells, leading to tumor clearance. In a variety of pre-clinical tumor models, administration of an anti-CTLA-4 antagonist antibody induced tumor rejection. The success of anti-CTLA-4 therapy takes interest in immunotherapy and resulted in the approval by the FDA in 2011 of anti-CTLA-4 mAb ipilimumab (Yervoy®, Bristol-Myers Squibb) [52].

Most of the clinical experience with ipilimumab has come from studies in patients with melanoma, but there is a Phase II monotherapy study of ipilimumab in ovarian cancer patients with platinum-sensitive ongoing [22].

## Vaccines

One of the main strategies used to generate systemic immune responses against cancer is the development of antitumor vaccine based therapy [21]. The vaccine is designed to induce an immune response specific to the tumor, enhancing the presentation of tumor-associated antigen (TAA) by antigen presenting cells (APCs) generate specific cytotoxic lymphocytes to the tumor antigen.

Unlike chemotherapy, surgery, radiotherapy, or antibody therapy, an effective immune response induced by the vaccine may establish a state of immunological memory, which persists and suppresses a new tumor growth. In recent decades, several therapeutic approaches to cancer vaccines have been developed and dendritic cell vaccines are recognized as efficacious in ovarian cancer [21, 53].

### Vaccines Dendritic Cells (DC)

Vaccines dendritic cells (DC) attempt to increase the uptake of efficient DC (and hence tumor specific T cells) and presentation of tumor-associated antigen (TAAs) in order to change the equilibrium toward immunosuppression immune surveillance or reprogram the immune system from the phase escape or tumor escape to balance or elimination phase [53]. The innate immune system is potentially capable of recognizing and mutant cells to induce an antitumor response, orchestrated in transition with acquired immune cells, especially DCs [54]. The immunotherapeutic strategy for dendritic cells is based on their ability to capture and present tumor proteins, triggering an effective immune response, through the activation and expansion of effector cells and Th1 lymphocytes, CTL lymphocytes and NK cells (61). The immune system is stimulated to generate a specific response and to discriminate their targets with great precision, making the attack mechanism is highly directed towards the neoplastic tissue. The cancer vaccine causes few side effects because it does not lead to immunosuppression, unlike chemotherapy [54].

Innate immunity trigger an initial response by releasing cytokines that target the abnormal cells lysis (lane NK cells), or by internalizing antigens (monocytes, macrophages or DCs) for subsequent presentation to T cells recognizing peptide complexes tumor cells via MHC-I through the TCR receptor, promotes the activation and release of CTL cytotoxin (perforin and granzyme), destroying malignant cells [55]. This anti-tumor immunotherapeutic strategy is based on the development of vaccines which, starting from DCs precursors are differentiated and subsequently loaded with autologous tumor antigens, favoring a targeted and effective immune response [55]. Immunosuppressive cells are attracted to the tumor microenvironment due to secretion of chemokines, cytokines and other mediators produced by the tumor and immune cells around the tumor. They will in turn start producing various mediators that will enhance their contributing to the escape of tumor cells. Among the groups of cells, the most relevant with regard to gynecological pelvic tumors are now the regulatory T (Treg) cells, suppressor cells derived from myeloid lineage (MDSC) and tumor associated macrophage (TAMs) [56]. The results of the first tests with DC vaccines were inconclusive since tumor regression was observed only sporadically [57].

## Adoptive Cell Therapy (ACT)

Recent advances in the application of immunotherapy based on the adoptive T cell transfer and its prospects for the treatment of EOC now offer a new opportunity to specifically modulate the number and activity of T cells in the EOC and mediate tumor regression [58].

The strategy of using primary human T cells genetically modified to express a co-stimulatory immune receiver provided with bispecific molecules provides the possibility of a simple method for distributing costimulatory signals to antigen-redirect cytotoxic T cells [59, 60]. Infusion of T-lymphocytes, referred to adoptive cell therapy (ACT), has the potential to enhance anti-tumor immunity, enhance vaccine efficacy, and eradicate the tumor. The adoptive transfer of TILs requires the isolation of fresh T cells from the patient biopsy samples and progressive expansion of specific T cells ex vivo tumor. Early studies identified methods for producing tumor-reactive polyclonal T cells or tumor ascites. The characteristics of tumor cells and immune components in the microenvironment EOC suggest that this cancer may be responsive to adoptive immunotherapy [61].

The population of tumor-infiltrating leukocytes differs between cancer and has been demonstrated that specific leukocyte at the site profile has a profound effect on tumor progression or regression. As the tumor microenvironment is typically immunosuppressant, efforts are underway to stimulate the immune population to recognize effectively and eliminate tumor cells [62].

The T lymphocytes redirection against tumor antigens can induce dramatic regression of malignancy at an advanced stage. The use of bispecific antibodies (BsAbs) which bind to both the T cell receptor (TCR) and a target antigen is a promising approach for the redirection of T cells [21]. Tumor cells expressing various proteins on their surfaces differing from those of healthy tissue, or by expression levels or to reveal new antigens.

In order to distinguish and mobilize T cells against cancer and maximize antibody targeted therapy, innovative methods are designed to permit T cells to be redirected against TAAs via the TAA-specific antibodies [21].

The adoptive cellular immunotherapy is the transfer of ex vivo activated immune cells with antitumor activity to a tumor bearing host. Examples of this strategy include the adoptive transfer of killer cells activated by lymphokines (LAK). In this approach, lymphoid cells derived from peripheral blood (primary NK cells) are obtained from cancer patients and subsequently activated and expanded in vitro by addition of IL-2.

Then, these cells are returned to the patient (usually accompanied by systemic IL-2 administration) [58, 61]. In a new study, researchers at the Perelman School of Medicine at the University of Pennsylvania showed that a personalized immunotherapy treatment in two phases - one dendritic cell vaccine with patients' own tumor, which was stored at the time of surgery, followed by adoptive therapy T cells - leads to anti-tumor immune responses in such patients. The researchers treated six women with advanced ovarian cancer. All cancers these women had progressed during chemotherapy care [63].

Of the six patients who received the vaccine dendritic cells, four developed an anti-tumor immune response, indicating that the approach was working. One of these patients had no measurable disease at study because it had been successfully removed during surgery. The other three who had an immune response to the vaccine still had residual disease and were taken to the second segment of treatment [63].

Once T-cells have been trained by the dendritic cell vaccine to attack tumor cells, adoptive transfer of T cells amplifies the antitumor immune response. Two women showed an immune response restored after T cell transfer One woman continued to have stable disease, while the other had a complete response to therapy [63].

## CONCLUSION

A significant problem in obtaining clinical benefit for women with ovarian cancer using immunotherapeutic approaches is immunosuppressive nature of the microenvironment of ovarian cancer. In general, the tumor microenvironment is composed of cancer cells together with normal cells (leucocytes, endothelial cells and fibroblasts) and extracellular matrix, which can have important effects on tumor progression. A better understanding of the impact of population of immunosuppressive leukocytes and the direct effect of tumor cells on the local immune function identified additional therapeutic target in ovarian cancer [64, 65].

The role of the immune system modulation, development and progression of cancer has been studied by many researchers, providing a strong reason to proceed foreword in the search for therapeutic strategies for disease. The recognition suppressive factors in the tumor environment will significantly improve the effectiveness of immune future protocols, together with an understanding of the impact of chemotherapeutic agents will allow for improved survival and quality of life of women with ovarian cancer.

## REFERENCES

[1] Jemal, A., Siegel, R., Xu, J. et al. Cancer statistics. *CA: A Cancer Journal for Clinicians*, 2010, 60, 277-300.

[2] Siegel, R., Ma, J., Zou, Z. et al. Cancer statistics. *CA: A Cancer Journal for Clinicians*, 2014, 64, 9-29.

[3] Gu, M., Shi, W. Current Research Management of Ovarian Cancer in China. *The Chinese German Journal of Clinical Oncology*, 2002, 4, 212-218.

[4] American Cancer Society. *Cancer Facts and Figures 2015*. Atlanta, 2015. Available from: www.cancer.org/acs/groups/content/@editorial/documents/document/acspc-044552.pdf.

[5] World Health Organization. *GLOBOCAN 2012: Estimated cancer incidence, mortality and prevalence worldwide in 2012*. France, 2015. Available from: www.globocan.iarc.fr/Default.aspx.

[6] Jemal, A., Bray, F., Center, M. M. et al. Global cancer statistics. *CA Cancer Journal for Clinicians*, 2011, 61: 69-90.

[7] Pylvas-Eerola, M., Karihtala, P., Puistola, U. Preoperative serum 8-hydroxydeoxyguanosine is associated with chemoresistance and is a powerful prognostic factor in endometrioid-type epithelial ovarian cancer. *BMC Cancer*, 2015, 15, 493.

[8] Tan, D. S., Agarwal, R., Kaye, S. B. Mechanisms of transcoelomic metastasis in ovarian cancer. *The Lancet Oncology*, 2006, 7, 925-34.

[9] Prislei, S. et al. Role and prognostic significance of the epithelial-mesenchymal transition factor ZEB2 in ovarian câncer. *Oncotarget, Advance Publications*, 2015 May 15.

[10] Murdoch, W. J., Martinchick, J. F. Oxidative damage to DNA of ovarian surface epithelial cells affected by ovulation: carcinogenic implication and chemoprevention. *Experimental Biology and Medicine*, 2004, 229, 546-552.

[11] Valko, M., Izakovic, M., Mazur, M. et al. Role of oxygen radicals in DNA damage and cancer incidence. *Molecular and Cellular Biochemistry*, 2004, 266, 37-56.

[12] Dubeau, L. The cell of origin of ovarian epithelial tumours. *Lancet Oncol.* 2008 Dec;9 (12):1191-7.

[13] Ali-Fehmi, R., Semaan, A., Sethi, S., Arabi, H., Bandyopadhyay, S., Hussein, Y. R. et al. Molecular typing of epithelial ovarian carcinomas using inflammatory markers. *Cancer*. 2011;15;117(2):301-9.

[14] Kurman, R. J., Shih Ie-Ming. The origin and pathogenesis of epithelial ovarian cancer: a proposed unifying theory. *Am. J. Surg. Pathol.* 2010; 34(3):433-43.

[15] Gardner, G. J., Jewell, E. L. Current and future directions of clinical trials for ovarian cancer. *Cancer Control*, 2011, 18, 44-51.

[16] Aghajanian, C. 1., Blank, S. V., Goff, B. A. et al. OCEANS: a randomized, double-blind, placebo-controlled phase III trial of chemotherapy with or without bevacizumab in patients with platinum-sensitive recurrent epithelial ovarian, primary peritoneal, or fallopian tube cancer. *J. Clin. Oncol.*, 2012, 10;30(17):2039-45.

[17] Jayson, G. C., Kohn, E. C., Kitchener, H. C. et al. Ovarian cancer. *Lancet*, 2014, 384 (9951), 1376-1388.

[18] Raja, F. A., Chopra, N., Ledermann, J. A. Optimal first-line treatment in ovarian cancer. *Annals of Oncology*, 2012, 23, 118-127.

[19] Wei, P., Wei, Z., Li, X., Li, L. et al. Evaluation of prognostic factors for secondary cytoreductive surgery in Chinese patients with recurrent epithelial ovarian carcinoma. *International Journal of Clinical and Experimental Medicine*, 2015, 8(1), 1066-1072.

[20] Chen, M., Jin, Y., Bi, Y. et al. Prognostic Significance of Lymphovascular Space Invasion in Epithelial Ovarian Cancer. *Journal Cancer*, 2015; 6(5): 412-419.

[21] Mocellin, S., Mandruzzato, S., Bronte, V. et al. Part I: vaccines for solid tumours. *Lancet Oncology*, 2004, 5, 681.

[22] Chester, C., Dorigo, O., Berek, J. S. et al. Immunotherapeutic approaches to ovarian cancer treatment. *Journal for ImmunoTherapy of Cancer*, 2015, 3, 7.

[23] Tse, B. W., Collins, A., Oehler, M. K. et al. Antibody-based immunotherapy for ovarian cancer: where are we at?. *Annals Oncology*. 2014, 25(2), 322-331.

[24] Chester, C., Marabelle, A., Houot, R. et al. Dual antibody therapy to harness the innate anti-tumor immune response to enhance antibody targeting of tumors. *Current Opinion in Immunology*, 2015, 33C, 1-8.

[25] Marchetti, C., Gasparri, M. L., Ruscito, I. et al. Advances in anti-angiogenic agents for ovarian cancer treatment: The role of trebananib (AMG 386). *Critical Reviews in Oncology/Hematology*, 2015, 94(3), 302-310.

[26] Hata, K., Watanabe, Y., Nakai, H. et al. Expression of the vascular endothelial growth factor (VEGF) gene in epithelial ovarian cancer: an approach to anti-VEGF therapy. *Anticancer Research*, 2011, 31, 731-737.

[27] Shim, W. S., Ho, I. A., Wong, P. E. Angiopoietin: a TIE(d) balance in tumor angiogenesis. *Mol. Cancer Res.* 2007 Jul;5(7):655-65.

[28] Pujade-Lauraine, E., Hilpert, F., Weber, B. et al. Bevacizumab combined with chemotherapy for platinum-resistant recurrent ovarian cancer: the AURELIA open-label randomized phase III trial. *Journal of Clinical Oncology*, 2014, 32, 1302-1308.

[29] Perren, T. J., Swart, A. M., Pfisterer, J. et al. A phase 3 trial of bevacizumab in ovarian cancer. *New England Journal of Medicine*, 2011, 365(26), 2484-2496.

[30] Burger, R. A., Brady, M. F., Bookman, M. A. et al. Incorporation of bevacizumab in the primary treatment of ovarian cancer. *New England Journal of Medicine*, 2011, 365(26), 2473-2483.
[31] Yap, T. A., Carden, C. P., Kaye, S. B. Beyond chemotherapy: targeted therapies in ovarian cancer. *Nature Reviews Cancer*, 2009, 9(3), 167-181.
[32] Lu, C., Thaker, P. H., Lin, Y. G. et al. Impact ofvessel maturation on antiangiogenic therapy in ovarian cancer. *American Journal of Obstetrics and Gynecology*, 2008 198 (4) 477.
[33] Nissen, L. J., Cao, R., Hedlund, E. M. et al. Angiogenicfactors FGF2 and PDGF-BB synergistically promote murine tumor neo-vascularization and metastasis. *The Journal of Clinical Investigation*, 2007, 117(10), 2766-2777.
[34] Gavalas Nikos, G., Liontos, M., Trachana, S. P. et al. Angiogenesis-Related Pathways in the Pathogenesisof Ovarian Cancer. *International Journal of Molecular Sciences*, 2013, 14, 15885-15909.
[35] Coxon, A., Bready, J., Min, H. et al. Context-dependent role ofangiopoietin-1 inhibition in the suppression of angiogenesis and tumorgrowth: implications for AMG 386, an angiopoietin-1/2-neutralizingpeptibody. *Molecular Cancer Therapeutics*, 2010, 9(10), 2641-2651.
[36] Karlan, B. Y., Oza, A. M., Richardson, G. E. et al. Randomized, double-blind, placebo-controlled phase II study of AMG 386 combined with weekly paclitaxel in patients with recurrent ovarian cancer. *Journal Clinical Oncology*, 2012, 30(4), 362-371.
[37] Hamanishi, J., Mandai, M., Ikeda, T. et al. Efficacy and safety of anti-PD-1 antibody (Nivolumab: BMS-936558, ONO-4538) in patients with platinum-resistant ovarian cancer. *Journal of Clinical Oncology*, 2014, 32, 5s.
[38] Fotopoulou, C., Vergote, I., Mainwaring, P. et al. Weekly AUC2 carboplatin in acquired platinumresistant ovarian cancer with or without oral phenoxodiol, a sensitizer of platinum cytotoxicity: the phase III OVATURE multicenter randomized study. *Annal of Oncology*, 2014, 25, 160-165.
[39] Liu, J., Matulonis, U. A. New strategies in ovarian cancer: translating the molecular complexity of ovarian cancer into treatment advances. *Clinical Cancer Research*, 2014, 20(20), 5150-5156.
[40] Crane, L. M., Arts, H. J., Van-Oosten, M. et al. The effect of chemotherapy on expression of folate receptor-alpha in ovarian cancer. *Cellular Oncology*, 2012, 35(1), 9-18.
[41] Serpe, L., Gallicchio, M., Canaparo, R. et al. Targeted treatment of folate receptor-positive platinum-resistant ovarian cancer and companion diagnostics, with specific focus on vintafolide and etarfolatide. *Pharmacogenomics and Personalized Medicine*, 2014, 29(7), 31-42.
[42] Tafe, L. J., Tsongalis, G. J. The human epidermal growth factor receptor 2 (HER2). *Clinical Chemistry and Laboratory Medicine*, 2012, 50(1), 23-30.
[43] Schmid, B. C., Oehler, M. K. New perspectives in ovarian cancer treatment. *Maturitas*, 2014, 77(2), 128-136.
[44] Takeda, K., Akira, S. TLR signaling pathways. *Seminars in Immunology*, 2004, 16, 3-9.
[45] Morse, M. A., Chapman, R., Powderly, J. Phase I study utilizing a novel antigen-presenting cell-targeted vaccine with toll-like receptor stimulation to induce immunity to self-antigens in cancer patients. *Clinical Cancer Research*, 2011, 17, 4844-4853.

[46] Zhou, M., Macfarland-Mancini, M. M., Funk, H. M. et al. Toll-like receptor expression in normal ovary and ovarian tumors. *Cancer Immunology, Immunotherapy*, 2009, 58, 1375-1385.

[47] Muccioli, M., Benencia, F. Toll-like Receptors in Ovarian Cancer as Targets for Immunotherapies. *Frontiers in immunology*, 2014, 22(5), 341.

[48] Wang, X., Deavers, M., Patenia, R. et al. Monocyte/macrophage and T-cell infiltrates in peritoneum of patients with ovarian cancer or benign pelvic disease. *Journal of Translational Medicine*, 2006, 4, 30.

[49] Ries, C. H., Cannarile, M. A., Hoves, S. et al. Targeting tumor-associated macrophages with anti-CSF-1R antibody reveals a strategy for cancer therapy. *Cancer Cell*. 2014, 25, 846-59.

[50] Cassier, P. A. Phase 1 study of RG7155, a novel anti-CSF1R antibody, in patients with locally advanced pigmented villonodular synovitis (PVNS). *Journal Clinical Oncology*, 2014, 32, 5s.

[51] Korman, A. J., Peggs, K. S., Allison, J. P. Checkpoint blockade in cancer immunotherapy. *Advances in Immunology*, 2006, 90, 297-339.

[52] Lipson, E. J., Drake, C. G. Ipilimumab: an anti-CTLA-4 antibody for metastatic melanoma. *Clinical Cancer Research*, 2011, 17, 6958-6962.

[53] Coosemans, A., Baert, T., Vergote, I. A view on dendritic cell immunotherapy in ovarian cancer: how far have we come?. *Facts, Views andVision in Obgyn*, 2015, 7(1), 73-78.

[54] Matias, B. F., Oliveira, T. M., Rodrigues, C. M. et al. Influence of immunotherapy with autologous dendritic cells on innate and adaptive immune response in cancer. *Clinical Medicine Insights: Oncology*, 2013, 28(7), 165-172.

[55] Koido, S. et al. Current Immunotherapeutic Approaches in Pancreatic Cancer. *Clinical and Developmental Immunology*, 2011, 2011, 1-15.

[56] Baert, T., Timmerman, D., Vergote, I. et al. Immunological parameters as a new lead in the diagnosis of ovarian cancer. *Facts, Views and Vision in Obgyn*. 2015, 7(1), 67-72.

[57] Sabado, R. L., Bhardwaj, N. Directing dendritic cell immunotherapy towards successful cancer treatment. *Immunotherapy*, 2010, 2(1), 37-56.

[58] Powell-Jr, D. J., Urbanska, K. Advances and prospects in adoptive cell transfer therapy for ovarian cancer. *Immunotherapy*, 2015, 7(5), 473-476.

[59] Urbanska, K., Lanitis, E., Poussin, M. et al. A universal strategy for adoptive immunotherapy of cancer through use of a novel T-cell antigen receptor. *Cancer Research*, 2012, 72, 1844-1852.

[60] Urbanska, K., Lynn, R. C., Stashwick, C. et al. Targeted cancer immunotherapy via combination of designer bispecific antibody and novel gene-engineered T cells. *Journal of Translational Medicine* 2014, 12, 347.

[61] Wick, D. A., Webb, J. R., Nielsen, J. S. et al. Surveillance of the tumor mutanome by T cells during progression from primary to recurrent ovarian cancer. *Clinical. Cancer Research*, 2014, 20(5), 1125-1134.

[62] Muccioli, M., Benencia, F. Toll-like Receptors in Ovarian Cancer as Targets for Immunotherapies. *Frontiers in immunology*, 2014, 22(5), 341.

[63] Kandalaft, L., Powell, D., Chiang, C. et al. Autologous lysate-pulsed dendritic cell vaccination followed by adoptive transfer of vaccine-primed ex vivo co-stimulated T cells in recurrent ovarian cancer. *OncoImmunology*, 2013, 2, 22664.

[64] Adams, S. F., Benencia, F. Immunotherapy for ovarian cancer: what are the targets of the future? *Future Oncology*. 2015, 11(9), 1293-1296.

[65] Hart, K. M., Byrne, K. T., Molloy, M J. et al. IL-10 immunomodulation of myeloid cells regulates a murine model of ovarian cancer. *Front. Immunology*. 2011, 2, 29.

In: Handbook on Ovarian Cancer
Editor: Bethany R. Collier
ISBN: 978-1-63483-874-0


*Chapter 5*

# DOPAMINE RECEPTOR: A TREATMENT TARGET FOR OVARIAN CANCER

***Min Yong, Jinyan Li, Lina Hu and Tinghe Yu****
Key Medical Laboratory of Obstetrics and Gynecology,
The Second Affiliated Hospital,
Chongqing Medical University, Chongqing, China

## ABSTRACT

The physiological actions of dopamine (DA) are mediated by five receptors (DR) that are divided into two major groups: D1 and D2. The D1-like subtypes (DR1 and DR5) can activate the adenylate cyclase thereby increasing the cAMP level, but the D2-like subtypes (DR2, DR3 and DR4) lead to the opposite effect (i.e., decreasing the cAMP level). The role of DA and DR in cancer therapy remains unclear. Human ovarian cancer cells express all DR except DR3. The DR2-mediated inhibition of the Src activation can reverse the permissive microenvironment for tumor growth attributable to chronic stress. DA favors the uptake of cisplatin via stabilizing tumor blood vessels, which results from DR1-mediated activation of the cAMP–kinase A signaling pathway. An antagonist of DR2 can inhibit tumor growth by targeting the VEGFR-2/PI3K/mTOR pathway. The blockage of D2-family proteins inhibits growth of cancer cells (including cancer stem cells). Therefore, DR2 can be a target for cancer treatments.

**Keywords:** Dopamine receptor, ovarian cancer, antagonist, treatment target

## 1. INTRODUCTION

The physiological functions of dopamine (a metabolite of the aminoacid tyrosine) have attracted an enormous amount of attention. Dopamine (DA) is a predominant catecholamine neurotransmitter in the mammalian brain. It controls various functions including the

* Correspondence: Tinghe Yu, E-mail: yutinghe@hotmail.com

locomotor activity, cognition, emotion, positive reinforcement, food intake and endocrine regulation in the central nervous system (CNS). In the periphery, DA plays an important role in modulation of the cardiovascular function, catecholamine release, hormone secretion, vascular tone, renal function and gastrointestinal motility.

The dysregulation of dopaminergic transmission is related to some pathological conditions such as Parkinson's disease, schizophrenia and hyperprolactinemia. Interestingly, some studies have shown that dopamine receptor (DR) is involved in the development of certain cancers. Schizophrenic patients receiving DR antagonists has a reduced incidence of cancers of the rectum, colon, prostate and uterine cervix. Parkinson's patients, characterized with dopaminergic deficient, also have a lower incidence of cancer.

Here we discuss the role of DR in ovarian cancer. The available findings suggest that DR may be a treatment target.

## 2. Classification, Gene and Structure of DR

DA can modulate the activity of adenylyl cyclase (AC) [1]. According to the effect of DA on the AC activity, DR is divided into two distinct populations: D1 and D2. The D1-subfamily can stimulate AC and the D2-subfamily has not such a role. The existence of specific peripheral DR was demonstrated in the late 1970s. After the introduction of gene cloning procedures, three novel DR subtypes have been identified as DR3, DR4 and DR5/D1b [2-4]. The individual members of D1- or D2-subfamily share a high homology in their transmembrane domains. It is commonly accepted that D1-class receptors (DR1 and DR5) activate the $G\alpha_{s/olf}$ family of G proteins to stimulate the cAMP production by AC. D2-class receptors (DR2, DR3 and DR4) couple to the $G\alpha_{i/o}$ family of G proteins, thereby inhibiting AC resulting in a decrease of the cAMP level.

The genomic organization of D1- and D2-class receptors supports the concept that they derive from two gene families that primarily differ in their coding sequences (i.e., absence or presence of introns). DR1 and DR5 genes do not contain introns in their coding regions, but D2-class receptors have several introns. The gene encoding D2-like receptors is interrupted by introns. The coding region of DR2, DR3 and DR4 contains 6, 5 and 3 introns, respectively [5]. The localization of introns is similar in three receptor genes. The presence of introns in the coding region of D2-class receptors allows the generation of receptor splice-variants. For instance, two DR2 variants $D_{2S}$ and $D_{2La}$ result from the alternative splicing of a 87-base-pair exon between the introns 4 and 5 [6-8].

The expression of DR can be self-modulated. In the striatum, chronic exposure to the neuroleptic drugs such as haloperidol and sulpiride increases the mRNA level of DR2, but DR1 is not affected [9-12]. Nigrostriatal dopaminergic neurons disrupted by 6-OHDA result in an increase in the DR2 mRNA level and a decrease in the DR1 mRNA. These two effects can be reversed by quinpirole and SKF-38393, respectively [13, 14]. Some factors other than DA or dopaminergic drugs can also modulate the expression of DR genes. Treatment with dibutyryl cAMP leads to the expression of DR2 in human retinoblastoma cells Y79, and epidermal growth factor (EGF) increases the mRNA levels of both $D_{2S}$ and $D_{2L}$ in $GH_3$ cells [15, 16].

DR is the member of seven-transmembrane (TM)-domain G protein-coupled receptor family, and shares certain distinct characteristics in the structure. DR1 and DR5 share 80% identity in their transmembrane domains. DR3 and DR4 have 75% and 53% identity in the transmembrane domain compared with DR2, respectively [17-19]. The NH2-terminal domain has a similar number of amino acids in all DR. However, the COOH-terminal for the D1-class receptors is seven times longer than that for the D2-class receptors [20, 21].

DR1 to DR5 differ in the affinity to various agonists and antagonists. A number of selective compounds have been developed for DR2, DR3 and DR4. The selectivity of a specific DR4 antagonist to DR4 is nearly 1000-fold higher than that of other subtypes. Compounds antagonizing DR3 show a selectivity of approximately 100-fold compared with DR2 [22-25]. However, it is impossible to pharmacologically differentiate DR1 and DR5, which have similar sensitivity to antagonists and agonists. The most efficient discriminating agent may be (+)-butaclamol, which shows a relatively higher affinity to DR1 [26, 27]. Additionally, some antagonists have negative effects on DR5. It seems that DR5 exhibits constitutive activity similar to various mutated G protein-coupled receptors [28, 29]. In contrast with DR1 and DR5, certain agonists and antagonists can distinguish DR3 from DR2. DA has 20 times higher affinity to DR3 than that to DR2, which may due to the sequence difference in the third intracellular loop [30, 31]. Although DR4 closely resembles to DR2 and DR3, its higher affinity for clozapine can distinguish it from DR2 or DR3 [32].

## 3. Function and Disease Related to DR

DR has a broad expression pattern in both the brain and periphery. In the brain, all subtypes of D1 and D2 receptors distribute in specific parts with different levels, depending on the physiological action of DA in that site. Many second messengers such as cAMP, calcium, potassium and arachidonic acid have been identified to participate in the signal transduction of DR. Recent findings indicate that D2-like receptors are involved in the mitogenesis and cell differentiation [33]. For cell growth and differentiation related to DR, the $Na^+/H^+$ exchanger and $Na^+$-$K^+$-ATPase play a pivotal role [34, 35].

DA is critically involved in a number of physiological processes. Controlling of the locomotor activity is connected with DR1, DR2 and DR3, which are also involved in the reward and reinforcement mechanisms [22, 36]. Animals lacking DR2 are with reduced spontaneous movement, akinetic and bradykinetic [37]. DR2 plays a role in the psychotic reactions observed in schizophrenia and bipolar disorder, because all clinically effective antipsychotics possess the ability to block DR2 [38, 39].

Treatment with neuroleptics that possesses the antipsychotic effect due to their action on DA in the mesolimbic system, has a major drawback termed the extrapyramidal syndrome including muscular rigidity and akinesia. Extrapyramidal side effects result from the blockage of DR2 in the striatum [40]. The high sequence homology between DR of the same subfamily makes it extremely laborious to develop a specific ligand that does not interact with other receptors. The function of DR4 and DR5 seems to be quite limited as revealed in pharmacological and genetic knockout studies [41].

Other DR-mediated functions outside the CNS include olfaction, vision and hormonal regulation. For example, DR2 is found in the anterior and intermediate lobes of pituitary gland, where they regulate the secretion of prolactin (PRL) and α-melanocyte-stimulating hormone (α-MSH) [41, 42]. The therapeutic application of DR2 agonists (e.g., bromocriptine) is management of hyperprolactinemia caused by the functional hypothalamus-pituitary defect or PRL-secreting tumors, because DR2 can inhibit the PRL secretion in anterior pituitary [43]. Although DR4 and its variant are found in the anterior pituitary, its physiology role remains unclear [44]. DR have other functions: DR1 in kidney mediating the renin secretion; DR1, DR2, and DR4 regulating the renal function; DR2 in adrenal gland regulating the aldosterone secretion; and regulating the sympathetic tone, blood pressure, vasodilation and gastrointestinal motility [45-48].

## 4. DR and Cancer

DR may have close connection with various cancers. Dalton et al. found that schizophrenic patients receiving DR antagonists had a relatively lower incidence of cancers of the rectum, colon, prostate and uterine cervix [49]. Driver et al. demonstrated that dopaminergic-deficient Parkinson's patients, functionally akin to disease-induced DR antagonism, had a lower incidence of cancer [50]. However, there yet lack direct evidences to verify the role of DR in cancers.

Sachlos et al. found that thioridazine, a DR2 blocker, can selectively target neoplastic cells and leukemic cancer stem cells (CSC), whilst having no effects on normal blood stem cells [51]. DR expresses on CSC and breast cancer cells, but hardly expresses on normal blood stem cells. These results suggest that DR may be a biomarker for malignancies. Similarly, Lu et al. found that hepatocellular carcinoma (HCC) expressed a lower level of DR1 and a higher level of DR5 compared with the adjacent nontumor tissues; DR2, DR3 and DR4 were not detected [52]. Blockage of DR with thioridazine inhibited the proliferation and sphere formation of HCC cell lines such as LM3, SNU449 and Huh7. Therefore, the expression of DR subtypes varies among cancer types and the inhibition of DR can be a strategy for cancer treatments.

A noticeable result was reported by Pornour et al. [53]. Bromocriptin can be used to treat breast cancer cells MCF-7. Aldosterone-producing adenoma (APA) expressed less DR2, where bromocriptin displayed an anti-proliferation effect via attenuating PKCμ and ERK phosphorylation [54]. The paradox suggest that the role of DR2 may depend on cancer type.

DR4 is involved in the early brain development, and therefore may be involved in the developmentally dependent tumors of CNS. Unland et al. demonstrated that DR4 was epigenetically suppressed in CNS tumors of children [55].

DA and DR may play a role in cancer immunotherapy. T cells express functional DR1 to DR5, but their levels and functions are dynamic. Wu et al. found that monocytic MDSC (myeloid-derived suppressor cell) induced by tumors led to inhibition of T cell proliferation and of the IFN-γ production; this effect could be attenuated by DA via DR1 [56]. These results suggest that DA can overcome tumor-induced immunosuppression, providing a strategy to overcome tumor-induced immunosuppression. Li et al. reported that silencing DR2 with si-/shRNAs suppressed the growth of glioblastoma cells in vitro and in vivo [57]. The combination inhibition of DR2 and epidermal growth factor receptor (EGFR) led to synergistic antitumor activity.

## 5. DR and Ovarian Cancer

Endothelial ovarian cancer cells express all DR except DR3. Those receptors may have intimate connection with the genesis, progression and treatment of ovarian cancer. Moreno-Smith et al. adopted a model of chronic stress to determine whether DA can block the effect of chronic stress on tumor growth [58]. DA blocked the stress-induced tumor growth and decreased the microvessel density, which can be reversed by the DR2 antagonist eticlopride. These findings indicate the tumor-inhibitory effect of DA is realized via DR2. DA or its agonist SKF 82958 can activate the pericyte cAMP-protein kinase A signaling pathway by coupling to DR1, thereby leading to a transient "normalization" of the vessels of ovarian tumor [59]. This effect produces a temporary increase in oxygen and nutrient delivery for cancer cells that surround these "normalized" vessels [60]. Such changes may enhance cell proliferation and accelerate tumor growth. On the other hand, the normalized vasculature that alleviate hypoxia favors the uptake of cisplatin, which increases the efficacy of cancer therapies. These two trends should be balanced in cancer treatment.

The action of DA mediated by DR has complicated effects on tumor vasculature and growth, so does a DR antagonist. Rho et al. using a gene signature-based approach, demonstrated that thioridazine was an inhibitor of the phosphatidylinositol-3'-kinase (PI3K)/AKT pathway in ovarian cancer cells [61]. The PI3K/Akt signal pathway plays a critical role in cell survival through suppressing apoptosis, promoting tumor invasion, and metastasis and antagonizing cell-cycle arrest [62]. Inhibition of the PI3K/Akt pathway can not only suppress tumor growth but also increase the action of chemotherapeutic agents. Park et al. found that thioridazine displayed both anti-tumor and -angiogenic activities in ovarian tumor xenografts in vivo. These effects are mediated by the VEGFR-2/PI3K/mTOR signal pathway [63]. Antagonizing DR2 by thioridazine specifically regulates the Wnt and Akt signaling pathway [64]. However, underlying mechanisms are only limited understood. The role of DR in ovarian cancer, therefore, needs further investigations.

## Summary

DR may play an important role in the development of ovarian cancer. Ovarian cancer expresses all DR except DR3. The DR antagonist thioridazine displays an anticancer effect through inducing apoptosis, and inhibiting angiogenesis and the survival pathway such as PI3K/AKT. A DR antagonist may be an adjuvant for cancer chemotherapy. Therefore, DR may be a target for treatment of ovarian cancer.

## Acknowledgments

The work in our laboratory was supported with grants from the Natural Science Foundation of China (34170822, 81300535) and the Sate Ministry of Education (SRFDP 20135503130002).

## REFERENCES


[1] Kebabian JW, Calne DB. Multiple receptors for dopamine. *Nature* 1979, 277, 93-96.

[2] Sokoloff P, Giros B, Martres MP, et al. Molecular cloning and characterization of a novel dopamine receptor (D3) as a target for neuroleptics. *Nature* 1990, 347, 146-151.

[3] Guan HC, Sunahara RK. Cloning of the gene for a human dopamine D4 receptor with high affinity for the antipsychotic clozapine. *Nature* 1991, 350, 610-614.

[4] Sunahara RK, Guan HC, O'Dowd BF, et al. Cloning of the gene for a human dopamine D5 receptor with higher affinity for dopamine than D1. *Nature* 1991, 350, 614-619.

[5] Gingrich JA, Caron MG. Recent advances in the molecular biology of dopamine receptors. *Annu. Rev. Neurosci.* 1993, 16, 299-321.

[6] Giros B, Sokoloff P, Martres MP, et al. Alternative splicing directs the expression of two D2 dopamine receptor isoforms. *Nature* 1989, 342, 923-926.

[7] Dal Toso R, Sommer B, Ewert M, et al. The dopamine D2 receptor: Two molecular forms generated by alternative splicing. *EMBO J.* 1989, 8, 4025-4034.

[8] Monsma FJ, McVittie LD, Gerfen CR, et al. Multiple D2 dopamine receptors produced by alternative RNA splicing. *Nature* 1989, 342, 926-929.

[9] Bernard V, Le Moine C, Bloch B. Striatal neurons express increased level of dopamine D2 receptor mRNA in response to haloperidol treatment: A quantitative in situ hybridization study. *Neuroscience* 1991, 45, 117-126.

[10] Buckland PR, O'Donovan MC, McGuffin P. Changes in dopamine D1, D2 and D3 receptor mRNA levels in rat brain following antipsychotic treatment. *Psychopharmacology* 1992, 106, 479-483.

[11] Jaber M, Tison F, Fournier MC, et al. Differential influence of haloperidol and sulpiride on dopamine receptors and peptide mRNA levels in the rat striatum and pituitary. *Mol. Brain Res.* 1994, 23, 14-20.

[12] Normand E, Popovici T, Fellmann D, et al. Anatomical study of enkephalin gene expression in the rat forebrain following haloperidol treatment. *Neurosci. Lett.* 1987, 83, 232-236.

[13] Brene S, Lindefors N, Herrera-Marschitz M, et al. Expression of dopamine D2 receptor and choline acetyltransferase mRNA in the dopamine deafferented rat caudate-putamen. *Exp. Brain Res.* 1990, 83, 96-104.

[14] Gerfen CR, Engber TM, Mahan LC, et al. D1 and D2 dopamine receptor-regulated gene expression of striatonigral and striatopallidal neurons. *Science* 1990, 250, 1429-1432.

[15] Monsma FJ, Barton AC, Sibley DR. Expression of functional D2 dopamine receptors following differentiation of Y79 human retinoblastoma cells. *J. Neurochem.* 1990, 54, 1200-1207.

[16] Missale C, Boroni F, Castelletti L, et al. Lack of coupling of D-2 receptors to adenylate cyclase in GH-3 cells exposed to epidermal growth factor. Possible role of a differential expression of Gi protein subtypes. *J. Biol. Chem.* 1991, 266, 23392-23398.

[17] Civelli O, Bunzow JR, Grandy DK. Molecular diversity of the dopamine receptors. *Annu. Rev. Pharmacol. Toxicol.* 1993, 33, 281-307.

[18] Gingrich JA, Caron MG. Recent advances in the molecular biology of dopamine receptors. *Annu. Rev. Neurosci.* 1993, 16, 299-321.

[19] Jackson DM, Westlind-Danielsson A. Dopamine receptors: Molecular biology, biochemistry and behavioural aspects. *Pharmacol. Ther.* 1994, 64, 291-370.

[20] O'dowd BF, Hnatowich M, Caron MG, et al. Palmitoylation of the human β2-adrenergic receptor. Mutation of Cys341 in the carboxyl tail leads to an uncoupled nonpalmitoylated form of the receptor. *J. Biol. Chem.* 1989, 264, 7564-7569.

[21] Packard MG, White NM. Dissociation of hippocampus and caudate nucleus memory systems by posttraining intracerebral injection of dopamine agonists. *Behav. Neurosci* 1991, 105, 295-306.

[22] Missale C, Nash SR, Robinson S, et al. Dopamine receptors: From structure to function. *Physiol. Rev.* 1998, 78, 189-225.

[23] Vallone D, Picetti R, Borrelli E. Structure and function of dopamine receptors. *Neurosci. Biobehav. Rev.* 2000, 24, 125-132.

[24] Sokoloff P, Diaz J, Foll BL, et al. The dopamine D3 receptor: A therapeutic target for the treatment of neuropsychiatric disorders. *CNS Neurol. Disord Drug Targets* 2006, 5, 25-43.

[25] Rankin ML, Marinec PS, Cabrera DM, et al. The D1 dopamine receptor is constitutively phosphorylated by G protein-coupled receptor kinase 4. *Mol. Pharmacol.* 2006, 69, 759-769.

[26] Self DW, Stein L. Receptor subtypes in opioid and stimulant reward. *Pharmacol. Toxicol.* 1992, 70, 87-94.

[27] Tiberi M, Jarvie KR, Silvia C, et al. Cloning, molecular characterization, and chromosomal assignment of a gene encoding a second D1 dopamine receptor subtype: Differential expression pattern in rat brain compared with the D1A receptor. *Proc. Natl. Acad. Sci.* 1991, 88, 7491-7495.

[28] Lefkowitz RJ, Cotecchia S, Samama P, et al. Constitutive activity of receptors coupled to guanine nucleotide regulatory proteins. *Trends Pharmacol. Sci.* 1993, 14, 303-307.

[29] Samama P, Cotecchia S, Costa T, et al. A mutation-induced activated state of the β2-adrenergic receptor. Extending the ternary complex model. *J. Biol. Chem.* 1993, 268, 4625-4636.

[30] Robinson SW, Jarvie KR, Caron MG. High affinity agonist binding to the dopamine D3 receptor: Chimeric receptors delineate a role for intracellular domains. *Mol. Pharmacol.* 1994, 46, 352-356.

[31] Sokoloff P, Giros B, Martres MP, et al. Molecular cloning and characterization of a novel dopamine receptor (D3) as a target for neuroleptics. *Nature* 1990, 347, 146-151.

[32] Guan HC, Sunahara RK. Cloning of the gene for a human dopamine D4 receptor with high affinity for the antipsychotic clozapine. *Nature* 1991, 350, 610-614.

[33] Lajiness ME, Chio CL, Huff RM. D2 dopamine receptor stimulation of mitogenesis in transfected Chinese hamster ovary cells: Relationship to dopamine stimulation of tyrosine phosphorylations. *J. Pharmacol. Exp. Ther.* 1993, 267, 1573-1581.

[34] Felder CC, Campbell T, Albrecht F, et al. Dopamine inhibits Na (+)-H+ exchanger activity in renal BBMV by stimulation of adenylate cyclase. *Am. J. Physiol.* 1990, 259, F297-F303.

[35] Yamaguchi I, Walk SF, Jose PA, et al. Dopamine D2L receptors stimulate Na+/K (+)-ATPase activity in murine LTK-cells. *Mol. Pharmacol.* 1996, 49, 373-378.

[36] Hyman SE, Malenka RC, Nestler EJ. Neural mechanisms of addiction: The role of reward-related learning and memory. *Annu. Rev. Neurosci.* 2006, 29, 565-598.

[37] Brene S, Lindefors N, Herrera-Marschitz M, et al. Expression of dopamine D2 receptor and choline acetyltransferase mRNA in the dopamine deafferented rat caudate-putamen. *Exp. Brain Res.* 1990, 83, 96-104.

[38] Snyder SH, Taylor KM, Coyle JT, et al. The role of brain dopamine in behavioral regulation and the actions of psychotropic drugs. *Am. J. Psychiatry* 1970, 127, 199-207.

[39] Roth BL, Sheffler DJ, Kroeze WK. Magic shotguns versus magic bullets: Selectively non-selective drugs for mood disorders and schizophrenia. *Nat. Rev. Drug Discov.* 2004, 3, 353-359.

[40] Hall AS, Bryson SE, Vaughan PF, et al. Pharmacological characterization of the dopamine receptor coupled to cyclic AMP formation expressed by rat mesenteric artery vascular smooth muscle cells in culture. *Br. J. Pharmacol.* 1993, 110, 681-686.

[41] Enjalbert A, Bockaert J. Pharmacological characterization of the D2 dopamine receptor negatively coupled with adenylate cyclase in rat anterior pituitary. *Mol. Pharmacol.* 1983, 23, 576-584.

[42] Cote TE, Eskay RL, Frey EA, et al. Biochemical and physiological studies of the beta-adrenoceptor and the D2 dopamine receptor in the intermediate lobe of the rat pituitary gland: A review. *Neuroendocrinology* 1982, 35, 217-224.

[43] Cunnah D, Besser M. Management of prolactinomas. *Clin. Endocrinol.* 1991, 34, 231-235.

[44] Van Tol HHM, Wu CM, Guan HC, et al. Multiple dopamine D4 receptor variants in the human population. *Nature* 1992, 358, 149-152.

[45] Aperia AC. Intrarenal dopamine: A key signal in the interactive regulation of sodium metabolism. *Annu. Rev. Physiol* 2000, 62, 621-647.

[46] Carlsson A. A paradigm shift in brain research. *Science* 2001, 294, 1021-1024.

[47] Witkovsky P. Dopamine and retinal function. *Doc. Ophthalmol.* 2004, 108, 17-39.

[48] Li ZS, Schmauss C, Cuenca A, et al. Physiological modulation of intestinal motility by enteric dopaminergic neurons and the D2 receptor: Analysis of dopamine receptor expression, location, development, and function in wild-type and knock-out mice. *J. Neurosci.* 2006, 26, 2798-2807.

[49] Dalton SO, Mellemkjær L, Thomassen L, et al. Risk for cancer in a cohort of patients hospitalized for schizophrenia in Denmark, 1969-1993. *Schizophrenia Res* 2005, 75, 315-324.

[50] Driver JA, Logroscino G, Buring JE, et al. A prospective cohort study of cancer incidence following the diagnosis of Parkinson's disease. *Cancer Epidemiol. Biomarkers Prev.* 2007, 16, 1260-1265.

[51] Sachlos E, Risueño RM, Laronde S, et al. Identification of drugs including a dopamine receptor antagonist that selectively target cancer stem cells. *Cell* 2012, 149, 1284-1297.

[52] Lu M, Li J, Luo Z, et al. Roles of dopamine receptors and their antagonist thioridazine in hepatoma metastasis. *Onco Targets Ther.* 2015, 8, 1543-1552.

[53] Pornour M, Ahangari G, H Hejazi S, et al. New perspective therapy of breast cancer based on selective dopamine receptor D2 agonist and antagonist effects on MCF-7 cell line. *Recent Pat Anticancer Drug Discov* 2015, 10, 214-223.

[54] Chang HW, Huang CY, Yang SY, et al. Role of D2 dopamine receptor in adrenal cortical cell proliferation and aldosterone-producing adenoma tumorigenesis. *J. Mol. Endocrinol.* 2014, 52, 87-96.

[55] Unland R, Kerl K, Schlosser S, et al. Epigenetic repression of the dopamine receptor D4 in pediatric tumors of the central nervous system. *J. Neurooncol.* 2014, 116, 237-249.

[56] Wu J, Zhang R, Tang N, et al. Dopamine inhibits the function of Gr-1+ CD115+ myeloid-derived suppressor cells through D1-like receptors and enhances anti-tumor immunity. *J. Leukoc. Biol.* 2015, 97, 191-200.

[57] Li J, Zhu S, Kozono D, et al. Genome-wide shRNA screen revealed integrated mitogenic signaling between dopamine receptor D2 (DRD2) and epidermal growth factor receptor (EGFR) in glioblastoma. *Oncotarget* 2014, 5, 882-893.

[58] Moreno-Smith M, Lu C, Shahzad MMK, et al. Dopamine blocks stress-mediated ovarian carcinoma growth. *Clin. Cancer Res.* 2011, 17, 3649-3659.

[59] Moreno-Smith M, Lee SJ, Lu C, et al. Biologic effects of dopamine on tumor vasculature in ovarian carcinoma. *Neoplasia* 2013, 15, 502-515.

[60] Winkler F, Kozin S V, Tong R T, et al. Kinetics of vascular normalization by VEGFR2 blockade governs brain tumor response to radiation: Role of oxygenation, angiopoietin-1, and matrix metalloproteinases. *Cancer Cell* 2004, 6, 553-563.

[61] Rho SB, Kim BR, Kang S. A gene signature-based approach identifies thioridazine as an inhibitor of phosphatidylinositol-3'-kinase (PI3K)/AKT pathway in ovarian cancer cells. *Gynecol. Oncol.* 2011, 120, 121-127.

[62] Franke TF, Hornik CP, Segev L, et al. PI3K/Akt and apoptosis: Size matters. *Oncogene* 2003, 22, 8983-8998.

[63] Park MS, Dong SM, Kim BR, et al. Thioridazine inhibits angiogenesis and tumor growth by targeting the VEGFR-2/PI3K/mTOR pathway in ovarian cancer xenografts. *Oncotarget* 2014, 5, 4929-4934.

[64] Sutton LP, Rushlow WJ. The dopamine D2 receptor regulates Akt and GSK-3 via Dvl-3. *Int. J. Neuropsychopharmacol.* 2012, 15, 965-979.

In: Handbook on Ovarian Cancer
Editor: Bethany R. Collier
ISBN: 978-1-63483-874-0


*Chapter 6*

# MALIGNANT OVARIAN GERM CELL TUMORS: TREATMENT AND PROGNOSIS

***R. Díaz-Murillo, M. Lombarte-García, J. de Santiago and I. Zapardiel****
Gynecologic Oncology Unit. La Paz University Hospital-IdiPAZ.
Madrid, Spain

## ABSTRACT

Malignant ovarian germ cell tumors are a very uncommon disorder. The incidence is estimated in 0.5/100000 women. They represent only a 5 percent of ovarian cancers overall. Mostly, ovarian germ cell neoplasms affect women aged between 10-30 years and they constitute in this collective the most frequent ovarian tumor (around 70%).

These type of neoplasms have their origin on the primordial ovarian cells. There are different hystological subtypes: they can be divided into embryo-like neoplasms (immature teratoma and dysgerminoma) and placenta-like neoplasms (similar than extraembrionic fetal-derived cell population), or a mixture. The main malignant ovarian germ cell are: *immature teratoma, dysgerminoma, endodermalsinus (yolksac) tumors, embryonalcell carcinoma, choriocarcinoma, polyembrioma and mixedgermcelltumors.*

Basically, patients present abdominal pain with abdominal enlargement, abnormal vaginal bleeding and/or precocious puberty.Tumor marker tester can be increased, as AFP, beta-HCG, inhibin, CA 125, LDH.

Malignant ovarian germ cell tumors are staged by the International Federation of Gynecology and Obstetrics (FIGO) into: stage I, confined to the ovarian; stage II extension into other pelvic organs; stage III, disease extended into the abdmen or retroperitoneal lymphnodes; stage IV, metastatic disease beyond the abdomen or affecting the liver. Frequently, the tumor is diagnosed at stage I.

Treatment involves primary surgery, depending on the preferences of the patient to conserve or not her fertility. Fertility-sparing surgery must be done laparoscopically with an intraoperative frozen section evaluation. At advanced stages, chemotherapy can be

* Correspondence: Ignacio Zapardiel, Gynecologic Oncology Unit, La Paz University Hospital, Madrid, Spain, ignaciozapardiel@hotmail.com.

involved to complete the treatment. Malignant ovarian germ cell tumors have an excellent prognosis: 5-years survival after complete suitable treatment is more than 85%.

In this chapter, treatment and prognosis are going to be explained, according to the official international guidelines.

## INTRODUCTION

Malignant ovarian germ cell tumors (MOGCTs) is a very unfrequent neoplasm, accounting for 2-5% of ovarian malignacies overall [1]. The incidence is estimated in 0.5-1/ 100000 women, and it has been constant during the las 30 years [2]. These neoplasms involve typically young women aged between 10 and 30 years, with a median age of 19 years, and represent the 70% of ovarian tumors in this group of age [3]. MOGCTs occur more frequently among Asian-Pacific Islander and Hispanic women, without clear reasons [3].

There is a broad espectrum of neoplasms included in this group. All of them are histollogically derived from primordial ovarian germ cells but differ in their clinical presentation, tumor biology and histology. Mainly, they can be divided into embryo-like neoplasms (immature teratoma and dysgerminoma) and placenta-like neoplasms (similar than extraembrionic fetal-derived cell population), or a mixture [3].

The most frequent MOGCTs are: *immature teratoma, dysgerminoma, endodermal sinus (yolk sac) tumors,* that represent the 90% overall. Other histological type are: *embryonal cell carcinoma, choriocarcinoma, polyembrioma and mixed germ cell tumors* [4]. Dysgerminomas are the most frequently subtype of MOGCT (32%), and compared with nondysgerminomas are very usually diagnosed at stage I and be bilateral [5].

Commonly, patients present clinical manifestations. Most of them suffer from abdominal enlargement due to the mass and/or ascites, and pain from rupture or torsion. These abdominal syptoms are found in 85% of the patients. Other signs and symptoms are related to the presence of bHCG, as precocious puberty, abnormal vaginal bleeding and other symptoms of pregnancy [3].

The diagnosis is suspected in the presence of an adnexal mass at the bimanual exploration and at the pelvic imaging test. The confirmation is made by histological study. Tumor marker tester can be increased: HCG and AFP (in the absence of pregnancy or neonatal period), CA 125, inhibin, LDH (mainly in dysgerminomas) [3, 5].

MicroRNAs that are non protein-coding RNAs with a significant role regulating the gene expression, are overexpressed in some histological subtypes that after successful treatment returned to normal levels (yolk sac tumor, embryonal carcinoma) and are potential new makers [5].

MOGCTs are staged by the International Federation of Gynecology and Obstetrics (FIGO), as epithelial ovarian cancers, into: stage I, confined to the ovarian; stage II, extension into other pelvic organs; stage III, disease extended into the abdomen or reroperitoneal lymph nodes; stage IV, metastatic disease beyond the abdomen or affecting the liver. Frequently, the tumor is diagnosed at stage I [3, 6].

# TREATMENT

## Surgery

In most of the cases, the first step of treatment is the surgery. To confirm the histological diagnosis it is needed to treat and stage the tumor. MOGCTs spread via the lymphatic channels very commonly, bloodstream to the liver and lung, and peritoneal surface dissemination. Lymph node involvement is considered an independent predictor of poor survival by some authors [7], however the lymph node involvement in these tumors is extremely rare and for that other authors defend that the addition of lymphadenectomy do not result in a significant survival benefit [5].

First of all, a pelvic and abdominal exploration must be properly done. Laparotomy incision or laparoscopic management are allowed. If ascites is noted, it should be collected and set for cytologic evaluation; if there is not ascites, cytologic washings must be obtained [1, 6, 7].

Many patients with these tumors are diagnosed at an early stage confined to one ovary. They are usually very young women and for this reason fertility conservative surgery by laparoscopy must be offered. If the result of the intraoperative frozen section evaluation of the specimen is positive for MOGCT and it is limited to the ovarian, fertility-sparing surgery can be performed. The options of primary surgery are salpingoophorectomy, oophorectomy, ovarian cystectomy or resection of the ovarian mass. Surgery should be avoided if the other ovarian has a normal aspect because postoperative adhesions can impair fertility. Completion surgery should be considered after finishing childbearing [5-7].

On the other hand, if the patient does not desire fertility preservation or have a clinical stage II, III or IV, a complete cytoreductive surgical staging surgery is the gold standard (hysterectomy, bilateral salpigoophorectomy, sample pelvic and paraaortic nodes, omentectomy, appendectomy). If desease is limited to the pelvis, peritoneal samples of both paracolic gutters, posterior cul-de-sac, sidewalls, vesicouterine fold and diaphragm could be performed but it is not mandatory [5-7].

Patients with advanced disease postoperative cwho have completely debulked have a longer remission rate after hemotherapy [1]. Second look surgery after chemotherapy with a normal computed tomography and/or MRI is unnecessary [5]; otherwise, is not indicated in women with initially completely resected disease or with persistently elevated serum tumor markers [7].

## Chemotherapy

After surgery, surveillance with radiological imaging and tumor markers is recommended without adjuvant treatment to follow-up patients with stage I dygerminoma or grade I immature teratoma [6]. Those patients with presumed stage I that have not been adequately staged, could be candidates for a second staging operation. Some MOGCTs at stage IA, observation or chemotherapy can be considered. Giving chemotherapy to all stage I patients will exposure most of them to unnecessary toxicity [5].

Many of the advances in combination chemotherapy have been tested previously in testicular carcinoma, which is 10 times more common. In the beginning, the first effective treatment was the VAC regimen, with a high response rate but a low survival rate. The introduction of cisplatin chemotherapy significantly improved the overall survival with currently ranges from 87-98% [8].

Patients with stage II to IV should receive adjuvant postopeative chemotherapy every 21 days for 3 to 4 cycles with blemomycin (30 units per week)/ etoposide (100mg/m² daily for days 1 to 5)/ cisplatin (20 mg/m² daily for days 1 to 5) (BEP), with a cure rate approching 98% [5]. Pulmonary function tests are recommended because of the use of bleomycin. In select patients with high risk of toxicity, 3 cycles of etoposide/carboplatin ca be used. If the patient presents adverse events as neutropenia, dose reduction or treatment delay are not recommended [6]. Recombinant hematopoietic growth factors can be appropriate as an alternative to dose reduction for patients with a prior episode of febrile neutropenia. Other common adverse events are alopecia, transient myelosupression, thrombocitopenia and mucocutaneous toxicity, and long term effects as infertility [7]. However, many studies support that reproductive function is unaffected after chemotherapy and the rate of infertility reported ranges from 5-10% similar than the normal population [8].

Other acceptable primary treatment in select patients to minimize toxicity (with preexisting neuropathy or renal disease), with stage IB to III dysgerminoma, is the use of etoposide (120mg/m² for days 1-3)/ carboplatin (400mg/m² on day 1) every 4 weeks for 3 courses [6, 7].

## Follow-up

Frequently recurrences will be developed within two first years of inital treatment; however dysgerminomas may recur later, after ten or more years [7].

Proper follow up for patients who have been diagnosed and treated of a MOGCT should be every 2-4 months the 2 first years with physical exam and serum tumor markers, and only the annual physical evaluation after that. If recurrence is suspected, CT-scan and tumor markers must be evaluated [6].

After finishing chemotherapy treatment, patient can present: complete clinical response; residual tumor on radiographic imaging with normal levels of tumoral markers; persistenly elevated markers with residual disease.

When the patient obtaines a complete clinical response after chemotherapy, clinical observation must be done every 2 to 4 months with AFP and bHCG levels for 2 years. During the observation, if the patient develops a recurrent disease or abnormal levels of tumor markers, treatment options are: high-dose chemotherapy or additional chemotherapy [6].

For patients with radiographic evidence of residual tumor wih normal AFP or bHCG, surgical resection of the tumor or observation are the two possible options. Additional chemotherapy must be considered if the result of the specimen study is residual malignancy [6].

Finally, the patient can present persistently elevated tumoral marker with definitive residual disease, recommendations include TIP (paclitaxel, ifosfamide, cisplatin) or high dose chemotherapy with stem cell support.

After multiple chemotherapic regimens, for patients having recurrent or residual disease without curative options considered possible may be treated with recurrence modality: TIP, VAC (vincristine, dactinomycin, cyclophosphamide), VeIp (vinblastine, ifosfamide, cisplatine), VIP (etoposide, ifosfamide, cisplaatin), cisplatin/etoposide, doetaxel/carboplatin, paclitaxel/ carboplatin, paclitaxel/gemtacitabine, paclitaxel/ifosfamide, docetaxel, paclitaxel, high-dose chemotherapy, radiotherapy or supportive care only [5, 6].

## Prognosis

Malignant ovarian tumors have in general poor prognosis, but the survival outlook of malignant germinal tumors has improved due to the appearance of new treatments with high effectiveness. The large majority of these tumors are chemosensitive, except mature teratomas with malignant disruption, which have a poor response to chemotherapy [9].

In spite of the sensitivity of these tumors to chemotherapy, one of the most important prognostic factors for outcome is volume tumor, and the prognosis is worse for patients with metastatic or incompletely resected disease [10].

## Pronostic Factors

The most important variable in the outcome of treatment and patient's survival is the FIGO stage: advanced stages present worse survival. Residual tumor volume after surgery is associated with the progression free-survival. Chemotherapy achieves better results as there is less residual tumor.

Other important pronostic factor is the age. The pronosis is better in young women because in these cases the disease occurs most often in early stages, with lower histological grades and less residual disease after initial surgery.

Furthermore, the incidence of different histological types varies depending on the age at the beginning of the tumor. MOGCT's are the most common type in women under the age of twenty. In addition, young women have a better overall condition (without comorbidities), respond better to chemotherapy and have a longer survival.

MOGCT's have the following five-year survival rate according to the stage at diagnose: stage I 72,8%, stage II 46,3%, stage III 17,2%, stage IV 4,8%.

These tumors have better prognosis due to having higher chemosensitivity. Each histologic subtype presents different survival rates. Five-year survival rates in dysgerminoma are: stage I 95-100% and stages II to IV 80-90%. However, immature teratomas, endodermal sinus (yolk sac) tumors, embryonal carcinomas and choriocarcinomas have quite worse rates: stage I 90-95% ad stages II to IV 50%. Endodermal sinus tumor is the most aggresive one, followed by choriocarcinoma, embryonal carcinoma and immature teratomas.

The overall prevalence of limph node metástasis in MOGCT varied by histology: dysgerminoma (28%), mixed germ cell tumors (16%), malignant teratoma (8%).

Lymph node involvement is an independent predictor of poor survival with a hazard ratio of 2.9 (95% CI, 1.4-5.7).

Grade of tumor differentiation, tumoral ploidy (diploid tumors have better survival) are described as prognosis factors.

Patients who achieve a complete response after neoadjuvant chemotherapy in advanced stages live longer than those that only reach a partial response. Moreover, a demonstrated chemosensitivity with complete remission of disease is a favourable prognostic factor to a second response in case of recurrence. Furthermore, the greater the disease-free interval, the better the prognosis [10-12].

In addition, tumor markers appear to have prognostic significance in this disease. In several trials it has been observed that patients who had elevations of both beta-HCG and AFP were almost five times more likely to die of their disease compared with those with initially normal levels of both markers [10].

## Recurrences

Most recurrences develop within two years of initial therapy. Dysgerminomas may recur later (after five years or more). Recurrences have worse prognosis if they appear less than six months after the treatment. Patients with persistent disease after two months of chemotherapy also have poor prognosis [9].

With modern cisplatin-based adjuvant chemottherapy, approximately 80% of patients who present with advanced disease will be long-term survivors, even if they have residual disease remaining after cytoreductive surgery [10].

## Postreatment Issues

Ovarian dysfunction or premature ovarian failure is an infrequent risk of chemotherapy. Premature menopause has been reported in women who previously received chemotherapy as children, adolescent or young adults. Also increases the frequency of secondary malignancies, both for solid tumors and for leukaemias. Etoposide in particular has been implicated in the development of treatment-related leukemias. The incidence of leukemias is less than 0.5% in patients receiving a typical three or four cycle course of BEP. There are other diseases that occur more frequently in these patients who received chemotherapy such as hypertension, hypercholesterolemia and hearing loss [3].

# References

[1] Abdul Razak AR, Li L, Bryant A, Diaz-Padilla I. Chemotherapy for malignant germ cell ovarian cancer in adult patients with early stage, advanced and recurrent disease. *Cochrane Database Syst* Rev. 2011 Mar 16;(3):CD007584.

[2] Solheim O, Kærn J, Tropé CG, Rokkones E, Dahl AA, Nesland JM, Fosså SD. Malignant ovarian germ cell tumors: presentation, survival and second cancer in a population based Norwegian cohort (1953-2009). *Gynecol. Oncol.* 2013 Nov; 131(2):330-5.

[3] Gershenson DM. Ovarian germ cell neoplasms: Pathology, clinical manifestasions, and diagnosis. *UpToDate* 2014 Jan.

[4] Park JY, Kim DY, Suh DS, Kim JH, Kim YM, Kim YT, Nam JH. Outcomcs of pediatric and adolescent girls with malignant ovarian germ cell tumors. *Gynecol. Oncol.* 2015 Jun;137(3): 418-22.

[5] Vazquez I, Rustin GJ. Controversies in the management of germ cell ovarian tumours. *Curr. Opin. Oncol.* 2013 Sep;25(5):539-45.

[6] NCCN Guidelines Version 1.2015 Ovarian Cancer. *National Comprehensive Cancer Network* 2015 Feb.

[7] Chalas E, Valea FA, Mann Jr WJ. Treatment of malignant germ cell tumors of the ovary. *UpToDate* 2014 Jan.

[8] Low JJ, Ilanceran A, Ng JS. Malignant ovarian germ-cell tumours. *Best. Pract. Res. Clin. Obstet. Gynaecol.* 2012 Jun; 26(3):347-55.

[9] Usandizaga-Berguiristáin JA, de la Fuente Pérez P. Obstetricia y Ginecología tomo 2, Marbán, 2011. 4ª Edición.

[10] Hoskins WJ, Bundy BN, Thigpen JT, Omura GA. The influence of cytoreductive surgery on recurrence-free interval and survival in small-volume stage III epithelial ovarian cancer: a Gynecologic Oncology Group study. *Gynecol. Oncol.* 1992 Nov; 47(2):159-66.

[11] Del Campo JM. Cáncer de Ovario. Sociedad Española de Oncología Médica. April 2015.

[12] Heintz AP. Carcinoma of the ovary. FIGO 26th Annual Report on the Results of Treatment in Gynecological Cancer. *Int. J. Gynaecol. Obstet.* 2006 Nov;95 Suppl. 1:S161-92.

[13] Sonmezer M, Oktay K. Fertility preservation in patients undergoing gonadotoxic treatment or gonadal resection. UpToDate 2015 Feb.

In: Handbook on Ovarian Cancer
Editor: Bethany R. Collier
ISBN: 978-1-63483-874-0


*Chapter 7*

# CONTROVERSIES IN THE MANAGEMENT OF OVARIAN CANCER

***Grace Hwei Ching Tan[1] and Melissa Ching Ching Teo[2*]***
[1]MBBS (London), MRCS (Edinburgh), Associate Consultant,
Division of Surgical Oncology, National Cancer Centre Singapore
[2]MBBS, FRCS (Edinburgh), MPH (Johns Hopkins),
Head & Senior Consultant Division of Surgical Oncology,
National Cancer Centre Singapore

## ABSTRACT

Ovarian cancer is one of the commonest malignancy in women worldwide and has an annual incidence of 239 000 [1, 2]. It is the most lethal of all the gynaecological malignancies, the fifth leading cause of cancer death, and claimed 151 917 lives in 2012 [1, 2]. Ovarian cancer often presents at an advanced stage, with the involvement of the peritoneal surface either at the initial diagnosis or at recurrence. Despite the advances made in the surgical techniques and chemotherapeutic options regarding agents, schedule, and route of administration, majority of the patients recur and eventually succumb to their disease. The change in the surgical approach, in a bid to attain optimal cytoreduction with no gross residual disease, has seen improvement in the survival, as has the use of intraperitoneal chemotherapy in combination with intravenous agents. Cytoreductive surgery (CRS) and hyperthermic intraperitoneal chemotherapy (HIPEC) provide the combined benefits of surgical eradication and effective chemotherapy, and can be performed with acceptable morbidity and mortality [7]. Further trials are being undertaken to examine its role in the primary, as well as recurrent settings of advanced ovarian cancer and to determine the ideal drug combinations and dosages [50-52]. We aim to discuss these increasing controversies.

* Correspondence: Adj. Associate Prof Melissa Teo Ching Ching, Email: Melissa.teo.c.c@nccs.com.sg, Address: 9 Hospital Drive, Singapore 169612, Tel:(65) 6436 8000, Fax: (65) 6225 6283

## Introduction

Ovarian cancer is one of the commonest malignancies in women [1, 2], the most lethal of all the gynaecological malignancies, and the fifth leading cause of cancer death worldwide [1, 2]. Most ovarian cancer patients present with non specific symptoms of abdominal bloatedness and discomfort, and hence are often only diagnosed at an advanced stage, with 60–70% of patients having stage 3 or 4 disease at diagnosis [3]. The standard approach to treatment, is optimal debulking and adjuvant chemotherapy with platinum-based and taxol-based chemotherapy. Even with optimal treatment, the median five-year survival is less than 50% [4] and in advanced ovarian cancer, this falls to less than 25% [4]. In a bid to attain optimal cytoreduction with no gross residual disease, changes in the surgical approach supporting more radical and extensive surgical procedures have been made. These changes have seen improvement in the survival, as has the use of intraperitoneal chemotherapy in combination with intravenous agents. Although peritoneal carcinomatosis has always been a poor prognostic factor, it ceases to be a factor of much importance if complete cytoreduction can be achieved [5, 6]. Cytoreductive surgery (CRS) and hyperthermic intraperitoneal chemotherapy (HIPEC) provide the combined benefits of surgical eradication and effective chemotherapy, and can be performed with acceptable morbidity and mortality [7]. In this paper, we aim to discuss these increasing controversies.

## Standard Treatment: Optimal Debulking

Surgery remains the core of the management of ovarian cancers, as it is often necessary initially to achieve a diagnosis, to stage the patient, and is the mainstay of treatment in the majority of diagnosed cases [8]. The definition of optimal cytoreduction has evolved over the years, but was originally defined as residual disease less than 2 cm in size. This was further changed with data establishing the significantly better survival of those with residual disease measuring less than 1 cm and subsequently 5 mm in size [9–11]. Even in patients with residual disease measuring less than 1 cm, the risk of death increases significantly when compared with those with no remaining disease [12]. Over the years, there has been a plethora of data concluding that complete cytoreduction, with no gross residual disease, yields the survival [13]. Patients with no gross residual disease, 0.1–2 cm residual disease, and more than 2 cm residual disease had five-year survivals of 60, 35, and less than 20%, respectively [14, 15].

## What Happens after Debulking?

Majority of patients receive adjuvant chemotherapy after surgery [16]. At the beginning, the chemotherapeutic agents of choice included a platinum-based chemotherapy and a classic alkylating agent. Common agents used were cisplatin and cyclophosphamide [17]. After the Gynaecological Oncology Group (GOG) 111 and OV10 trials, looking specifically at the combinations of cisplatin with either cyclophosphamide or paclitaxel, the standard of care following surgery for stage 3 and 4 ovarian cancer was a combination of a platinum-based agent and a taxane, with intravenous (i.v.) cisplatin and paclitaxel being the agents of choice. Subsequently, a combination of paclitaxel and carboplatin showed similar results for response and survival rates, and did not have the toxicity often related to cisplatin treatment, and with a better quality of life. Hence, the standard approach is now six cycles of paclitaxel 175mg/m$^2$ administered every three weeks, in combination with carboplatin area under the curve (AUC) 5–6 [18].

The response and survival rates vary between the different histological types, with the endometrioid and clear cell subtypes having the best and worst prognoses, respectively, and mucinous and serous subtypes having intermediate prognoses [19, 20]. High-grade features also affect the prognosis adversely and such diseases often take on a much more aggressive course [19, 20].

In order to improve response rates to chemotherapy, and progression-free and overall survivals, dose intense and dose-dense chemotherapy were initiated. The former refers to the increase of dosages with each drug delivery, whereas the latter implies increasing the frequency of drug administration. These methods were introduced, because of observations of tumour growth escalating in the initial phase but slowing down as the tumour volume increased; hence, delivering higher doses of chemotherapy from the start and at close intervals would increase tumour cell death. This theory was confirmed in a large meta-analysis studying the effects of dose-intense and dose-dense chemotherapy for ovarian cancer [21]. The results of the JGOG trial, with first-line dose-dense chemotherapy, are also encouraging, with an improvement of median progression-free survival from 17.5 to 28.2 months and an overall survival that was not reached [22].

Controversy #1: Intraperitoneal (IP) chemotherapy versus intravenous (IV) chemotherapy (not sure if we should call it "controversy")

The route of administration of chemotherapy for ovarian cancer has traditionally been i.v. In the1960s, intraperitoneal (i.p.) chemotherapy was introduced with the purpose of controlling malignant ascites. It was found that certain drugs such as cisplatin were cleared from the peritoneal cavity gradually, which meant that a high concentration of the drug could be delivered intraperitoneally without resulting in a systemic overdose of the drug.

Drugs that are particularly suited for i.p. delivery, have high molecular weights and are water soluble, leading to a delayed peritoneal but high systemic clearance, and so having a pharmacological advantage for treating peritoneal disease.

The underlying rationale behind i.p. chemotherapy is the delivery of high concentrations of the appropriate drug to the site that is most likely to develop recurrences, at the opportune moment where tumour burden is at its minimum, i.e., after the performance of complete cytoreduction, with eradication of all macroscopic disease. It is critical that no gross residual disease is present, as penetration of i.p. chemotherapy is up to a depth of 2.5 mm [23-25]; hence, there is an inherent risk that larger volumes of tumour deposits will not be sufficiently treated by the intraperitoneal chemotherapy.

Ovarian cancer is a model cancer for treatment via an i.p. route. The majority of cases present with peritoneal disease, in the absence of extra-peritoneal metastases [3]. Even in patients who have undergone seemingly curative surgery and adjuvant chemotherapy, up to 70% develop recurrent disease, which often remains confined to the peritoneal cavity. The tendency for the peritoneum as the only site of disease makes this cancer the ideal candidate for such loco-regional treatment. I.p. chemotherapy has also been used with success in mucinous tumours of the appendix and peritoneum [26], colon cancers [27], and has even been shown to provide improved survival in gastric cancers [28].

There have been numerous studies examining the results of i.p. chemotherapy in the management of ovarian cancer. Amongst the first few randomized controlled trials (RCTs) was that conducted by the Southwest Oncology Group (SWOG) and GOG 104 trial, in which patients with cytoreduction of less than 2 cm residual disease were administered i.v. cyclophosphamide and either i.v. or i.p. cisplatin. The patients who received the i.p. chemotherapy, had significantly increased median overall survival [29]. The GOG 111 trial that combined i.v. paclitaxel with i.v. or i.p. cisplatin reached similar conclusions, in support of the i.p. treatment. Other RCTs produced progression-free and overall survivals of 28 and 63–66 months, respectively. In the GOG 172 trial, the median overall survival was 65.6 and 49.7 months for the combination i.p./i.v. and cytoreductive surgery (CRS) and i.v. chemotherapy alone arms, respectively. There were criticisms of these trials as the i.p. arm in GOG 114 and GOG 172 received two cycles of carboplatin at AUC 9 and i.p. paclitaxel on day 8, respectively; consequently, we expect the results of additional RCTs that attempt to study the effect of i.p. chemotherapy and establish the ideal algorithm for the management of ovarian cancer [30].

## Recurrent Ovarian Cancer

Despite receiving treatment, up to 70% of all patients diagnosed with ovarian cancer still suffer from relapse. Historically, early detection of persistent disease by second-look laparotomies was often performed, but as it was found to make no difference in the GOG-0158 trial, it is no longer practiced [31]. Presently, close follow-up of patients by serial CA-125 levels at intervals of one to three months is practiced, and an increase in CA-125 from initial levels is the most frequent method for which disease relapse is detected. However, the MRC-OV05 trial [32], which examined the consequences of early treatment for recurrence versus treatment delayed until clinical symptoms appeared, showed that there was no benefit in the detection of the early presence of disease by CA-125, with only a 1.4 month benefit in survival for the early treatment group.

In patients with clinically evident relapse, treatment options include secondary cytoreduction with or without hyperthermic intraperitoneal chemotherapy (HIPEC), and systemic chemotherapeutic regimes.

Systemic treatment is dependent on the platinum sensitivity of the disease. When platinum-sensitive, retreatment with a platinum or platinum-containing combination is advocated, and in platinum-resistance disease, clinical trials involving topotecan, docataxel, gemcitabine, paclitaxel, pemetrexed and bevacizumab should be considered.

Controversy #2: Cytoreductive surgery (CRS) and hyperthermic intraperitoneal chemotherapy (HIPEC)

Hyperthermic intraperitoneal chemotherapy (HIPEC) was first introduced in the early 1980s for the treatment of peritoneal carcinomatosis, and Dr. Sugarbaker popularized CRS and HIPEC for the management of peritoneal surface malignancies in the 1990s [27]. The addition of hyperthermia to the i.p. chemotherapy, has been shown to enhance penetration of the chemotherapy and increase its absorption into the tumour cells, escalating the intracellular accumulation of the drug [33]. The cytotoxic effect also appears to be potentiated by the hyperthermia, secondary to an impairment of the cells' ability to perform DNA repair [5, 33]. The drugs selected for HIPEC use, must be heat stable, with a high molecular weight and a low water solubility to be optimally used in the process of HIPEC. Cisplatin, mitomycin-C, oxaliplatin and doxorubicin are the frequently employed drugs.

HIPEC is carried out intraoperatively, as the patient is under general anaesthesia, via a pump that maintains the temperature and circulation of the drug solution. The advantages of administering HIPEC during the surgery include an ability to ensure that the entire peritoneal surface is submersed in the chemotherapeutic agent, before the development of obstructing adhesions that may form in the postoperative period. If HIPEC were administered in an opened-abdomen fashion, the surgeon would be able to manually swirl the chemotherapy to achieve this target. The most crucial prognostic factor remains the completeness of cytoreduction, with a 5.5% increase in the median overall survival for every patient undergoing optimal cytoreduction [8], which also affirms that the shifting surgical paradigm for ovarian cancer embracing complete cytoreduction has resulted in significantly better survival results [34].

The combination of CRS and HIPEC for ovarian cancer has shown promising results, with median overall and progression-free survivals of up to 64 and 57 months, respectively [33, 35, 36]. With optimal cytoreduction, five-year survivals of 12–66% can be attained [36]. These results are compatible with those of the author's institution [37]. A meta-analysis examining i.p. versus i.v. trials also showed the superiority of the i.p. over the i.v. regime, with hazard ratios of 0.79 for both disease-free and overall survivals [38]. Patients with platinum-sensitive disease have better response rates of 20–77% compared with up to 28% in those with platinum-resistant disease [39].

Controversy #3: If we agree for CRS and HIPEC, when do we do it?

The time points at which CRS and HIPEC have been used in the management of advanced ovarian cancer include the primary setting, after neoadjuvant chemotherapy, at the point of recurrence, and as a second-line treatment [40]. In the Milan 2006 consensus statement, it was concluded that CRS and HIPEC could be feasible at all of these time points.

The morbidity and mortality for this procedure range from 0 to 40 and 0 to 10%, respectively [36, 37], and hence, the key is in patient selection. It is essential that patients with good functional status, and an ability to tolerate such a radical procedure be chosen. The best candidates have long disease-free intervals and low volume disease that can be confidently optimally cyto-reduced.

Many of the studies included reviews of CRS and HIPEC for advanced ovarian cancer show the usage of this modality of treatment in the recurrent setting. However, evidence supporting the use of i.p. chemotherapy in the initial setting of advanced ovarian cancer [41] suggests that there is sound rationale behind CRS and HIPEC, even in the primary setting. There are more than 40 studies that have reported on the role of HIPEC in the management of ovarian cancer, but many of these studies are small in number and heterogeneous in their design. Further trials such as the Italian HORSE study (http://clinicaltrials.gov/show/NCT01539785) that randomizes patients with platinum-sensitive disease to CRS and HIPEC with cisplatin 75mg/m$^2$ and CRS alone, and the French CHIPOR study (http://clinicaltrials.gov/show/NCT01376752) that randomizes patients with recurrent platinum-sensitive disease (relapse beyond six months) after they have received platinum-based chemotherapy and optimal cytoreduction (less than 2.5 mm residual disease) to HIPEC with i.p. cisplatin 75mg/m$^2$ and no HIPEC [39] will provide answers about the role of HIPEC in patients with platinum-sensitive disease. There is a need for phase 3 randomized trials to elucidate which timing and cohort of patients would be most beneficial for CRS and HIPEC.

# FUTURE DIRECTIONS

## CRS and HIPEC

It is evident that complete cytoreduction, with no residual disease, yields the best clinical outcome. However, in a significant proportion of patients recurrence in the peritoneal cavity occurs, and CRS and HIPEC are considered. Perhaps the role of CRS and HIPEC as an adjuvant treatment should be considered an upfront treatment option for primary ovarian cancers, especially with improved morbidity results for this treatment modality. A randomized trial examining the overall and disease-free survivals of patients managed with CRS and adjuvant i.v. chemotherapy and those who undergo CRS and HIPEC, with adjuvant i.v. chemotherapy, for ovarian cancer in the primary setting would enable these questions to be addressed.

## Intraperitoneal Bevacizumab

The role of vascular endothelial growth factor (VEGF) in ovarian cancer has received much attention because VEGF increases vascular permeability and enhances angiogenesis [42]. Overexpression of VEGF has been reported in ovarian cancer [43-45] and several studies have indicated that VEGF-regulated angiogenesis is an important component of ovarian cancer growth [46, 47]. Microvessel density and level of VEGF expression in ovarian cancer directly correlate with poor prognosis, suggesting that angiogenesis, possibly mediated at least in part by VEGF, influences disease progression [46, 47]. Currently, vascular endothelial growth factor receptor (VEGFR) antibody, bevacizumab, is given intravenously for select patients with ovarian cancer.

The role of intraperitoneal VEGF inhibition using bevacizumab has been explored for the treatment of malignant ascites [48]. In a mouse peritoneal model of human ovarian cancer, the author demonstrated that the administration of i.p. bevacizumab and rapamycin not only reduced ascites, but was also able to suppress the development of peritoneal carcinomatosis [49]. This is an indication that this therapy may potentially be useful for the treatment of peritoneal carcinomatosis and may also be a novel, efficient strategy for reducing recurrence of ovarian cancers.

# CONCLUSION

Ovarian cancer often presents at an advanced stage, with the involvement of the peritoneal surface either at initial diagnosis or at recurrence. Despite the advances made in surgical techniques and chemotherapeutic options regarding agents, schedule, and route of administration, the majority of the patients still relapses and eventually succumbs to their disease. A alteration in the surgical approach, supporting more radical and extensive surgical procedures in an attempt to attain optimal cytoreduction with no gross residual disease, has seen an improvement in survival, as has the use of i.p. chemotherapy in combination with i.v. agents. Although peritoneal carcinomatosis has always been a poor prognostic factor, it ceases to be a factor of much importance if complete CRS can be achieved [5, 6]. CRS and HIPEC provide the combined benefits of surgical eradication and effective chemotherapy, and can be performed with acceptable morbidity and mortality [7]. Further trials are being undertaken to examine its role in the primary as well as recurrent settings of advanced ovarian cancer, and to determine the ideal drug combinations and dosages [50–52].

## REFERENCES

[1] Ferlay J, Soerjomataram I, Ervik M, et al. GLOBOCAN 2012 v1.0, Cancer incidence and mortality worldwide: IARC CancerBase No. 11 [Internet]. Lyon, France: International Agency for Research on Cancer; 2013. Available from: http://globocan.iarc.fr

[2] Bernard W. Stewart and Christopher P. Wild. *World cancer report* 2014. IARC publication; 2014.

[3] Coleman RL, Monk BJ, Sood AK, et al. Latest research and treatment of advanced-stage epithelial ovarian cancer. *Nat. Rev. Clin. Oncol.* 2013; 10: 211–224. doi: 10.1038/nrclinonc.2013.5.

[4] Horner MJ, Ries LA, Kracho M, et al. SEER cancer statistics review, 1975-2006. Bethesda, MD: National Cancer Institute; 2009. http://seer.cancer.- AQ5 gov/csr/1975_2006/.

[5] Deraco M, Baratti D, Laterza B, et al. Advanced cytoreduction as surgical standard of care and hyperthermic intraperitoneal chemotherapy as promising treatment in epithelial ovarian cancer. *Eur. J. Surg. Oncol.* 2011; 37:4–9.

[6] Herter P, Hahmann M, Lueck HJ, et al. Surgery for recurrent ovarian cancer: role of peritoneal carcinomatosis: exploratory analysis of the DESKTOP 1 trial about risk factors, surgical implications, and prognostic value of peritoneal carcinomatosis. *Ann. Surg. Oncol.* 2009; 16:1324–1330.

[7] Chan DL, Morris DL, Rao A, Chua TC. Intraperitoneal chemotherapy in ovarian cancer: a review of tolerance and efficacy. *Cancer Manag Res.* 2012; 4:413–422.

[8] Kang S, Park SY. To predict or not to predict? The dilemma of predicting the risk of suboptimal cytoreduction in ovarian cancer. *Ann. Oncol.* 2011; 22 (Suppl. 8): viii23–viii28. doi: 10.1093/annonc/mdr530.

[9] Bookman MA, Brady MF, McGuire WP, et al. Evaluation of new platinum based treatment regimens in advanced-stage ovarian cancer: a Phase III Trial of the Gynecologic Cancer Intergroup. *J. Clin. Oncol.* 2009; 27: 1419–1425.

[10] Chang SJ, Bristow RE. Evolution of surgical treatment paradigms for advanced-stage ovarian cancer: redefining 'optimal' residual disease. *Gynecol. Oncol.* 2012; 125: 483–492. doi: 10.1016/j.ygyno.2012.02.024.

[11] Chang SJ, Bristow RE, Ryu HS. Impact of complete cytoreduction leaving no gross residual disease associated with radical cytoreductive surgical procedures on survival in advanced ovarian cancer. *Ann. Surg. Oncol.* 2012; 19: 4059–4067.

[12] Elattar A, Bryant A, Winter-Roach BA, et al. Optimal primary surgical treatment for advanced epithelial ovarian cancer. *Cochrane Database Syst. Rev.* 2011; CD007565.

[13] Gavin S, Henry K, Monica B, et al., on behalf of the participants of the 4th Gynaecological Ovarian Cancer Consensus Conference (OCCC) 2010. Gynaecologic Cancer Intergroup (GCIC) consensus statement on clinical trials in ovarian cancer: report from the Fourth Ovarian Cancer Consensus Conference. *Int. J. Gynaecol. Cancer* 2011; 21: 750–755.

[14] Fotopoulou C, Savvatis K, Kosian P, et al. Quaternary cytoreductive surgery in ovarian cancer: does surgical effort still matter? *Br. J. Cancer* 2013; 108: 32–38.

[15] Chang SJ, Hodeib M, Chang J, Bristow RE. Survival impact of complete cytoreduction to no gross residual disease for advanced-stage ovarian cancer: a meta-analysis. *Gynecol. Oncol.* 2013; 130: 493–498.

[16] NCCN Practice Guidelines in Oncology (NCCN Guidelines). http://www.nccn.org/professionals/physician_gls/pdf/ovarian.pdf. [Accessed 6 September 2013].

[17] Kroep JR. Advances in epithelial ovarian cancer. *Curr. Pharmaceut Des.* 2012; 250: 3735–3740.

[18] Thigpen T, duBois A, McAlpine J, et al. First-line therapy in ovarian cancer trials. *Int. J. Gynaecol. Cancer* 2011; 21: 756–762.

[19] Mackay HJ, Brady MF, Oza AM, et al. Prognostic relevance of uncommon ovarian histology in women with stage III/IV epithelial ovarian cancer. *Int. J. Gynecol. Cancer* 2010; 20: 945–952.

[20] Landrum LM, Java J, Mathews CA, et al. Prognostic factors for stage III epithelial ovarian cancer treated with intraperitoneal chemotherapy: a Gynecologic Oncology Group study. *Gynecol. Oncol.* 2013; 130: 12–18.

[21] Boere IA, van der Burg ME. Review of dose-intense platinum and/or paclitaxel containing chemotherapy in advanced and recurrent epithelial ovarian cancer. *Curr. Pharmaceut Des.* 2012; 18: 3741–3753.

[22] Katsumata N, Yasuda M, Isonishi S, et al. Long-term results of dose-dense paclitaxel and carboplatin versus conventional paclitaxel and carboplatin for treatment of advanced epithelial ovarian, fallopian tube, or primary peritoneal cancer (JGOG 3016): a randomised, controlled, open-label trial. *Lancet Oncol.* 2013; 14: 1020–1026.

[23] Van der Speeten K, Govaerts K, Stuart OA, Sugarbaker PH. Pharmacokinetics of the perioperative use of cancer chemotherapy in peritoneal surface malignancy patients. *Gastroenterol. Res. Pract.* 2012; 2012: 378064.

[24] De Bree E, Helm CW. Hyperthermic intraperitoneal chemotherapy in ovarian cancer: rationale and clinical data. *Expert Rev. Anticancer Ther* 2012; 12: 895–911.

[25] Dedrick RL, Flessner MF. Pharmacokinetic problems in peritoneal drug administration: tissue penetration and surface exposure. *J. Natl. Cancer Inst.* 1997; 89: 480–487.

[26] Schomas DA, Miller RC, Donohue JH et al. Intraperitoneal treatment for peritoneal mucinous carcinomatosis of appendiceal origin after operative management: long-term follow-up of the Mayo Clinic experience. *Ann. Surg.* 2009 Apr; 249(4): 588-95.

[27] Mohamed F, Cecil T, Moran B, Sugarbaker P. A new standard of care for the management of peritoneal surface malignancy. *Curr. Oncol.* 2011; 18: e84–e96.

[28] Sun J, Song Y, Wang Z. Benefits of hyperthermic intraperitoneal chemotherapy for patients with serosal invasion in gastric cancer: a meta-analysis of the randomized controlled trials. *BMC Cancer* 2012; 12: 526.

[29] Echarri Gonzalez MJ, Green R, Muggia FM. Intraperitoneal drug delivery for ovarian cancer: why, how, who, what, and when? *Oncology* (Williston Park) 2011; 25: 156–165.

[30] Gujiwara K, Nagao S, Aotani E, et al. Principle and evolving role of intraperitoneal chemotherapy in ovarian cancer. *Expert Opin Pharmacother* 2013; 14: 1797–1806.

[31] Ozols RF, Bundy BN, Greer BE, et al. Phase III trial of carboplatin and paclitaxel compared with cisplatin and paclitaxel in patients with optimally resected stage III ovarian cancer: a Gynecologic Oncology Group study. *J. Clin. Oncol.* 2003; 21 (17): 3194-3200.

[32] Rustin GJ1, van der Burg ME, Griffin CL et al. Early versus delayed treatment of relapsed ovarian cancer (MRC OV05/EORTC 55955): a randomised trial. *Lancet*. 2010 Oct 2; 376 (9747): 1155-1163.

[33] Saladino E, Flere F, Irato S, et al. *The role of cytoreductive surgery and hyperthermic intraperitoneal chemotherapy in the treatment of ovarian cancer relapse* 2014 Jun;66(2):109-13.

[34] Chi DS, Eisenhauer EL, Zivanovic O, et al. Improved progression-free and overall survival in advanced ovarian cancer as a result of a change in surgical paradigm. *Gynaecol. Oncol.* 2009; 114: 26–31.

[35] Biliatis I, Haidopoulos D, Rodolakis A, et al. Survival after secondary cytoreduction for recurrent ovarian cancer: which are the prognostic factors? *J. Surg. Oncol.* 2010; 102: 671–675. doi: 10.1002/jso.21686.

[36] Chua TC, Robertson G, Liauw W, et al. Intraoperative hyperthermic intraperitoneal chemotherapy after cytoreductive surgery in EOC peritoneal carcinomatosis: systematic review of current results. *J. Cancer Res. Clin. Oncol.* 2009; 135: 1637–1645.

[37] Teo MC, Tan GH, Tham CK, et al. Cytoreductive surgery and hyperthermic intraperitoneal chemotherapy in Asian patients: 100 consecutive patients in a single institution. *Ann. Surg. Oncol.* 2013; 20: 2968–2974.

[38] Cascales Campos P. Morbidity and mortality outcomes of cytoreductive surgery and hyperthermic intraperitoneal chemotherapy in patients with primary and recurrent advanced ovarian cancer. *Eur. J. Surg. Oncol.* 2013. S0748-7983(13)00752-X.

[39] Furet E, Chereau E, Lambaudie E, et al. Feasibility, morbidity and survival of surgery combined with HIPEC in the management of recurrent ovarian cancer. *Gynecol. Obstet Fertil* 2013; 41: 493–498.

[40] Mulier S, Claes JP, Dierieck V, et al. Survival benefit of adding hyperthermic intraperitoneal chemotherapy (HIPEC) at the different time points of treatment of ovarian cancer: review of evidence. *Curr. Pharmaceut Des.* 2012; 18: 3793–3803.

[41] Rowan K. Intraperitoneal chemotherapy for ovarian cancer: why has it not become standard? *J. Natl. Cancer Inst.* 2009; 101: 775–777.

[42] Mutch DG, Williams S. Biology of epithelial ovarian cancer. *Clin. Obstet Gynecol.* 1994; 37: 406–422.

[43] Boocock CA, Charnock-Jones DS, Sharkey AM, et al. Expression of vascular endothelial growth factor and its receptors flt and KDR in ovarian carcinoma. *J. Natl. Cancer Inst.* 1995; 87: 506–516.

[44] Dvorak HF, Brown LF, Detmar M, Dvorak AM. Vascular permeability factor/vascular endothelial growth factor, microvascular hyperpermeability, and angiogenesis. *Am. J. Pathol.* 1995; 146: 1029–1039.

[45] Paley PJ, Staskus KA, Gebhard K, et al. Vascular endothelial growth factor expression in early stage ovarian carcinoma. *Cancer* 1997; 80: 98–106.

[46] Hu L, Hofmann J, Jaffe RB. Phosphatidylinositol 3-kinase mediates angiogenesis and vascular permeability associated with ovarian carcinoma. *Clin. Cancer Res.* 2005; 11: 8208–8212.

[47] Pourgholami MH, Yan CZ, Lu Y, Wang L, Morris DL. Albendazole: a potent inhibitor of vascular endothelial growth factor and malignant ascites formation in OVCAR-3 tumor-bearing nude mice. *Clin. Cancer Res.* 2006; 12: 1928–1935.

[48] Kobolda S, Hegewisch-Beckerb S, Oechsle K et al. Intraperitoneal VEGF inhibition using bevacizumab: a potential approach for the symptomatic treatment of malignant ascites? *The Oncologist* 2009; 14(12): 1242–1251.

[49] Huynh H, Teo M, Soo KC. Bevacizumab and rapamycin inhibit tumor growth in peritoneal model of human ovarian cancer. *Mol. Cancer Ther.* 2007; 6(11): 2959–2966.

[50] Chia TC, Liauw W, Robertson G, et al. Towards randomized trials of cytoreductive surgery using peritonectomy and hyperthermic intraperitoneal chemotherapy for ovarian cancer peritoneal carcinomatosis. *Gynaecol. Oncol.* 2009; 114: 137–139.

[51] Classe JM, Muller M, Frenel JS, et al. Intraperitoneal chemotherapy in the treatment of advanced ovarian cancer. *Mem A´ cad Nat Chir* 2009; 8: 86–90.

[52] OVHIPEC trial. ClinicalTrials.gov identifier. NCT0042657. http://clinical-trials.gov/ct2/show/nct0042657.

In: Handbook on Ovarian Cancer
Editor: Bethany R. Collier

ISBN: 978-1-63483-874-0


*Chapter 8*

# SPLENECTOMY AS PART OF CYTOREDUCTIVE SURGERY FOR ADVANCED STAGE AND RELAPSED OVARIAN CANCER

***N. Bacalbasa*[1,*] *and Irina Balescu*[2]**

[1]"Carol Davila" University of Medicine and Pharmacy, Bucharest
[2]Ponderas Hospital, Bucharest, Romania

## ABSTRACT

Ovarian cancer is the second most common gynecologic malignancy among women worldwide after endometrial cancer and the most common cause of death in women with gynecologic malignancies. Because of the increasing life expectancy experienced worldwide it is estimated that the incidence of this aggressive disease will significantly increase in the next few decades. Among all cases diagnosed with ovarian cancer the histopathological subtype consisting of epithelial tumors represents the largest part and has been widely studied. However, there is still an important number of patients who are diagnosed in an advanced stage of the disease, when disseminated bulky tumors are already present. It has been demonstrated that the most frequent patterns of spread are represented by the peritoneal, hematogenous and lymphatic route, all of them being responsible in different proportions for the presence of upper abdominal burden which sometimes is present from the moment of initial diagnosis. In all these cases the therapeutic mainstay remains cytoreductive surgery, followed by taxanes and platinum based adjuvant chemotherapy. When it comes to long term outcomes, among various prognostic factors such as age, stage at diagnosis, histopathological subtype, differentiation grade and residual disease, only residual disease has been widely demonstrated to strongly impact survival; at the same time, the amount of residual tumor burden at the end of debulking surgery is the only parameter which is influenced by the treating physician's experience. The presence of upper abdominal disseminations has been considered for a long period of time to be the sign of a tumor with a more aggressive biology and was considered as a poor prognostic factor. The main invaded organs in the upper abdomen consist of liver and porta hepatis, diaphragm, and less

* Corresponding author: Nicolae Bacalbasa, Address: Dimitrie Racovi'ă Street, no. 2, Bucharest, Romania. Phone number: +40723540426. Mail address: nicolae_bacalbasa@yahoo.ro

common, the spleen. While in cases presenting hepatic involvement the presence of hematogenous disease has been accepted as a poor prognosis factor and was classified the disease as FIGO stage IV, there was no explicit specification whether parenchimatous splenic involvement should be classified as part of the same FIGO stage. Initially a poorer outcome was reported for patients submitted to splenectomy as part of debulking surgery for advanced stage epithelial ovarian cancer, this fact being related to a more aggressive biological behaviour of the tumor. Other studies have stipulated the fact that the presence of splenic metastases is an independent poor prognosis factor but they could not distinguish whether the poorer outcome is related to the presence of hematogenous involvement of the upper abdominal parenchimatous viscera or to the co-existence of bulky left quadrant upper abdominal tumoral burden.

However, the initial results were strongly influenced by the small number of cases included and by the different characteristics of the included patients. For example patients submitted to splenectomy as part of primary and secondary cytoreduction were included in the same study so the results were also influenced by the moment of performing the surgery.

More recently, a significant difference in terms of survival was reported for hematogenous versus peritoneal splenic metastases and concluded that their presence should be considered as an explicit criterion for FIGO stage IV disease. Although it is a safe and effective surgical procedure, performing a splenectomy as part of cytoreductive surgery for advanced stage or relapsed ovarian cancer might associate a higher rate of postoperative morbidity rather due to the fact that in these cases ovarian cancer becomes a systemic disease with multiple visceral involvements, imposing multiple visceral resections in order to achieve an R0 resection; in all these cases the postoperative outcomes are influenced by a cumulative postoperative risk related to each performed resection in part.

However, since splenectomy can be safely performed with acceptable rates of postoperative complications it should be routinely performed in cases presenting splenic tumoral involvement in order to increase the rate of complete cytoreduction. This chapter focuses on the patterns of spread, prognostic factors of patients with splenic involvement, safety and effectiveness of splenectomy as part of cytoreductive surgery for advanced stage and relapsed epithelial ovarian cancer.

## INTRODUCTION

Splenic tumors usually develop in the context of lymphoreticular malignancies, while most commonly splenic involvement from solid tumors occurs in breast, lung, melanoma, colorectal, gastric and ovarian cancer [1, 2, 3]. In the majority of cases splenic metastases from solid tumors occur in the context of disseminated hematogenous spread and are associated with other visceral tumoral lesions [1]. The prevalence of splenic metastases from solid tumors is mainly obtained from large autopsy studies and range between 2.3-7.4%, the largest investigated series being conducted by Berge who reported 312 splenic metastases among 7165 autopsies for cancer [1]. In the last decades large studies on living patients have been conducted and reported that the splenic tumoral involvement (determined by histopathological studies of the splenectomy specimen) occurs in 1.1-1.3% of cases while the incidence of splenic metastases at preoperative imagistic studies is up to 0.15% (in a Japanese study conducted on 24761 patients 37 cases were diagnosed ultrasonographically with splenic involvement) [4, 5]. The rarity of splenic tumoral involvement is explained through multiple mechanisms: inhibitory influence of the splenic microenvironment on neoplastic cells, the sharp angle and tortuosity of the splenic artery which associates a modified blood flow through the splenic vasculature, the lack of splenic lymphatic afferents, the rhythmic contractility and the role of barrier of the splenic capsule [2, 3, 6-8].

When it comes to splenic involvement in advanced stage ovarian cancer, three patterns of spread have been advocated: hematogenous, peritoneal and lymphatic way. However, tumor cell metastasis involves multiple mechanisms including disconnection of the tumor cell from the solid tumor, invasion of the malignant cells into the blood, lymphatic flow or ascites, escape from the immunological filters, adhesion to endothelial cells, extravasation from the blood or lymphatic flow and angiogenesis induction [9].

## Pathways of Splenic Involvement

Ovarian cancer metastasizes more likely via intraperitoneal dissemination followed by the hematogenous and lymphatic route. Intraperitoneal spread is influenced by growth factors and cytokines which will induce the epithelial – mesenchymal transition, responsible for the increased motility and invasion ability of the tumoral cells [9]. This transition consists of dramatic phenotypic changes which will provide epithelial to mesenchymal cell conversion. Once malignant cells acquire mesenchymal properties, they will express a higher capacity of adhesion and an increased motility leading to a higher capacity of inducing distant metastases [9]. Recently the epithelial-mesenchymal transition was classified into three distinct categories, only type 3 of transition being considered as part of tumor progression; the other two types are considered to be part of embryogenesis (type 1) and inflammation and tissue damage repair respectively (type 2) [10]. Once a type 3 epithelial-mesenchymal transition occurs, distant metastases are expected. After evading from the ovarian capsule, the malignant cells will become part of the peritoneal fluid and will follow its' normal route into the peritoneal cavity [11]. In the study conducted by Carmingani et al. it has been demonstrated that the malignant cells will be transported by the peritoneal fluid according to physical forces such as intraperitoneal fluid hydrodynamics and gravity; according to this study, preferential tumor seeding will develop in the pelvic space, near the ileocecal valve, along the right paracolic gutter, diaphragm and greater omentum. The diaphragmatic and omental involvement were explained by the presence at this level of lymphatic lacunae on the diaphragmatic peritoneal surface and lymphoid tissue of the greater omentum respectively [12]. In contrast, if the intraperitoneal fluid is reduced, malignant cells are restricted in motion and will implant nearby the primary tumor leading to rectal or urinary bladder invasion [13]. Although it is not a common site of involvement, the spleen can be interested by the development of isolated peritoneal nodules or by contiguity from the greater omentum. In the latter situation involvement occurs by contiguous spread to the attached colon, spleen, gastroc-colic ligament, stomach and even pancreas and necessitates performing of extended left upper quadrant resections in order to provide a local control of the disease [14].

Another pattern of spread is the lymphatic route; however it has been demonstrated that this pathway is rather a secondary route which develops later in the evolution of the disease leading to pelvic and para-aortic lymph node metastases. When it comes to the upper abdomen lymphatic involvement, Feki et al. demonstrated that once the malignant cells disseminate into the greater omentum and diaphragmatic peritoneum, they will migrate through the milky spots which are mainly found at these levels, pass through the mesothelial barrier and get into the lymphatic flow. The authors also hypothesized that ovarian malignant cells migrate primarily via lymphatics and block the lymphatic clearance of the peritoneum [11]. However the presence of distant lymphatic metastases has been considered as a poor prognostic factor and cases diagnosed with lymph node metastases have been classified as FIGO stage IIIC [15].

As for the hematogenous route of dissemination, although it is less frequently seen, it is associated with the poorest prognostic. Hematogenous route is incriminated whenever parenchymal organ involvement is encountered and has been widely studied in patients with ovarian cancer liver metastases. Hematogenous liver metastases are usually associated with decreased survival even if the principles of radical surgery are applied; these findings enabled the International Federation of Gynecology and Obstetrics to classify these cases as stage IV disease status [16, 17]. When it comes to splenic hematogenous involvement, initially there was no explicit mention whether these patients should be classified as FIGO stage IV, especially due to the low number of cases diagnosed with parenchimatous splenic involvement [18], the reported incidence of splenic metastases at the time of primary cytoreduction ranging between 0 and 41% [19-22]. However, FIGO classification presented in 2014 clearly distinghuished between parenchymatous and peritoneal seeding and classified capsular splenic lesions as stage IIIC of the disease while the parenchymatous lesions were classified as FIGO stage IV.

## Splenectomy As Part of Debulking Surgery in Advanced Stage Ovarian Cancer with Bulky Upper Abdominal Involvement

It has been widely demonstrated that the best therapeutic option to achieve an increased long term survival in advanced stage ovarian cancer is obtaining a complete cytoreduction with no residual disease. In Bristow's meta-analysis involving 6885 patients diagnosed with advanced stage ovarian cancer each 10% increase in the proportion of patients undergoing maximal cytoreduction was associated with a concomitant 5.5% increase in median cohort survival time [23]. The same study reported that the percentage of patients submitted to optimal cytoreduction widely varies in the literature reported data from 15% to 85%; these differences are mostly related to the presence of extended upper abdominal disease at the time of diagnosis [23]. According to the study conducted by Eisenkop in 2001, the disease sites which are usually associated with incomplete cytoreduction are the diaphragm (in 76.3% of cases), portal triad (in 77.1% of cases), mesentery (in up to 82% of cases) and omentum, spleen and pancreas (in 13% of cases) [24]. The authors included in their study 393 physicians and questioned them regarding the therapeutic strategy and the number of performed procedures in order to achieve complete cytoreduction; in the meantime the responders were asked to define the notion of optimal cytoreduction. A median of 95% of patients were reported to be submitted directly to cytoreductive surgery while in the other 5% of cases neoadjuvant chemotherapy followed by surgery was the treatment of choice. At the question regarding the number of performed procedures as part of debulking surgery, a median value of nine procedures (range 0-15) was reported. When it comes to the definition of optimal cytoreduction, 12% of the responders defined it as no residual disease, 13.7% used a 5 mm threshold, and 60.8% used a 1 cm threshold while 12.6% used a 1.5 – 2 cm threshold.

When questioned about the possibility of performing upper abdominal resections in order to maximize the cytoreductive effort, 60.1% of respondents declared that they excise the omentum en bloc with splenectomy and distal pancreatectomy if necessary, 16.2% do not perform this type of surgery due to the lack of experience and 23.7% do not perform it due to an unacceptable risk of postoperative complications or due to the lack of data establishing the efficacy of the procedure. In the meantime 83.9% of the respondents favoured the development of post-fellowship training in debulking surgery. Those who voted against post-fellowship training also invoked concerns related to the efficacy of multiple resections ($p = 0.01$) [24].

However, due to the improvement achieved in surgical techniques regarding the upper abdominal resections and in the postoperative management of the patients submitted to extended hepato-bilio-pancreatic surgery, these type of surgical procedures were successfully implemented in the armamentarium of the oncologic surgeon. It has been widely demonstrated that addition of upper abdominal resection provides a significant increase of the rate of complete resection to no residual disease cytoreduction with acceptable rates of postoperative morbidity, so radical surgery in the upper abdomen is widely performed nowadays [25-28].

In the study conducted by Oliver Zivanovic between 1989 and 2005, 490 patients submitted to surgery for FIGO stage IIIC ovarian cancer at Memorial Sloan Kettering Center were introduced [29]. The patients were classified according to the presence of upper abdominal disease in three groups: group 1 – no upper abdominal disease and included 116 cases, group 2 – upper abdominal disease < 1cm and included 161 cases and group 3 – bulky upper abdominal disease and included 197 cases. Optimal cytoreduction was considered whether residual disease was < 1cm and was achieved in 81%, 63% and 39% of cases in groups 1, 2, and 3 respectively ($p < 0.001$). The patients were also stratified according to the time of surgery: before 2001 and after 2001. The distribution of the upper abdominal involvement was similar for both time periods ($p = 0.289$); however the majority of surgical procedures involving upper abdomen resections were performed after 2001 (66 cases were submitted to upper abdominal resections after 2001 compared to 12 cases submitted to upper abdominal procedures before 2001, $p < 0.001$). The rate of optimal cytoreduction was significantly higher after 2001 (40% before 2001 versus 78% after 2001, $p < 0.001$), this effect being more pronounced in patients with bulky upper abdominal disease (11% before 2001 versus 70% after 2001, $p < 0.001$) [29]. In another study conducted by the same author involving 526 patients with stage IIIC ovarian cancer 158 cases had minimal upper abdominal involvement, 243 cases had bulky abdominal involvement while the other 125 cases had no upper abdominal involvement [30]. The authors demonstrated that the long term outcomes were not influenced by the location of the tumoral burden; the most important predictor for an improved outcome remained the completion of the resectional process: patients submitted to suboptimal cytoreductive surgery reported comparable low median progression free survivals (14 months for cases with no upper abdominal disease, 11 months for cases with minimal upper abdominal disease and 13 months for patients with bulky abdominal disease respectively). Although in cases submitted to complete cytoreduction to no residual disease patients with bulky upper abdominal involvement had a poorer outcome when compared to those with no upper abdomen involvement, the benefits of radical surgery were still present, underlining the necessity to maximize the debulking effort whenever is possible [30].

Initially large studies have been conducted on the issue of upper abdominal surgery in advanced stage ovarian cancer and discussed about the benefits of multiple visceral resections including hepatic, diaphragmatic, splenic, pancreatic and upper abdomen lymph node dissection; it has been demonstrated that all these surgical procedures can be safely performed, with acceptable rates of postoperative complications and in the meantime with increased rates of long term survivors [14, 16, 28].

The necessity to perform splenectomy in order to achieve an R0 resection and the complications related to this surgical procedure widely vary between the existing studies. The largest studies which include splenectomy as part of upper abdominal resections are summarized in Table 1.

These data come to suggest that splenectomy was increasingly associated as part of debulking surgery in the last two decades leading to an increased rate of cytoreduction to no residual disease; in the meantime association of splenectomy does not seem to increase the postoperative complications. For example, in the study conducted by Pierluigi Beneditti Panici regarding the predictors of postoperative morbidity after cytoreduction for advanced stage ovarian cancer 121 patients were included, submitted to 212 surgical procedures [33]. At diagnosis 96 patients were diagnosed with FIGO stage IIIC disease while the other 25 cases had FIGO stage IV disease. Upper abdominal metastatic sites included diaphragmatic involvement in 62 cases, liver involvement in 43 cases, stomach in 16 cases, biliary tract and porta hepatis in 24 cases, spleen in 53 cases and pancreatic tail in 14 cases. The main associated resections were diaphragmatic peritonectomies in 28.9% of cases, diaphragmatic resections in 31.4% of cases, glissonian resections in 15.7% cases, liver resections in 13.2% of cases, partial gastrectomies in 9.9% of cases, distal pancreatectomies in 13.2% of cases and splenectomies in 39.6% of cases. When it comes to the extent of cytoreduction, an R0 resection was achieved in 75.1% of cases, while in other 20.7% of cases a residual disease < 1 cm; in the other 4.1% of cases an R2 resection (defined as residual disease > 1 cm) was performed. At univariate analysis diaphragmatic, pancreatic, gastric and splenic resections were associated to a prolonged hospital in stay while in multivariate analysis only diaphragmatic resections and pancreatic resections were associated with a longer hospitalization. Intraoperative and postoperative complications occurred in 29.7% of cases. Intraoperatively the main complication consisted of severe blood loss and was observed after multiple liver resections for disseminated hepatic lesions while postoperatively the complication rate was influenced by the number of associated resections. In multivariate analysis diaphragmatic resections, diaphragmatic peritonectomies, pancreatectomies and hepatic surgery were associated with an overall increased risk of postoperative complications while diaphragmatic, hepatic, pancreatic and biliary tract resections were independent predictors of severe complications. When studying the risk of developing a pleural effusion it was significantly influenced by performing diaphragmatic surgery, hepatic and pancreatic surgery. Although splenectomy was associated with an increased postoperative hospitalization, splenic resection did not predispose to a higher rate of postoperative complications; moreover, the authors also concluded that the surgical procedure with the most severe postoperative complications remains pancreatic resections [33].

Based on the observation that a significant number of patients present bulky upper abdominal disease at the time of diagnosis and necessitate multivisceral en bloc resections, Hoffman et al. conducted a study on six patients submitted to en bloc resection in the left upper abdominal quadrant [14].

**Table 1. Studies in which splenectomy was included as part of upper abdomen debulking surgery**

| Author | Period of the study | Year of publishing the study | No. of cases | No. of performed splenectomies (%) | R0 definition | R0 resection (%) | Postoperative complications | Splenectomy related complications | 30 days postoperative mortality |
|---|---|---|---|---|---|---|---|---|---|
| Cliby et al. [31] | 1998-2001 | 2004 | 41 | 7 (17%) | Largest residual tumor <1cm | 90% | 19.6% | NR | 2.4% |
| Chi et al. [27] | 1998-2002 | 2004 | 140 | 9 (6.4%) | Residual tumor <1cm | 62.8% | 5% (Clavien Dindo grade 3-5 complications) | NR | 0.71% |
| Eisenhauer et al. [16] | 1998-2003, splenectomy was performed after May 2000 | 2006 | 262 | 17 (6.4%) | No visible residual disease | 19.08% | 12% | NR | NR |
| Hoffman et al. [14] | 2002-2004 | 2007 | 6 | 6 (100%) | No residual disease | 33% | 50% | NR | 0 |
| Chi et al. [32] | January 2001-December 2006 | 2010 | 141 | 45 (32%) | No gross residual disease | 30% | 22% | NR | 1.4% |
| Panici et al. [33] | September 2006-May 2014 | 2015 | 121 | 53 (43.8%) | No visible residual disease | 75% | 29.7% | NR; however splenectomy was not a predictor of severe complications | 0 |

Starting from the hypothesis that almost all women with advanced stage ovarian cancer already have omentum tumor burden which might spread via the ligaments to the surrounding viscera, the authors proposed a en bloc technique of the involved organs in order to achieve an R0 resection: after an initial phase of exploration of the peritoneal cavity mobilization of the involved colic segment is required in order to determine which is the length of bowel which will be resected and how many anastomoses will by necessary. If the splenic flexure is involved by contiguous spread, it will be not mobilized. Than the gastrocolic ligament is dissected close to the stomach providing a good access in the omental bursa; the anterior surface of the pancreas and the splenic vessel are explored. Bulky left abdominal tumor will be removed en bloc with the spleen, pancreatic tail, splenic flexure and parcelar gastrectomy if the stomach is involved. Postoperative complications were described in three patients and consisted of pulmonary embolism associated with a small anastomotic leak in one case, left quadrant abscess in one case and gastric leak requiring re-operation in the third case. The reported disease free survival ranged between 2-12 months, one patient refusing adjuvant chemotherapy. The authors demonstrated the efficacy of en bloc resection in these cases underlining the advantage of a more complete apparent clearance of the tumor compared to piecemeal resection and secondarily a benefit in terms of survival [14].

However, although surgical technique continued to improve in the last decades, there are still cases in which a complete resection to no residual tumor cannot be reached. In the study conducted by Francesco Raspagliesi, 37 patients with advanced stage ovarian cancer with upper abdominal dissemination were included. In 67% of cases omental bursa was involved, consisting of anterior pancreatic surface, caudate lobe, supra-gastric lesser sac, porta hepatis or celiac trunk involvement [28]. Debulking surgery consisted of omental removal en bloc with the lesser omentum, gastro-colic ligament, surface of the pancreas, caudate lobe, celiac lymph nodes and portal nodes. Other associated procedures consisted of splenectomy in 35% of cases, diaphragmatic resections in 21.6% of cases, large bowel resections in 54% of cases or small bowel resections in 18.9% of patients. Splenic spread was present in 12 of the 25 cases presenting omental bursa involvement. In three cases residual disease < 5 mm was present at the end of debulking surgery due to the presence of deep infiltration of porta hepatis or celiac trunk. No postoperative complication was related to the association of splenic resection. The authors demonstrated the importance of omental bursa exploration at the time of cytoreductive surgery in order to achieve a complete resection and concluded that this region could be the "sanctuary" of residual disease which might be responsible to splenic hylum tumoral spread [28].

In a similar study conducted by A. Martinez involving 28 patients with upper abdominal tumor burden complete cytoreduction to no residual disease was achieved in all but one patient who was cytoreduced to millimetric residual disease. Splenectomy was safely associated in 10 cases; major postoperative complications occurred in 35.7% of cases, none of them being related to the association of splenic resection [34].

Other reported factors associated with an improved outcome after cytoreductive surgery for stage IIIC ovarian malignancies with splenic involvement were the histological grade and the adjuvant chemotherapic treatment. In the study conducted by Zheng et al. on 32 patients with epithelial ovarian cancer submitted to splenectomy as part of debulking surgery at Zhejiang Cancer Hospital between 1998 and 2006 the univariate analysis revealed the influence of the histological grade, residual tumor and cycles of chemotherapy on the overall survival ($p < 0.05$) while in multivariate analysis only residual tumor and association of adjuvant chemotherapy impacted on survival. After a median follow up of 38 months the estimated 2 year and 5 year survival were 70% and 36% enabling the authors to consider that splenectomy can be successfully associated as part of debulking surgery [35].

## Splenectomy As Part of Cytoreductive Surgery in Advanced Stage and Relapsed Ovarian Cancer

Once the benefits of extended upper abdominal resections in advanced stage ovarian cancer were widely demonstrated, further studies were conducted on the issue of splenectomy as part of cytoreductive surgery. However, due to the fact that splenic involvement is not such a frequent situation, initially only case reports or case series have been described, leading to conflicting results regarding the benefits and postoperative complications [36-38]. One of the first series reported on this subject was conducted by Paul Matigbay and involved 112 patients submitted to splenic resections during primary and secondary cytoreductive surgery for advanced stage and relapsed ovarian cancer at Mayo Clinic between 1983 and 2003 [39]. At the time of the study 66 patients were submitted to primary cytoreduction while the other 46 cases underwent secondary cytoreduction for recurrent disease. Splenectomy was performed for direct splenic involvement in 46% of cases, while an en-bloc resection to facilitate the removal of peri-splenic disease was performed in 41% of cases; in other 13 per cents splenectomy was imposed by the intraoperative trauma leading to an uncontrollable haemorrhage. Other associated visceral resections consisted in intestinal resections (performed in 52% of cases at the time of primary cytoreduction and in 48% of cases at the time of secondary cytoreduction) and urinary tract resections (performed in 3% of patients at the moment of primary cytoreduction and 7% of patients at the moment of secondary cytoreduction). Intraoperatively the median number of units of packed red blood cells was 2 units while on the whole in stay period the median number of transfused red blood cells was 4. Reoperation due to postoperative bleeding was needed in two cases: one case developed a severe intravascular coagulopathy with diffuse bleeding areas including the splenic bed while in the second case the bleeding originated from the pelvic sidewall. Postoperatively 6,3% of cases developed wound infection, 4.5% developed postoperative pneumonias, 8% experienced thromboembolic events and 4.5% developed a septic status due to fungal infection (in two cases), anastomotic leak (in one case) and of unknown origin (in other two cases). However none of these septic complications could be directly attributed to the splenectomy; the 30-days postoperative mortality rate was 5% and was associated to septic shock due to an anastomotic leak in one case and due to respiratory failure secondary to pneumonia in other two cases. Other causes of early postoperative mortality were thromboembolic events in two cases while in another case the death cause remained unknown. No postoperative pancreatic leakage was reported. When it comes to the long term outcomes, the primary cytoreduction group reported an overall median survival time of 21.6 months with an estimated 2-year survival of 46.2% while the median overall survival and the estimated 2 year survival in the secondary cytoreduction group were 20.3 months and 42.3% respectively. The strongest predictor for long term survival remained the completion of the resection; when it comes to the various patterns of spread, no difference in terms of survival was obtained in parenchimatous versus peritoneal seeding of the spleen. This was the largest reported series regarding the safety of splenectomy as part of debulking surgery for advanced and relapsed ovarian cancer; however the study failed to identify other prognostic factors and which patients could mostly benefit from splenectomy as part of debulking surgery in advanced stage and recurrent ovarian cancer. This fact could be explained by the heterogeneity of the studied cohort, which included patients at different moments of disease evolution. Moreover, the study also included a number of 15 cases in which splenectomy was necessary for haemostatic purpose due to an intraoperative uncontrollable haemorrhage [39].

In a similar study conducted by Gemignani et al. and published in 1997 the authors included six patients submitted to splenectomy during cytoreductive surgery for isolated parenchymal splenic metastasis [40]. The study retrospectively reviewed data of patients submitted to surgery between 1991 and 1997. The single reported complication was a diaphragmatic tear which necessitated chest tube placement. At a median follow-up of 25.5 months all patients were alive and free of recurrent disease [40].

In order to determine if the presence of splenic metastases is the reflection of a more biologically aggressive disease and if performing a splenic resection could increase survival, Scott Eisenkop et al. conducted a study on 356 patients submitted to complete cytoreduction for stage IIIC ovarian cancer; in 49 cases splenectomy was required in order to maximize the cytoreductive effort while in the other 307 patients an R0 resection was feasible without requiring splenectomy [41]. Patients requiring splenectomy were older ($p$ = 0.05), had a poorer general status ($p < 0.001$), a higher volume of ascites ($p < 0.001$) and a larger maximal diameter of metastatic disease ($p$ = 0.004); in the meantime cases in which splenectomy was required necessitated more often other extended resections such as pelvic exenteration ($p < 0.001$), diaphragm stripping ($p < 0.001$), diaphragm resection ($p < 0.001$) and gross pelvic or para-aortic lymph nodes ($p$ = 0.006) when compared to cases in which splenectomy was not required. Regarding the intraoperative and postoperative outcomes, patients in whom splenectomy was performed had a significantly longer operative time (238 minutes versus 192 minutes, $p$ = 0.004), a higher blood loss (1663 ml versus 1167 ml, $p$ = 0.001), a higher number of transfused red blood cells (5.3 units versus 3.2 units, $p$ = 0.002) and a longer hospitalization (16.1 days versus 12.2 days, $p$ = 0.001). However the rates of postoperative complications and 30 days mortality were similar between the two groups. When it comes to the long term outcomes, patients requiring splenectomy had a median overall survival rate of 56.4 months and an estimated 5 year survival of 48% while cases in which splenectomy was not necessary had a median survival rate of 76.8 months and an estimated 5 year survival rate of 58%. However these data did not reach statistical significance ($p$ = 0.4). The authors underlined that, although a less favourable outcome was observed among patients submitted to splenectomy when compared to those who did not necessitate it, the presence of splenic involvement should not be considered an indicator of a biologically aggressive disease which could contraindicate the surgical approach. The authors also considered that a stratification of the overall survival according to the type of splenic involvement (contiguous spread of the omental disease, confluent metastases, parenchimatous or lymphatic hylar involvement) could not be feasible due to the small number of cases in each subgroup and suggested that a large multi-institutional prospective observational study is needed to determine whether there are prognostic differences between the hematogenous, peritoneal and lymphatic pattern of spread [41].

## Differences in Terms of Prognosis According to the Pattern of Spread

Once it has been demonstrated that the presence of parenchimatous liver metastases is a poor prognostic factor compared to peritoneal seeding and was considered as an inclusion criteria of FIGO stage IV disease, attention was focused to determine if the presence of other parenchimatous lesions should also be considered as a criterion of FIGO stage IV disease. One of the first authors which suggested that FIGO stage IV should be extended in order to include parenchimatous splenic lesions was J. L. Nicklin in 1995. The author conducted a study on 18 patients submitted to splenectomy as part of primary cytoreduction for advanced stage ovarian cancer between 1989 and 1994; among these cases, three patients were found to have splenic parenchimatous lesions. Due to the poorer outcome of these patients, the authors proposed an extension of FIGO classification in order to include splenic parenchimatous metastases as a criterion for stage IV disease. In the meantime the reported rates of postoperative complications enabled the authors to consider that splenectomy should be performed only in selected cases [42].

Another study in which the authors investigated if a difference in terms of survival should be expected according to the pattern of splenic involvement was conducted by Ayhan et al. The authors reported a series of 34 patients submitted to cytoreductive surgery to < 1 cm residual disease over 12 years in whom splenectomy was performed as part of primary debulking effort [20]. Among these cases the hematogenous pattern of spread was incriminated in 18 cases. Although patients with splenic metastases reported a trend to a poorer prognosis when compared to those who did not have splenic involvement this fact did not reach statistical significance ($p > 0.05$) and the authors concluded that splenectomy should be performed whenever is needed in order to maximize the cytoreductive effort even if parenchimatous lesions are present. The authors reported a postoperative morbidity rate of 29.4% and a 30-days postoperative mortality rate of 8.8%, none of the complications being directly related to the splenectomy procedure [20].

The first study which came to demonstrate that parenchimatous splenic metastases is an independent poor prognostic factor and should be considered as a criterion for FIGO stage IV of disease is the one conducted by Eduard Tanner and published in 2013 [18]. The study involved 576 patients submitted to cytoreductive surgery for FIGO stage IIIB-IV at Memorial Sloan Kettering Cancer Center between 2001 and 2010. Splenectomy was performed in 97 patients while optimal cytoreduction (defined as residual disease as less than or equal to 1 cm) was achieved in 87.6% of them. The histopathological studies of the specimens revealed the presence of parenchimatous lesions in 20.8% of cases, capsular lesions in 67% of cases, splenic hylum in in 47.4% of cases and attached fat in 69.1% of cases. Among the patients with parenchimatous lesions, six of them had other evidence of stage IV disease: hepatic parenchimatous metastases in three cases, supradiaphragmatic adenopathy in two cases and malignant pleural effusion in one case. Patients requiring splenectomy were more likely to be diagnosed in an advanced stage of the disease ($p = 0{,}014$), including bulky upper abdominal tumors ($p < 0.0001$). In the meantime patients in whom splenectomy was performed were more likely to necessitate other visceral resection such as: rectal resections ($p < 0.0001$), colic resections ($p < 0.0001$), distal pancreatectomies ($p < 0.0001$), hepatic resections ($p < 0.0001$), or diaphragmatic resections ($p < 0.0001$). In order to quantify the complexity of the surgical procedure the authors used the Surgical Complexity Score introduced by Aletti; according to this score, the patients were classified into low ($\leq 3$), intermediate (4-7) and high ($> 7$) complexity scores. Based on this classification, patients submitted to splenectomy were more likely to be considered as having a high complexity score ($p < 0.0001$). When studying the long term outcomes, cases in which a complete cytoreduction was achieved had a significantly better outcome (with a reported progression free survival of 26.3 months and an overall survival of 69.7 months) when compared to those with residual disease < 1 mm (with a reported progression free survival of 16.5 months and an overall survival of 45.7 months) and to those with residual disease >1 mm (with a reported progression free survival of 12.7 months and an overall survival of 35.3 months). The presence of parenchimatous splenic metastases was another poor prognostic factor, inducing a 21 months decrease in overall survival (the reported overall survival was 28.5 months for patients with parenchimatous lesions versus 49.9 months for cases in which the hematogenous splenic involvement was not present). Other prognostic factors which reached statistical influence in univariate analysis were the age at diagnosis ($p < 0.0001$), preoperative albumin levels ($p < 0.0001$), FIGO stage ($p = 0.001$), histopathological subtype ($p = 0.028$), presence of bulky upper abdominal disease ($p < 0.0001$), the absence of residual disease ($p < 0.0001$), and association of intraperitoneal chemotherapy ($p < 0.0001$). In multivariate analysis the presence of parenchimatous splenic lesions maintained a significant association with a decreased overall survival (OR=0.506; 95% CI, 0.272–0.944) [18].

Another study conducted on this issue involved patients with advanced stage ovarian cancer submitted to splenectomy at the moment of primary cytoreduction in „Dan Setlacec" Center of Gatrointestinal Disease and Liver Transplantation, Fundeni Clinical Institute, Bucharest [43]. Sixty-six patients were eligible for the study, in 55 cases the upper abdominal tumor burden being limited to the spleen while in the other 11 cases bulky abdominal disease being reported. Preoperatively 47 patients were diagnosed in FIGO stage IIIC while the other 19 cases were diagnosed in FIGO stage IV. The most often associated visceral resections included colorectal resections (37 cases), diaphragmatic resections (9 cases), gastric resections (9 cases), distal pancreatectomies (3 cases) and atypical hepatectomies (1 case). The histopathological studies of the specimens described a hematogenous pattern of spread in 19 cases, capsular involvement in 35 cases and hilar involvement in 12 cases. The median hospital in stay was 12 days while the main postoperative complications were pancreatic leakage (in four cases), abdominal abscess (in four cases, two of them necessitating re-operation), pleural effusion (three cases), bronchopneumonia (three cases) and neurologic disorders (three cases). The overall morbidity rate was 30% while the 30-day postoperative mortality rate was 7%; death occurred in five cases: two due to abdominal abscess (originating from an enteral anastomosis in one case and pancreatic leakage in the other case), one case due to a severe bronco-pneumonia, one patient developed a cerebral ischemic stroke, while the fifth patient (with important preoperative cardiac and respiratory dysfunctions) developed a severe uncontrollable metabolic acidosis leading to a multiple organ failure. The authors compared the results to a control group including 272 patients with advanced stage ovarian cancer submitted to cytoreductive surgery in the same period of time and by the same surgical teams but in whom splenectomy was not necessary. The rates of postoperative morbidity and 30 days mortality were similar between the two subgroups: while the postoperative morbidity was 30% among patients submitted to splenectomy and the 30 days postoperative mortality rate was 7%, in the control group which did not necessitate performing a splenectomy, complications developed in 27% of cases and the early postoperative mortality rate was 5%. Similarly to Tanner's study, a significant difference in terms of survival was obtained between the three patterns of spread: while patients diagnosed with peritoneal seeding reported an overall survival of 58.4 months, patients with parenchimatous lesions had a median overall survival of 24.5 months ($p = 0.0126$); in the meantime the overall survival of cases diagnosed with hylar involvement was 40.6 months. When studying the differences in terms of survival between hylar and parenchimatous lesions and respectively hylar versus peritoneal seeding no significant difference was obtained ($p = 0.362$ and respectively $p = 0.457$). However the study demonstrated the feasibility of the procedure and demonstrated that the presence of hematogenous splenic involvement is an independent negative prognosis factor [43].

## SPLENECTOMY AS PART OF CYTOREDUCTION FOR RELAPSE OVARIAN CANCER

After demonstrating the benefits in terms of survival after splenectomy at the time of primary cytoreduction for advanced stage ovarian cancer, studies went even further and tried to demonstrate the feasibility of the procedure as part of secondary and even tertiary cytoreduction. The main studies investigating this issue are summarized in Table 2.

In the study conducted by Hanprasertpong et al. six patients were sumitted to splenectomy as part of interval debulking surgery and secondary cytoreduction respectively [49]. Among the three patients submitted to splenectomy as part of secondary cytoreduction in two cases an isolated splenic recurrence was diagnosed while in the third case the splenic lesion was associated to an inguinal lymph node metastasis.

The postoperative course was uneventful in all cases, splenectomy being well tolerated. The histopathological findings revealed the presence of parenchimatous splenic lesions in two cases and a capsular lesion in the third case. When it comes to the long term survival, none of the patients presented evidence of recurrent disease at the moment of ending the study [49].

In a more recent study, twenty-eight patients submitted to splenectomy at the time of secondary, tertiary and even quaternary cytoreduction were introduced [50]. All cases were submitted to surgery in the same center („Dan Setlacec" Center of Gastrointestinal Disease and Liver Transplantation, Fundeni Clinical Institute, Bucharest) between 2002 and 2014. Splenectomy was performed at the time of secondary cytoreduction in 21 cases, at tertiary cytoreduction in six cases and at quaternary cytoreduction in one case. In all cases the specimen of splenectomy was sent to histopathological study in order to determine if the splenic involvement had a peritoneal, hematogenous or lymphatic origin. At the time of secondary cytoreduction the main associated visceral resections consisted of colic resections (42.86% of cases), rectosigmoidian resections (33.33% of cases), distal pancreatectomy (19.05% of cases), atypical hepatectomy (14.29% of cases) and partial frenectomy (14.29% of cases). The histopathological studies revealed a hematogenous pattern of spread in 42.85% of cases and peritoneal lesions in 52.38% of cases, while the hilar involvement was reported in a single case.

**Table 2. Splenectomy as part of debulking surgery in relapsed ovarian cancer**

| Author | Period of the study | Year of publishing the study | Type of cytoreduction | No. of cases | No. of performed splenectomies (%) | R0 definition | R0 resection (%) | Postoperative complications | Splenectomy related complications | 30 days post-operative mortality |
|---|---|---|---|---|---|---|---|---|---|---|
| Fagotti et al.[44] | May 2005-September 2008 | 2009 | secondary | 25 | 8 (32%) | No visible residual disease | 92% | Overall: 44%; severe complications: 28% | NR | 0 |
| Schorge et al.[45] | January 1998-January 2008 | 2010 | secondary | 40 | 4(10%) | No residual disease | 55% | 23% - severe complications | NR | 0 |
| Petrillo et al.[46] | January 1995-December 2010 | 2013 | secondary | 73 | 4(5.4%) | 1 cm | 100% | NR | NR | NR |
| Tang et al. [47] | May 1999-November 2010 | 2013 | tertiary | 83 | 2 (2.4%) | Microscopic residual disease | 34.9% | 15% | NR | 0 |
| Magrina et al. [48] | January 2006-December 2010 | 2013 | secondary | 52 | 5 (9.6%) | No visible residual disease | 75% | 36.5% (overall complication rate) | NR | 0 |

The median duration of hospitalization was 14 days (range 2-89 days). Early postoperative complications were reported in six cases, in half of them re-operation being needed; in one case re-operation was imposed by a high-flow enteral fistula, in the second case the indication of re-operation was given by an unresponsive to conservative treatment pancreatic fistula while in the third case early postoperative hemoperitoneum occurred. The early postoperative mortality rate was 9.5%; death occurred in two cases, due to uncontrolled septic shock in one case and haemorrhagic shock with disseminated intravascular coagulopathy in the second case. Although it did not reach statistical significance, the median overall survival of patients with peritoneal seeding was longer when compared to cases with parenchimatous lesions (35 months versus 12 months, $p = 0.2$). When it comes to patients submitted to splenectomy in the setting of tertiary cytoreduction, the main associated visceral resections were: colic resections (in 3 cases), rectosigmoidian resections (in two cases), distal pancreatectomy (in one case) and atypical hepatectomy (in one case).

The histopathological studies revealed a peritoneal pattern of spread in four cases while in the other two cases the hematogenous route was incriminated, the splenic metastases being entirely surrounded by normal parenchyma. Postoperatively two patients developed complications – an abdominal abscess and a biliary fistula, both cases being successfully managed conservatively. The long term outcomes revealed an improved survival for patients with peritoneal seeding (21 month) versus parenchimatous lesions (4 months). However, the results were not statistically significant ($p = 0.08$). As for the patient submitted to splenectomy as the time of the third relapse, quaternary cytoreduction was performed at 102 months after the initial diagnosis and also associated an atypical hepatectomy, partial gastrectomy and extended pelvic resections for a large pelvic recurrence. The histopathological studies revealed a hematogenous liver lesion associated with a peritoneal splenic seeding. The postoperative outcome was uneventful; however the patient died of disease 20 months after quaternary cytoreduction.

This study came to underline that also not statistically significant, a poorer outcome should be expected in patients with parenchimatous lesions at secondary and even tertiary cytoreduction. However, splenectomy was safely associated whenever it was needed in order to maximize the debulking effort [50].

## The Role of Laparoscopic Splenectomy in Advanced Stage and Relapsed Ovarian Cancer

In order to improve the early postoperative outcome, to provide a faster recovering and secondarily a more rapid association of adjuvant chemotherapy, attention was focused in performing laparoscopic resections for advanced stage and recurrent ovarian cancer. The first hand-assisted splenectomy for isolated splenic metastases was first reported in 1998 by Klinger demonstrating the feasibility of the procedure [51].

In the study conducted by Dennis Chi et al. the authors included six patients submitted to laparoscopic or hand assisted splenectomy between 1996 and 2005; in five of the six cases laparoscopic or hand assisted resection was performed while in the sixth case conversion to laparotomy was imposed by the presence of peritoneal carcinomatosis [52]. In four of the six cases the histopathological examinations confirmed the presence of splenic tumoral involvement while in the other case a benign splenic cyst was found. In one of the cases residual tumor < 1 cm was reported, all the other cases being cytoreduced to no residual disease. The estimated blood loss ranged between 50 and 300 ml while the postoperative hospitalization ranged between 3 and 5 days. Postoperatively all five cases in which recurrent disease was diagnosed were submitted to adjuvant therapy with platinum based salts and taxanes (in four cases) while the fifth patient underwent aromatase inhibitor therapy. At 2084 months after surgery all patients were free of any recurrent disease. The study came to demonstrate the effectiveness of the procedure and underlined the fast recovery of the patient; however the authors considered that this procedure should be performed only by specialized surgeons and in selected cases [52].

In the meantime, Pedro Ramirez published a paper focusing on the technique of open versus totally laparoscopic splenectomy in cases with advanced or recurrent ovarian cancer. The author demonstrated the feasibility of total laparoscopic splenectomy by a lateral approach using a four ports technique. After complete mobilization, the specimen of splenectomy is placed in an Endobag and extracted through the 12 mm trocar after extending the incision line. According to the same author after laparoscopic splenectomy a pancreatic leak rate of 6% is expected while the thromboembolic events occur in up to 10% of cases [53].

In another similar study Fagotti introduced 10 patients with relapsed ovarian cancer who were submitted to laparoscopic or robotic surgery associated with intraperitoneal hypertemic chemotherapy (HIPEC) for isolated recurrences [54]. In seven cases debulking was performed on the laparoscopic route while in the other three cases a robotic approach was chosen. As for the chosen chemotherapic agent for HIPEC, nine patients received cisplatin while the tenth patient received oxaliplatin. In two cases splenectomy was needed while in the other eight cases location of the recurrence necessitated radical omentectomy or selective splenectomy. The operative time ranged between 95 and 140 minutes while the estimated blood loss ranged between 50 and 100 ml. All patients were discharged after 3-7 days while systemic chemotherapy was administrated after a median interval of 21 days (19-32 days). A single patient developed postoperative complications consisting of a low frequency atrial fibrillation. When it comes to long term outcomes, no recurrence or death was reported after 10 months (range 6-37 months). The authors demonstrated the safety and efficacy of laparoscopic surgery for isolated relapse from ovarian cancer in association with HIPEC, a shorter convalescence interval and a faster administration of systemic chemotherapy being achieved [54].

One of the most suggestive studies regarding the benefits of minimally invasive surgery in relapsed ovarian cancer comes from Javier Magrina et al. and involved a retrospective analysis of 52 patients submitted to secondary cytoreduction for relapsed ovarian cancer at Mayo Clinic Arizona between January 2006 and December 2010 [48]. Among these cases laparoscopic resection was performed in 9 cases, robotics in 10 cases, while the other 33 patients were benefited from a classic approach. Splenectomy was performed in 11.1% of patients submitted to laparoscopy and 12.1% of patients submitted to laparotomy. The perioperative outcomes were similar between the three subgroups in terms of operating time, rate of complete debulking surgery, intra- and postoperative complications, while the estimated blood loss and postoperative hospital in stay were significantly lower in the minimally invasive subgroup. In the meantime there was no significant difference in regard to the long term outcomes, the reported overall survival being similar among the three subgroups [48].

## Association of Pancreatic Resections to Splenectomy As Part of Cytoreductive Surgery in Advanced Stage and Relapsed Ovarian Cancer

In a significant number of cases the presence of the bulky left quadrant abdominal disease will force the surgeon to perform multiple visceral resections en bloc with the tumor in order to achieve negative resection margins and an R0 resection. One of the most frequent associated visceral resection to splenectomy remains distal pancreatectomy [14]. Although initially it has been considered that a pancreatic resection predisposes to an unacceptable risk regarding the postoperative morbidity rate, progression achieved in hepat-bilio-pancreatic surgery offered the possibility to safely include pancreatic resection as part of debulking surgery for advanced and relapsed ovarian cancer. However, at this moment the reported experience regarding pancreatic surgery as part of debulking is still limited, most of the reported cases including small series of patients.

In the study conducted by Pieluigi Benediti Panici involving 121 patients with advanced stage ovarian cancer distal pancreatectomy was associated in 16 cases while splenectomy was performed in 48 cases. After performing an aggressive surgical approach the rate of complete cytoreduction (defined as no residual disease) was 75.1%. When studying the short term outcomes, the authors reported that performing pancreatic resection was associated with a longer length of hospitalization in both univariate and multivariate analysis. In the meantime pancreatic surgery was associated with the higher rate of postoperative complications, with a reported rate of pancreatitis and abscess formation secondary to a pancreatic leak of 13% among cases submitted to pancreatic resections [33].

Most often complications related to pancreatic surgery are related to the exocrine pancreatic secretion as pancreatic leaks and their rate ranges between 30-60% while the mortality rate is up to 5% [55-57]. However, the rate of reported pancreatic leaks widely varies in literature data due to the absence of a standard definition of the pancreatic leak. While Rodriguez *et al.* defined pancreatic fistula as a daily output of at least 30ml/day with amylase levels three times higher compared to amylase serum levels after the fifth postoperative day [57], Grobmyer defined it as clinical signs or radiological confirmation of a collection with increased levels of amylase (more than 50 ml/day) beyond the fifth postoperative day [58]. The first standardized definition came from the International Study Group of Pancreatic Fistula: according to their opinion, pancreatic leak was defined as a left upper quadrant fluid collection present after the third postoperative day with a fluid amylase level>3 times the level of serum amylase [59].

In order to determine the incidence and management of pancreatic leaks after splenectomy en bloc with distal pancreatectomy during primary cytoreduction Siobhan Kehoe et al. conducted a study on 17 patients; all cases were submitted to splenectomy en bloc with distal pancreatectomy as part of primary cytoreduction between January 2001 and December 2006 [60]. In the meantime splenectomy without pancreatic resection was performed in other 24 cases. Pancreatic leaks were defined accordingly to the International Study Group of Pancreatic Fistula. Optimal cytoreduction was defined as residual tumor of less than 1 cm. In all cases distal pancreatectomy was performed for left quadrant bulky disease invading the

[15] FIGO Cancer Committee (1986). Staging announcement, *Gynecol Oncol* 25: 5.
[16] Eisenhauer EL, Abu-Rustum NR, Sonoda Y, Levine DA, Poynor EA, Aghajanian C, Jarnagin WR, DeMatteo RP, D'Angelica MI, Barakat RR, Chi DS (2006). The addition of extensive upper abdominal surgery to achieve optimal cytoreduction improves survival in patients with stages IIIC-IV epithelial ovarian cancer, *Gynecol Oncol* 103: 1083-1090.
[17] Elattar A, Bryant A, Winter-Roach BA, Hatem M, Naik R (2011). Optimal primary surgical treatment for advanced epithelial ovarian cancer, *Cochrane. Database. Syst. Rev.* CD007565.
[18] Tanner EJ, Long KC, Feffer JB, Leitao MM, Jr., Abu-Rustum NR, Barakat RR, Chi DS, Gardner GJ (2013). Parenchymal splenic metastasis is an independent negative predictor of overall survival in advanced ovarian, fallopian tube, and primary peritoneal cancer, *Gynecol Oncol* 128: 28-33.
[19] Chen LM, Leuchter RS, Lagasse LD, Karlan BY (2000). Splenectomy and surgical cytoreduction for ovarian cancer, *Gynecol Oncol* 77: 362-368.
[20] Ayhan A, Al RA, Baykal C, Demirtas E, Ayhan A, Yuce K (2004). The influence of splenic metastases on survival in FIGO stage IIIC epithelial ovarian cancer, *Int. J. Gynecol Cancer* 14: 51-56.
[21] McCann CK, Growdon WB, Munro EG, Del Carmen MG, Boruta DM, Schorge JO, Goodman A (2011). Prognostic significance of splenectomy as part of initial cytoreductive surgery in ovarian cancer, *Ann. Surg. Oncol* 18: 2912-2918.
[22] Bilgin T, Ozerkan K, Ozan H (2005). Splenectomy in cytoreductive surgery for advanced ovarian cancer, *Arch. Gynecol Obstet.* 271: 329-331.
[23] Bristow RE, Tomacruz RS, Armstrong DK, Trimble EL, Montz FJ (2002). Survival effect of maximal cytoreductive surgery for advanced ovarian carcinoma during the platinum era: a meta-analysis, *J. Clin. Oncol* 20: 1248-1259.
[24] Eisenkop SM, Spirtos NM (2001). What are the current surgical objectives, strategies, and technical capabilities of gynecologic oncologists treating advanced epithelial ovarian cancer?, *Gynecol Oncol* 82: 489-497.
[25] Lim MC, Kang S, Lee KS, Han SS, Park SJ, Seo SS, Park SY (2009). The clinical significance of hepatic parenchymal metastasis in patients with primary epithelial ovarian cancer, *Gynecol Oncol* 112: 28-34.
[26] Song YJ, Lim MC, Kang S, Seo SS, Park JW, Choi HS, Park SY (2009). Total colectomy as part of primary cytoreductive surgery in advanced Mullerian cancer, *Gynecol Oncol* 114: 183-187.
[27] Chi DS, Franklin CC, Levine DA, Akselrod F, Sabbatini P, Jarnagin WR, DeMatteo R, Poynor EA, Abu-Rustum NR, Barakat RR (2004). Improved optimal cytoreduction rates for stages IIIC and IV epithelial ovarian, fallopian tube, and primary peritoneal cancer: a change in surgical approach, *Gynecol Oncol* 94: 650-654.
[28] Raspagliesi F, Ditto A, Martinelli F, Haeusler E, Lorusso D (2013). Advanced ovarian cancer: omental bursa, lesser omentum, celiac, portal and triad nodes spread as cause of inaccurate evaluation of residual tumor, *Gynecol Oncol* 129: 92-96.
[29] Zivanovic O, Eisenhauer EL, Zhou Q, Iasonos A, Sabbatini P, Sonoda Y, Abu-Rustum NR, Barakat RR, Chi DS (2008). The impact of bulky upper abdominal disease cephalad to the greater omentum on surgical outcome for stage IIIC epithelial ovarian, fallopian tube, and primary peritoneal cancer, *Gynecol Oncol* 108: 287-292.

[30] Zivanovic O, Sima CS, Iasonos A, Hoskins WJ, Pingle PR, Leitao MM, Jr., Sonoda Y, Abu-Rustum NR, Barakat RR, Chi DS (2010). The effect of primary cytoreduction on outcomes of patients with FIGO stage IIIC ovarian cancer stratified by the initial tumor burden in the upper abdomen cephalad to the greater omentum, *Gynecol Oncol* 116: 351-357.
[31] Cliby W, Dowdy S, Feitoza SS, Gostout BS, Podratz KC (2004). Diaphragm resection for ovarian cancer: technique and short-term complications, *Gynecol Oncol* 94: 655-660.
[32] Chi DS, Zivanovic O, Levinson KL, Kolev V, Huh J, Dottino J, Gardner GJ, Leitao MM, Jr., Levine DA, Sonoda Y, Abu-Rustum NR, Brown CL, Barakat RR (2010). The incidence of major complications after the performance of extensive upper abdominal surgical procedures during primary cytoreduction of advanced ovarian, tubal, and peritoneal carcinomas, *Gynecol Oncol* 119: 38-42.
[33] Benedetti PP, Di D, V, Fischetti M, Casorelli A, Perniola G, Musella A, Marchetti C, Palaia I, Berloco P, Muzii L (2015). Predictors of postoperative morbidity after cytoreduction for advanced ovarian cancer: Analysis and management of complications in upper abdominal surgery, *Gynecol Oncol* 137: 406-411.
[34] Martinez A, Pomel C, Mery E, Querleu D, Gladieff L, Ferron G (2011). Celiac lymph node resection and porta hepatis disease resection in advanced or recurrent epithelial ovarian, fallopian tube, and primary peritoneal cancer, *Gynecol Oncol* 121: 258-263.
[35] Zheng AW, Zheng F, Chen YQ, Zhu HN, Qian JH (2008). [Splenectomy in epithelial ovarian cancer: analysis of 32 cases], *Zhonghua Fu Chan Ke.Za Zhi.* 43: 197-200.
[36] Koh YS, Kim JC, Cho CK (2004). Splenectomy for solitary splenic metastasis of ovarian cancer, *BMC. Cancer* 4: 96.
[37] Lauro S, Trasatti L, Capalbo C, Conti A, Ricci F, Mingazzini PL, Vecchione A (2002). Solitary splenic recurrence of epithelial ovarian cancer: a case report and review, *Anticancer Res.* 22: 3643-3645.
[38] Minagawa Y, Kanamori Y, Ishihara H, Morishita K, Kigawa J, Ito T, Maeda K, Saito S (1991). Solitary metastatic ovarian carcinoma of the spleen: a case report, *Asia Oceania J.Obstet.Gynaecol.* 17: 45-48.
[39] Magtibay PM, Adams PB, Silverman MB, Cha SS, Podratz KC (2006). Splenectomy as part of cytoreductive surgery in ovarian cancer, *Gynecol Oncol* 102: 369-374.
[40] Gemignani ML, Chi DS, Gurin CC, Curtin JP, Barakat RR (1999). Splenectomy in recurrent epithelial ovarian cancer, *Gynecol Oncol* 72: 407-410.
[41] Eisenkop SM, Spirtos NM, Lin WC (2006). Splenectomy in the context of primary cytoreductive operations for advanced epithelial ovarian cancer, *Gynecol Oncol* 100: 344-348.
[42] Nicklin JL, Copeland LJ, O'Toole RV, Lewandowski GS, Vaccarello L, Havenar LP (1995). Splenectomy as part of cytoreductive surgery for ovarian carcinoma, *Gynecol Oncol* 58: 244-247.
[43] Bacalbasa N, Balescu I, Dima S, Brasoveanu V, Popescu I. Hematogenous Splenic Metastases as an Independent Negative Prognosis Factor at the Moment of Primary Cytoreduction in Advanced Stage Epithelial Ovarian Cancer – A Single Center Experience. Anticancer Research *35*: xxx-xxx (2015).

[44] Fagotti A, Paris I, Grimolizzi F, Fanfani F, Vizzielli G, Naldini A, Scambia G (2009). Secondary cytoreduction plus oxaliplatin-based HIPEC in platinum-sensitive recurrent ovarian cancer patients: a pilot study, *Gynecol Oncol* 113: 335-340.

[45] Schorge JO, Wingo SN, Bhore R, Heffernan TP, Lea JS (2010). Secondary cytoreductive surgery for recurrent platinum-sensitive ovarian cancer, *Int. J. Gynaecol. Obstet.* 108: 123-127.

[46] Petrillo M, Fagotti A, Ferrandina G, Fanfani F, Costantini B, Vizzielli G, Pedone AL, Nero C, Margariti PA, Scambia G (2013). Ovarian cancer patients with localized relapse: clinical outcome and prognostic factors, *Gynecol Oncol* 131: 36-41.

[47] Tang J, Liu DL, Shu S, Tian WJ, Liu Y, Zang RY (2013). Outcomes and patterns of secondary relapse in platinum-sensitive ovarian cancer: implications for tertiary cytoreductive surgery, *Eur. J. Surg. Oncol* 39: 786-791.

[48] Magrina JF, Cetta RL, Chang YH, Guevara G, Magtibay PM (2013). Analysis of secondary cytoreduction for recurrent ovarian cancer by robotics, laparoscopy and laparotomy, *Gynecol Oncol* 129: 336-340.

[49] Hanprasertpong J, Ohishi R, Iwasa N, Nagao S, Okamoto K, Fujiwara K (2010). Splenectomy during secondary cytoreductive surgery for epithelial ovarian cancer, *Asian Pac. J. Cancer Prev.* 11: 413-416.

[50] Bacalbasa N, Balescu I, Dima S, Brasoveanu V, Popescu I. Splenectomy as Part of Cytoreductive Surgery in Recurrent Epithelial Ovarian Cancer. Anticancer Research *35*: xxx-xxx (2015).

[51] Klingler PJ, Hinder RA, Menke DM, Smith SL (1998). Hand-assisted laparoscopic distal pancreatectomy for pancreatic cystadenoma, *Surg. Laparosc. Endosc.* 8: 180-184.

[52] Chi DS, Abu-Rustum NR, Sonoda Y, Im HB, Jhamb N, D'Angelica M, Rim M, Dupont J, Barakat RR (2006). Laparoscopic and hand-assisted laparoscopic splenectomy for recurrent and persistent ovarian cancer, *Gynecol Oncol* 101: 224-227.

[53] Ramirez PT, Dos RR (2007). Splenectomy in patients with advanced or recurrent ovarian cancer: open and laparoscopic surgical techniques and clinical outcomes, *Gynecol Oncol* 104: 29-32.

[54] Fagotti A, Petrillo M, Costantini B, Fanfani F, Gallotta V, Chiantera V, Turco LC, Bottoni C, Scambia G (2014). Minimally invasive secondary cytoreduction plus HIPEC for recurrent ovarian cancer: a case series, *Gynecol Oncol* 132: 303-306.

[55] Gouma DJ, van Geenen RC, van Gulik TM, de Haan RJ, de Wit LT, Busch OR, Obertop H (2000). Rates of complications and death after pancreaticoduodenectomy: risk factors and the impact of hospital volume, *Ann. Surg.* 232: 786-795.

[56] Connor S, Raraty MG, Howes N, Evans J, Ghaneh P, Sutton R, Neoptolemos JP (2005). Surgery in the treatment of acute pancreatitis--minimal access pancreatic necrosectomy, *Scand. J. Surg.* 94: 135-142.

[57] Rodriguez JR, Germes SS, Pandharipande PV, Gazelle GS, Thayer SP, Warshaw AL, Fernandez-del Castillo C (2006). Implications and cost of pancreatic leak following distal pancreatic resection, *Arch. Surg.* 141: 361-365.

[58] Grobmyer SR, Pieracci FM, Allen PJ, Brennan MF, Jaques DP (2007). Defining morbidity after pancreaticoduodenectomy: use of a prospective complication grading system, *J. Am. Coll. Surg.* 204: 356-364.

[59] Pratt WB, Maithel SK, Vanounou T, Huang ZS, Callery MP, Vollmer CM, Jr. (2007). Clinical and economic validation of the International Study Group of Pancreatic Fistula (ISGPF) classification scheme, *Ann. Surg.* 245: 443-451.

[60] Kehoe SM, Eisenhauer EL, Abu-Rustum NR, Sonoda Y, D'Angelica M, Jarnagin WR, Barakat RR, Chi DS (2009). Incidence and management of pancreatic leaks after splenectomy with distal pancreatectomy performed during primary cytoreductive surgery for advanced ovarian, peritoneal and fallopian tube cancer, *Gynecol Oncol* 112: 496-500.

[61] Bacalbasa N, Balescu I, Dima S, Brasoveanu V, Popescu I (2015). Pancreatic Resection as Part of Cytoreductive Surgery in Advanced-stage and Recurrent Epithelial Ovarian Cancer - A Single-center Experience, *Anticancer Res.* 35: 4125-4129.

In: Handbook on Ovarian Cancer
Editor: Bethany R. Collier

ISBN: 978-1-63483-874-0


*Chapter 9*

# LIVER SURGERY IN OVARIAN CANCER LIVER METASTASES

***N. Bacalbasa[1,*] and Irina Balescu[2]***
[1]"Carol Davila" University of Medicine and Pharmacy, Bucharest, Romania
[2]Ponderas Hospital, Bucharest, Romania

## ABSTRACT

Ovarian cancer is one of the most aggressive gynecologic malignancies and represents a major cause of death for women worldwide. This aggressive behavior is especially related to the fact that most patients are diagnosed in an advanced stage of the disease when disseminated tumoral burden is already present. Although the intraperitoneal route seems to be the most common pattern of spread, ovarian cancer can also develop distant metastases by hematogenous route and throughout lymphatic channels, the most commonly affected sites by hematogenous spread including the lungs and liver. Historically, patients with liver involvement have been considered as having a systemic, uncontrollable disease and were considered as candidates for supportive care or palliative chemotherapy.

Although the presence of liver metastases at the moment of diagnosis is usually associated with an altered tumor biology and aggressive disease, there was no convincing evidence that cytoreduction in the presence of liver metastases is less efficacious. Starting from this hypothesis, hepatic resection for ovarian cancer liver metastases has been proposed.

However, at this moment it is estimated that the number of patients submitted to liver resection for hepatic metastases from gynecological cancer represent less than 1% of the total resected liver metastases, the role of surgery in patients with ovarian cancer liver metastases being still in question. The main reason for this paucity of hepatectomies in ovarian cancer liver metastases is related to the fact that usually these kinds of tumors develop liver metastases in the settings of obvious systemic or regional dissemination which is not suitable for a complete macroscopic resection. Patients presenting resectable, isolated and limited to liver metastases are rather an exception than a rule in

* Corresponding author: Nicolae Bacalbasa, Address: Dimitrie Racovi'ă Street, no. 2, Bucharest, Romania. Phone number: +40723540426. Mail address: nicolae_bacalbasa@yahoo.ro

the setting of ovarian cancer. However this small subgroup of patients with isolated hepatic lesions has been initially considered to suit best to liver resection.

According to this principle, initially the main indication for resection in ovarian cancer liver metastases was the presence of solitary liver lesions with no extrahepatic tumoral burden as the best results in terms of survival had been obtained in such cases. More recently, it has been demonstrated that the presence of extrahepatic tumoral burden does not represent a significant prognostic factor for a poorer outcome in all patients and allowed to identify the subsets of patients with extrahepatic tumor burden who could benefit most from liver resections.

A crucial step in studying the long term outcomes after liver resection for ovarian cancer hepatic metastases was demonstrating the different outcomes between the two distinct patterns of hepatic involvement: peritoneal and hematogenous spread. Metastases originating from peritoneal seeding with parenchimatous invasion of at least 2 cm were classified as peritoneal lesions while lesions entirely surrounded by liver parenchyma were considered to have hematogenous origins. Significant differences in terms of survival between patients with peritoneal versus hematogenous lesions submitted to complete resections were observed. Based on these findings, it has been largely accepted that the presence of peritoneal seeding involving the liver included the case in FIGO stage IIIC while the presence of hematogenous liver involvement should be classified as FIGO stage IV.

When it comes to the role of liver resection as part of secondary or even tertiary cytoreduction, literature data is even scarcer, the presence of liver metastases being considered for long time as an exclusion criterion when establishing whether a patient is a candidate for optimal cytoreduction at the moment of surgery for recurrent disease. In time, improved understating of hepatic anatomy in association with the improvement of surgical techniques and postoperative care transformed hepatic resection in a more frequent associated surgical procedure in serial resections for ovarian cancer relapse. Once liver resection has been successfully associated as part of cytoreduction for relapsed ovarian cancer, attention was focused on determining other potential prognostic factors which might influence survival such as initial FIGO stage, disease free survival or histopatologic subtype of the tumor.

This chapter focuses on the subject of liver resection as part of cytoreductive surgery for advanced stage or relapsed ovarian cancer. The influence of different patterns of spread, the safety and effectiveness of performing anatomical or extended liver resections are also presented.

## INTRODUCTION

Ovarian cancer remains one of the most common and aggressive malignancies worldwide, with an estimated incidence of 225,500 new cases per year and a reported mortality of 140,200 deaths per year [1]. Unfortunately, the majority of patients are diagnosed in an advanced stage of the disease when disseminated lesions are already present; most of these cases will experience recurrent disease; only 20-25% of patients being expected to experience a long term survival despite an initial good response to primary therapeutic strategy [2-4]. However, in the last decades the reported survival even in patients diagnosed in an advanced stage of the disease significantly increased due to the progressive incorporation of more extended surgical resections in order to maximize the debulking effort [5]. When it comes to the optimal residual disease, the definition of optimal cytoreduction has modified from remnant tumor < 1cm to no gross residual disease [5]. The redefinition of optimal residual disease was proposed by Chang and Bristow and was based on the results of Bristow's meta-analysis conducted on 6885 patients with advanced stage ovarian cancer. The author demonstrated that each 10% increase in the proportion of patients undergoing maximal cytoreduction was associated with a 5.5% increase of the median cohort survival time. The authors concluded that one of the strongest factors influencing the long terms outcomes was performing a maximal cytoreductive surgery [6]. However, in patients diagnosed in an advanced stage of the disease, presenting disseminated lesions multiple visceral resections might be needed. In cases with pelvic extension association of surgical procedures such as pelvic peritonectomy, rectosigmoidian resection, colic or enteral resections or even urinary tract resections have been successfully implemented in the armamentarium of the oncologic gynecologist increasing the rate of resection to no visible residual disease [7-10]. Although these procedures have been introduced as part of the standard surgical procedures which might be needed in order to achieve a complete cytoreduction, the percentage of patients benefiting from a maximal debulking effort widely varies in the literature data from 15% to 85% [6]. It has been advocated that studies in which the reported rate of optimal cytoreduction surpasses 50% usually incorporate extensive upper abdominal resections [11-13]. Chi et al. demonstrated that association of upper abdominal extended resections leads to a significant improvement of disease free survival and overall survival, so they recommended that surgeons should consider including these therapeutic gestures as part of the standard treatment in patients presenting upper abdominal involvement [14].

When it comes to hepatic metastases in ovarian cancer, the presence of liver involvement at the time of diagnosis or during the evolution of the disease is usually considered as a poor prognosis factor with devastating effects on the long term outcomes [15].

## MECHANISMS OF LIVER INVOLVEMENT IN ADVANCED STAGE AND RELAPSED OVARIAN CANCER

When it comes to the most common patterns of spread in advanced stage ovarian cancer, it has been widely demonstrated that the main pathways of spread are represented by the peritoneal route, followed by lymphatic and hematogenous route. While the presence of peritoneal spread is usually conditioned by the apparition of the epithelial –to – mesenchymal transition in association with the presence of growth factors and cytokines, the hepatic involvement via hematogenous route usually occurs via portal flow [16, 17]. However, the presence of ovarian cancer liver metastases is common events since Rose et al. reported in their study that nearly one half of the patients with ovarian cancer have liver metastases at the time of death. The study presenting the autopsy findings in 428 patients with various histological subtypes of ovarian cancer also reported that while the peritoneum was most commonly involved (in up to 100% of cases), lymph node metastases were reported in up to 60% of cases [17]. In the study conducted by Cormio et al. the liver was reported as the most common site of distant metastases [15]. The different outcomes reported after liver resections of peritoneal versus hematogenous liver metastases is also suggested by the inclusion of the two patterns of spread as two separate criteria in FIGO classification: while the presence of capsular hepatic lesions is considered as IIIC stage of the disease while the presence of hematogenous lesions (defined as hepatic parenchymatous lesions) is considered as an inclusion criteria for FIGO stage IV of disease [18]. In conclusion, a clear distinction between the different pathways of liver involvement needs to be made in all cases.

## Safety and Effectiveness of Hepatic Resections in Ovarian Cancer Liver Metastases

Initially it has been considered that liver resection is not justified due to the fact the hepatic involvement usually develops in the context of a systemic disease and therefore, systemic chemotherapy should be the treatment of choice [19-21]. However, the reported success after hepatic resections in colorectal and neuroendocrine malignancies quantified by increasing the rate of long term survivors up to 25% at ten year follow up encouraged the surgeons worldwide to study the effectiveness and benefits in long term outcomes for liver resection in non-colorectal non-neuroendocrine liver metastases [19-23]. Although the groups of patients involved in these studies are small in number and heterogeneous in regard to the primary tumor, the general conclusion is that hepatic resection could improve the long term outcomes [21-23]. Among cases included in these studies, patients with advanced stage or relapsed ovarian cancer were involved and a benefit in terms of survival was achieved. The most important studies focused on this issue are summarized in Table 1.

All these reported results showing increased rates of survival after resection of liver metastases enabled the surgeons worldwide to include it in the standard treatment for hepatic metastases from other primaries including gynecological cancers.

In the study conducted by Sarah Kamel et al. the authors introduced 87 patients diagnosed with liver metastases from gynecological malignancies submitted to hepatic resections at John Hopkins Hospital between 1990 and 2010. Most patients included in the study had a primary tumor located in the ovary (67 cases, 77%) and were classified with FIGO stage III disease. Other involved primaries were uterus/endometrium (in 17% of patients), cervix (in 4% of cases) and fallopian tube (in 2% of cases). The main surgical procedure consisted of total hysterectomy with bilateral adnexectomy (81%), concurrent lymph node dissection (61%) and peritoneal debulking (81%). Up to 34% of cases were found to have positive lymph nodes.

Synchronous liver involvement was reported in 30 patients (34% of cases) while in the other 57 patients metachronous lesions were found after a median disease free interval of 25 months.

Among patients with synchronous liver metastases 24 cases (80%) were submitted to concomitant liver resections. Among patients diagnosed with metachronous liver lesions 45 patients had been submitted to neoadjuvant chemotherapy; furthermore, 23 patients were submitted to liver resections. When studying the completeness of resection, negative resections margins were seen in 63% of cases, while 15% of specimens revealed microscopic disease on the specimen's margins; in a single case macroscopic residual disease was reported. The postoperative mortality rate was 0. Recurrence was found in 39 cases after a median follow up of 13 months: in six cases the recurrence was limited to the liver, in 13 cases only an extrahepatic recurrent disease was found, while in the other 18 cases both intrahepatic and extrahepatic recurrences were reported; in other two cases the site of recurrence remained unknown.

**Table 1. Studies conducted on the issue of hepatic resections in non-colorectal non-neuroendocrine liver metastases including subjects with ovarian cancer**

| Author, year of the study | Period of the study | No. of cases | No of patients with ovarian cancer (%) | 5-year overall survival of the entire cohort | Median survival after resection of cases with ovarian primaries (months) |
|---|---|---|---|---|---|
| Slotta et al. 2014 [21] | 7 years | 101 | 5 (15.84%) | 30% | 15.84 |
| Reddy et al. 2007 [22] | 1995-2005 | 82 | 11 (13.4%) | 37% | NR |
| Martel et al. 2105 [24] | 1990-2012 | 52 | 3 (5.7%) | 58% | 89.9 |
| Lendoire et al. 2007 [25] | 1989-2006 | 106 | 14(13.2%) | 19% | NR, 5-year OS for genitor-urinary tumors (renal, ovarian) 30% |
| Adam et al. 2006 [26] | 1983-2004 | 1452 | 65 (4.47%) | 36% | 98 |

Of the six patients diagnosed with intrahepatic recurrent disease three cases were submitted to re-operation. The median overall survival after resection of liver metastases with ovarian origin was similar to the other non-ovarian primaries (21 versus 22 months respectively, $p = 0.53$). Although patients diagnosed with parenchimatous lesions had a poorer outcome, this fact did not reach statistical significance ($p = 0.12$) [27].

One year later Jose Ramia et al. published a literature review suggestively entitled: "Liver Metastases from Gynecological cancers: Time to Resection?" in which the author included the published articles between 1990 and 2011 based on a PubMed Search. A total of 20 articles including case-reports were reviewed; however the authors referred only to hematogenous metastases. When it came to ovarian cancer, liver resection was mainly proposed for isolated lesions, the presence of concomitant extra-hepatic burden being even considered as an absolute contraindication by some authors [28, 29]. However, most studies considered that primary debulking surgery followed by adjuvant chemotherapy is the treatment of choice, although relapse might occur [30-32]. Moreover, a second debulking surgery has been proposed, especially in patients with a reported disease free survival of at least 12 months. Although an important percentage of patients is expected to be submitted to secondary cytoreduction, liver resection is performed only in a low percentage of cases ranging between 0 and 9%. When it comes to prognostic factors, negative resection margins, the absence of extrahepatic burden, slow-growing tumors, a longer disease free survival (> 12 months) and a good clinical status were associated with improved survival [33].

## Liver Resection As Part of Upper Abdominal Surgery in Advanced Stage and Relapsed Ovarian Cancer

In an attempt to improve the rates of complete cytoreductive surgery Dennis Chi et al. introduced in the therapeutic armamentarium extensive upper abdominal surgical procedures as part of primary cytoreduction for advanced stage ovarian cancer from 2001. In order to demonstrate the feasibility and safety of these procedures, the authors compared the results with those obtained before the year of 2001 in the same hospital. The first study group consisted of 168 patients submitted to cytoreductive surgery between 1996-1999 while the second group consisted of 210 patients submitted to cytoreductive surgery between 2001 and 2004. Both study groups included patients with FIGO stage IIIC and IV; however, upper abdominal surgery was performed only in the second group. Extended upper abdominal surgery included diaphragmatic peritonectomy and/or resection, splenectomy, distal pancreatectomy, cholecistectomy, hepatectomy and porta hepatis tumor resection. Optimal residual disease was defined as no residual tumor larger than 1 cm. The two subgroups were similar in regard to age at diagnosis, tumor stage, tumor grade or clinical status according to the American Society of Anesthesiologists class. Among the patients submitted to extended upper abdominal resections, hepatectomy was performed in 13 patients (6% of cases) while resection of porta hepatis lesions was performed in 11 patients (5% of cases). The rate of complete cytoreduction was significantly higher among the second group (80% versus 46% in the first group, $p < 0.01$). In the meantime the estimated blood loss, intraoperative transfusion rates, operative time and major complications were more frequently present in the second group. However none of these aspects influenced the administration of adjuvant chemotherapy while the mortality rate was similar between the two groups (0.6% in the first group versus 0.6% in the second group). When it comes to long term outcomes, the 5 year overall survival rate was 31% in the second group, significantly higher when compared to the first group (with a 5 year overall survival rate of 14%, $p = 0.001$). The reported median overall survival was 54 months for the second group and only 43 months for the first group ($p = 0.03$) [14].

In another similar study focused on the issue of extended upper abdominal resections in patients with stage IIIC and IV ovarian cancer, Eisenhauer et al. introduced 262 patients divided in three groups: the first group included 57 patients who required extended upper abdominal resection to achieve complete cytoreduction, the second group included 122 patients in which upper abdominal procedures were not necessary while the third group included 83 patients with advanced stage disease but who were submitted to incomplete cytoreduction. Among cases submitted to extended upper abdominal procedures liver resection was performed in 9 cases (16%) while porta hepatis tumor was resected in 8 cases (14%). The first group reported a longer operative time and a higher median blood loss while the complication rate was similar between the different groups. In the meantime, although patients from the first group were submitted to the adjuvant chemotherapy later on when compared to the other two groups, similar doses of chemotherapic agents were administrated and the response to chemotherapy was significantly improved. As for the long term outcomes, comparable rates of survival were obtained for the first two groups and were significantly higher when compared to the third group (at the end of the study the median overall survival was not yet reached for group 1, was 84 months for group 2 and 37 months for group 3). The similar reported outcomes between the first two groups come to demonstrate the efficiency of extended resections. In the meantime comparable rates of postoperative complications enabled the surgeons to consider that addition of upper abdominal resections is a safe procedure [34].

Once it has been widely demonstrated that completion of the resection is one of the strongest predictors for long term survival, few authors focused on determining the specific involvement sites which could predict the presence of unresectable disease. For example, Francesco Raspagliesli studied the influence of upper abdominal tumor burden involving the omental bursa, lesser omentum, celiac, portal and triad nodes spread as cause of incomplete cytoreduction. A total of 37 consecutive patients with advanced stage ovarian cancer and upper abdomen involvement were introduced in the study: 29 cases were diagnosed with FIGO stage IIIC disease while the other 8 patients were classified as FIGO stage IV. Cytoreduction to no residual disease was achieved in 34 cases, while in the other 3 cases residual disease of 5 mm was reported. The main location of the residual nodules was at the level of hepatic pedicle, demonstrating that the involvement of the areas surrounding the vital anatomic structures in the upper abdomen might still be a reason for incomplete cytoreduction [35].

While most studies focus on the possibility of obtaining a complete cytoreduction and an improved long term survival, only few studies have been conducted on the issue of the early postoperative complications and their predictors. One of the largest studies regarding this subject was conducted by Pierluigi Beneditti Panici and involved 121 patients submitted to 212 surgical procedures including upper abdominal resections. Upper abdominal sites of involvement included: diaphragm (51.2%), the liver (33.5%), the stomach (13.3%), the biliary tract and porta hepatis (19.8%), the spleen (43.8%) and the pancreatic tail (11.6%). The main performed upper abdominal procedures included diaphragmatic peritonectomies (28.9%), diaphragmatic resections (31.4%), glissonian resections (15.7%), liver resections (13.2%), gastric resections (9.9%), distal pancreatectomies (13.2%), splenectomy (39.6%) and biliary tract surgery (19.8%). In univariate analysis performing diaphragmatic, pancreatic, gastric and splenic resections was associated with longer postoperative hospital in stay. Hepatic surgery was associated with a minimal increase of the length of hospitalization (9.2 days for patients submitted to liver resections versus 8.8 days for cases in which liver resection was not necessary, $p = 0.757$).

Despite this fact, liver surgery was associated with a higher rate of complications. In two cases a severe blood loss was observed after resection of nine and seven respectively liver metastases, while postoperatively hepatic surgery was significantly associated with an increased rate of both overall and severe complications ($p = 0.037$ and $p = 0.004$ respectively). The reported 90 days mortality rate was 0.8%. The authors concluded that extended upper abdominal resections should be performed in selected cases and by selected surgical teams, in centers with a high capacity to manage life-threatening complications [36].

## Liver Resection At the Moment of Primary Cytoreduction for Advanced Stage Ovarian Cancer

At the time of primary cytoreduction, liver resection for ovarian cancer is most often presented as integrative part of the maximal cytoreductive effort in association with other extrahepatic resections.

In order to evaluate the role of debulking surgery in patients with stage IV ovarian cancer, Bristow et al. conducted a study on 84 patients with a median age at diagnosis of 61 years. Forty-four percents were diagnosed with parenchymal liver metastases while 38% had malignant pleural effusion. Optimal cytoreduction (defined as residual disease < 1 cm) was achieved in 30% of cases and was associated with a median overall survival of 38.4 months, while patients with suboptimal residual disease reported an overall survival of 10.3 months ($p = 0.0004$).

Optimal resection of both intrahepatic and extrahepatic disease was achieved in 16% of cases and reported an overall survival of 50.1 months, significantly higher when compared to patients with optimal extrahepatic disease but suboptimal residual hepatic tumor (with a median survival rate of 27 months) and with those with suboptimal extrahepatic and hepatic disease who had a median overall survival rate of 7.6 months [37].

The benefits of multiple visceral resections in the setting of FIGO stage IIIC and IV ovarian cancer were also reported in the study conducted by Heinz Scholz over a five year period, on 101 patients in Nurnberg, Germany. Among these cases, 54% of patients were submitted to surgery as primary therapeutic option while the other 46% of cases had been previously submitted to neoadjuvant chemotherapy. In all cases cytoreduction to no gross residual disease was attempted and was achieved in 82% of cases submitted to surgery as first therapeutic option and in 85% of cases in which neoadjuvant chemotherapy had been performed ($p = 0.793$).

Partial hepatectomy was performed in 11% of cases while Glisson capsule resection was performed in 39% of cases; the 30 days postoperative mortality rate was 0. Long term outcomes revealed a median survival of 47 months while the five year survival rate was 33% for the entire group. Patients submitted directly to surgery reported a better outcome in terms of survival comparatively to those submitted to neoadjuvant chemotherapy and interval debulking surgery ($p = 0.046$). The authors demonstrated the effectiveness of debulking surgery even if hepatic metastases are present and revealed the superiority of primary surgical treatment comparatively to interval debulking surgery [38].

Another German study comes from Ulf Neumann and discusses the benefits of liver resections as part of primary cytoreductive surgery in advanced stage ovarian cancer. The study was conducted between 1991 and 2007 and included 70 patients with advanced stage disease submitted to surgery in Charite, Virchow Clinic. Liver resection was performed in 41 out of the 70 patients, the other 29 cases presenting unresectable disease. Additional surgical procedures included total hysterectomy (in 14.3% of cases), bilateral adnexectomy (in 24.3% of cases), omentectomy (in 32.9% of cases), partial colectomy (in 51.4% of cases), partial small bowel resection (in 32.9% of cases), partial gastrectomies (in 5.7% of cases) and partial pancreatectomies (in 4.3% of cases).

In all cases submitted to liver resection a residual tumor volume < 5 mm was achieved. The 3- months postoperative mortality rate was 14.6% in the subgroup submitted to liver resection and 41% in the subgroup in which liver resection was not feasible ($p = 0.025$), while the morbidity rate was similar between the two groups. Regarding the long term outcomes, the median survival rate was significantly higher among patients submitted to liver resection: patients submitted to an R0 resection reported a median survival rate of 42 months while cases in which liver resection was not feasible reported a median overall survival of 4 months ($p < 0.001$).

Other poor prognostic factors were represented by the presence of ascites and bilobular liver metastases. When it came to establishing the predictors of resecability of hepatic metastases, only the presence of ascites was associated with a poorer resecability rate. The authors concluded that liver resection should be part of the standard therapeutic protocol whenever a residual disease of less than 5 mm can be achieved and demonstrated that performing hepatic resections in ovarian cancer liver metastases does not increase the early postoperative mortality rate [39].

## The Significance of Hematogenous Hepatic Metastases in the Setting of Advanced Stage Ovarian Cancer

Based on the postoperative outcome, liver involvement in advanced stage ovarian cancer is classified as FIGO stage IIIC when peritoneal seeding involving the liver parenchyma is diagnosed and stage IV respectively when hematogemous spread is the pathogenic mechanism. Thus, hepatic hematogenous involvement is based on the postoperative pathologic diagnosis. In an attempt to determine if there is a survival difference between parenchimatous and peritoneal hepatic involvement in cases in which an R0 resection is achieved large studies have been conducted.

In the study conducted by Lim et al. data of 117 patients submitted to primary cytoreduction for advanced stage ovarian cancer with liver involvement were retrospectively reviewed. Sixteen of the 117 patients were diagnosed with parenchimatous lesions and were included in FIGO stage IV group; however, in two cases the tumors proved to be unresectable and liver surgery consisted only in liver biopsy, confirming the ovarian origin. The remaining 14 cases were underwent hepatic resections and the histopathological studies confirmed the presence of hematogenous liver involvement. In all cases negative resection margins were achieved. The remnant 101 patients were diagnosed with FIGO stage IIIC disease. In the two cases in which liver resection could not be performed, although 3rd line chemotherapy was initiated, the reported survival was of inly 9 and 10 months respectively. Among patients diagnosed with FIGO stage IIIC disease 44 cases were submitted to neo-adjuvant chemotherapy. When it comes to the preoperative and intraoperative findings, there were no significant differences regarding the age, histology or grade, median CA 125 levels or the administration of neo-adjuvant chemotherapy. Optimal cytoreduction was achieved in 94% and 93% respectively in patients diagnosed in FIGO stage IIIC and IV while no visible residual disease was reported in 47 and 43% of patients with FIGO stage IIIC and IV respectively. The main types of liver resection included wedge resections in 50% of cases, segmentectomies in 36% of cases and hemi-hepatectomies in 14% of cases. There was no significant difference regarding the operative time, estimated blood loss, transfusion, postoperative hospital stay, largest residual disease or time to adjuvant chemotherapy. No liver-related surgery complication such as bile leakage or bleeding occurred. The most common complications in the both group were febrile morbidity, ileus, pancreatic fistula and pleural effusion. In regard to the long term outcomes, the 5-year overall survival rates were 55% and respectively 51% for the two subgroups $p = 0.5671$). The authors concluded that if an R0 resection is achieved in cases with parenchimatous lesions, a similar overall survival to cases with peritoneal lesions should be expected and suggested that a possible revision of FIGO classification might be taken in consideration [40].

In a similar study conducted at "Dan Setlacec" Center of Gastrointestinal Disease and Liver Transplantation, Fundeni Clinical Institute, Bucharest 11 patients submitted to liver resection at the time of primary cytoreduction were included. Neoadjuvant chemotherapy was administrated in two cases. Postoperatively the rate of severe complications in 25% patients, all of them being diagnosed with stage IV disease; however, the 30 days postoperative mortality was 0. Although it did not reach statistical significance the overall survival was consistently higher among patients with peritoneal seeding (34.33 months versus 15.63 months, $p = 0.702$) [41].

## LIVER RESECTION AS PART OF SECONDARY CYTOREDUCTIVE SURGERY

The benefits of secondary cytoreduction in the setting of relapsed ovarian cancer have been widely demonstrated with maximal effects in cases with a long disease free interval after completion of the primary therapeutic protocol and if isolated recurrences are found at the time of relapse [42]. However, even if multiple recurrences are found at the time of diagnosis, an aggressive surgical approach in order to maximize the debulking effort is perfectly justified in order to improve survival [43-46]. In the study conducted by Niu et al. the authors included both patients with no history of extrahepatic disease as well as patients with extrahepatic burden. Although patients with liver confined disease had an improved outcome (median overall survival of 41.42 months) when compared to those with both intrahepatic and extrahepatic disease (median overall survival of 36.99 months), the benefit in terms of survival was consistent when compared to the results of the patients submitted to chemotherapy alone [46]. In a similar study conducted by Roh et al. the outcomes of 18 patients submitted to hepatic resections for ovarian cancer liver metastases with the reported results of 25 cases with unresectable liver metastases; although extrahepatic resections were similar between the two groups, in the second subgroup no liver procedure (including surgery, radiofrequency ablation or ethanol injection) was performed. The overall survival rate was significantly improved in the hepatectomy group - 38 months, comparatively to the non-hepatectomy group - 10 months ($p$ = 0.0232) [47]. The largest studies conducted on the issue of liver resection at the moment of secondary resection are summarized in Table 2. As for the early postoperative outcomes, improvement of surgical technique of hepatic resections has led to acceptable postoperative rates of liver related surgery complications and an early postoperative mortality rate almost null [51, 52]. In the meantime the actual surgical techniques in association with the postoperative management provided the possibility of resecting up to 70% of the liver parenchyma with mortality rates of up to 5% [53]. All these aspects encouraged surgeons to perform more extended resections for liver metastatic disease. When it comes to the long term outcomes, association of liver resection as part of cytoreductive surgery has significantly improved the overall survival. The most suggestive results in regard to the short and long term outcomes are summarized in Table 3.

## Prognostic Factors after Liver Resection at the Moment of Secondary Cytoreduction

### Association of Extrahepatic Tumor Burden and Diameter of the Residual Tumor

The strongest predictor for long term survival remains the completeness of the resection. In Bosquet's study optimal cytoreduction was defined as hepatic or extra-hepatic residual disease < 1cm in the greatest diameter was consistently associated with improved survival: the median disease specific survival was significantly higher in patients submitted to optimal cytoreduction when compared to those in which optimal cytoreduction was not feasible: 41.3 months versus 5.7 months, $p < 0.0001$) [42].

Similar results were reported by Kolev et al. at the same cut-off of 1 cm [49]. In the study conducted by Niu et al. involving 60 patients submitted to liver resection for metachronous liver metastases the completion of the resection was achieved by studying the resection margins of the specimen. The absence of tumor involvement on the resection margins was defined as R0 resection and associated a significantly improved outcome when compared to patients with R1 resection (defined as microscopic involvement of the resection margins of the specimen) (51.9 months versus 22.01 months, $p$ = 0.039) [46]. Although not statistical significant, extrahepatic tumor burden was associated with a poorer outcome in Niu's study (41.42 months for patients with liver confined disease versus 36.99 months for cases with both intra- and extrahepatic lesions ($p$ = 0.290).

**Table 2. Studies regarding the role of hepatic resections as part of secondary cytoreduction in relapsed ovarian cancer**

| Author, year | Period of the study | No. of cases | Median DFI from initial diagnosis to liver rmetastases (months) | Extent of liver resection | Type of resection(definition of optimal cytoreduction) | Residual disease | Associated visceral resections |
|---|---|---|---|---|---|---|---|
| Bosquet et al., 2006 [42] | 1976-2003 | 35 | NR | NR | Residual disease< 1cm | < 1cm: 29pts<br>> 1cm: 6 pts | Bowel resection: 34.3%<br>Other associated resections: 80% |
| Niu et al., 2012 [46] | 2000-2011 | 60 | 34 | Wedge resection: 46.7%<br>Lobectomy: 11.7%<br>Trisegmentectomy: 11.7%<br>-Bisegmentectomy:20%<br>-RFA:10% | R0= negative resection margins on the specimen of liver resection<br>R1= microscopic involvement of the margins | Negative resection margins: 54 pts<br>Microscopic disease at margins: 6 pts | 0 |
| Abood et al., 2008 [48] | 1998-2006 | 10 | 48 | Trisegmentectomy: 40%<br>Lobectomy: 50%<br>Bisegmentectomy: 10% | R0= negative resection margins on the specimen of liver resection<br>R1= microscopic involvement of the margins | Negative resection margins:5 pts<br>Microscopic disease at margins: 5 pts | Diaphragmatic resection: 60%<br>Bowel resection: 30%<br>Adrenalectomy: 10% |
| Kolev et al., 2014 [49] | 1988-2012 | 27 | 27 | Multisegmentectomy: 11.1%<br>Lobectomy: 14.8%<br>Segmentectomy:40.7%<br>Wedge resections: 33.3% | Residual disease < 1cm | < 1cm: 25pts<br>> 1cm: 2 pts | Diaphragmatic resections: 33.3%<br>Bowel resection: 7.4%<br>Splenectomy: 7.4% |
| Yoon et al., 2003 [30] | 1988-2001 | 24 | 68.5 | Trisegmentectomy: 8.3%<br>Lobectomy: 8.3%<br>Segmentectomy: 70.8%<br>Wedge resection:12.5% | Residual disease < 1cm | R0: 88% of cases<br>R1: 12% of cases | |

| Author, year | Period of the study | No. of cases | Median DFI from initial diagnosis to liver rmetastases (months) | Extent of liver resection | Type of resection (definition of optimal cytoreduction) | Residual disease | Associated visceral resections |
|---|---|---|---|---|---|---|---|
| | | | | | | | Resection of extrahepatic disease: 66%<br>Diaphragmatic resections: 50%,<br>Cholecystectomy: 54.16%<br>Colectomy: 16.6%<br>Lung resection: 12.5%<br>Nephrectomy: 8.3%<br>Pericardial resection: 8.3%<br>Adrenalectomy: 4.16%<br>Splenectomy: 4.16%<br>Pancreatectomy: 4.16%<br>Gastrectomy: 4.16% |
| Roh et al., 2011 [47] | 1991-2008 | 18 | 33 | Bisegmentectomy: 5.5%<br>Segmentectomy:72.2%<br>Wedge resections: 22.2% | Residual disease < 1cm | < 1cm: 12pts<br>>1cm: 6 pts | Resection of extrahepatic disease, multiple sites: 100% |
| Pekmezci et al., 2010 [50] | 2003-2008 | 8 | 64.5 (5.38 years) | Right hepatectomy: 12.5%<br>Left lateral sectorectomy: 25%<br>Segmentectomy: 37.5%<br>Wedge resection: 25% | Macroscopic residual disease | No macroscopic residual disease and no microscopic invasion of the resection margins were achieved in all cases | Upper abdomen lymph node dissection: 25%<br>Resection of intra-abdominal peritoneal nodules: 25% |
| Merideth et al., 2003 [32] | 1976-1999 | 26 | 29.4 | Right hepatectomy: 15.4%<br>Left hepatectomy: 3.8%<br>Segmentectomy: 69.2%<br>Trisegmentectomy: 11.5% | Intra- and extrahepatic residual disease < 1cm | R0: 21 pts<br>R1: 5 pts | Bowel resection: 42.3%<br>Diaphragmatic resection: 50%<br>Splenectomy: 7.7%<br>Lung resection: 7.7%<br>Lymph node dissection:15.4%<br>Cholecystectomy: 9.2% |

DFI: disease free interval; RFA: radiofrequency ablation.

**Table 3. Early postoperative outcomes and long term results after liver resection for ovarian cancer liver metastases as part of secondary cytoreduction**

| Author, year | Period of the study | No. of cases | Postoperative complications | Hepatic surgery related complications | 30 days postop. mortality rate | Median overall survival (months) |
|---|---|---|---|---|---|---|
| Bosquet et al. 2006 [42] | 1976-2003 | 35 | 2.9% of patients required reoperation (small bowel fistula) | 0 | 0 | 27.4 |
| Niu et al. 2012 [46] | 2000-2011 | 60 | 10% (pulmonary complications, wound infections) | 0 | 0 | 39 |
| Abood et al. 2008 [48] | 1998-2006 | 10 | 10% (anemia requiring transfusion occurred in one case) | 10% | 0 | 33 |
| Kolev et al. 2014 [49] | 1988-2012 | 27 | 11% (two anastomotic leaks requiring reoperation and one postoperative sepsis) | NR | 0 | 56 months – from the time of the diagnosis |
| Yoon et al. 2003 [30] | 1988-2001 | 24 | 21% (two bilomas, one case of ileus, one case of urinary tract infection, one case of pneumonia | 8.3% | 0 | 62 |
| Roh et al. 2011 [47] | 1991-2008 | 18 | The rate of major complication was 5.6% (one case of transverse colon perforation). Five other patients experienced minor complications (ileus, wound infection, bile leakage, transient abnormality liver function or pleural effusion) | NR | 0 | 38 |
| Pekmezci et al. 2010 [50] | 2003-2008 | 8 | 0 | 0 | 0 | NR, disease free survival after liver resection=39 months |
| Merideth et al., 2003 [32] | 1976-1999 | 26 | 7.6% (wound infection in one case and small bowel perforation requiring reoperation in the second case | 0 | 0 | 26.3 |

In the study conducted by Roh et al. including 18 patients resection margins of the hepatectomy specimen and residual disease were both associated with an improved survival.

Patients presenting negative resection margins experienced a significantly improved survival when compared to those with positive resection margins (40 months versus 9 months, $p = 0.0196$) while patients submitted to an optimal cytoreduction (defined as residual disease < 1cm) reported a median overall survival of 40 months, significantly higher when compared to those with suboptimal cytoreduction (median overall survival of 9 months, $p = 0.0004$) [47]. Optimal cytoreduction (defined as extrahepatic and intrahepatic residual disease < 1 cm) was also associated with an improved survival (27.3 months versus 8.6 months, $p = 0.031$) in Melissa Meredith's study conducted at Mayo Clinic, Rochester between 1976 and 1999 [32].

Based on these findings, the authors concluded that hepatic resection should only be considered if optimal cytoreduction is feasible [32, 47]. Similar results were also obtained by other studies, demonstrating that the tumoral burden as well as the diameter of the metastatic tumor are important prognostic factors and patients submitted to cytoreduction in the presence of extrahepatic disease should be carefully selected [47, 48].

## Disease Free Survival

It has been advocated that patients with an increased disease specific survival from the primary surgery for ovarian cancer to the moment of liver resection have an improved outcome. In Bosquet's study patients with disease specific survival longer than one year also experienced an improved survival after liver resection (31.7 months versus 15.1 months, $p = 0.01$) [42]. Similar results were also reported by Niu's study, with a significantly improved median overall survival for patients with disease free survival of more than 12 months between ovarian cancer surgery and diagnosis of liver metastases (50.96 months versus 30.94 months, $p = 0.018$). The same authors stated that the improved results obtained after liver resections in patients with an initial linger disease free survival might be a reflection of a biologically indolent tumor [46]. In Kolev's study involving 27 patients a disease free survival after the initial treatment of 24 months was found to be statistically significant ($p = 0.044$) [49]. One of the most suggestive studies which demonstrates that the patient selection is crucial comes from S.S. Yoon et al. and was conducted at Memorial Sloan Kettering Cancer Center between June 1988 and December 2001. All patients included in this study had a relatively slow tumor progression and initially chemosensitive disease; this fact is demonstrated by the long disease free survival between the diagnosis of ovarian cancer and the apparition of liver metastases (with a median reported disease free interval of 68.5 months). In the meantime, the reported median overall survival was 62 months, although 75% of patients had extrahepatic tumoral burden [30]. Pekmezci et al. also considered that a longer disease free survival after the initial surgery for ovarian cancer is the mark of a good biological tumor behavior and considered these cases as the ideal candidates for secondary cytoreduction; the authors included in their study eight patients who developed liver metastases after a median disease free survival of 5.38 years; in the meantime the authors reported a secondary disease free survival after liver resection of 39 months which also favors the hypothesis of a less aggressive biology of the tumor [50]. Mayo Clinic reported similar results with a median overall survival of 27.3 months for patients with initial disease free survival longer than 12 months versus 5.7 months for patients with a shorter initial disease free survival ($p = 0.004$) [32]. Oppositely to these results, in Hyun Jin Roh's study conducted on 18 patients, time from initial diagnosis to liver resection did not significantly impacted on survival [47].

## Number and Distribution of the Hepatic Lesions

The benefits of liver resection in patients presenting multiple lesions have been widely studied in colon cancer. In a study conducted by Bolton et al. patients submitted to liver resection for colorectal hepatic metastases were divided in to subgroups: cases with fewer than three liver metastases and cases with more lesions. The authors demonstrated that if all the lesions were resected, there was no difference in terms of survival between the two groups [54]. More recently, in order to find out if there is any limit regarding the maximum number of metastases which could be resected in liver metastases from colorectal cancer, an international panel of multidisciplinary experts decided that there is no limitation in regard to the number of excised lesions [55].

When it comes to ovarian cancer, although a higher number of hepatic lesions and a bilobar distribution might be considered as a poor prognosis factor, the reported results are inconstant. In Bosquet's study neither the number nor the distribution of the hepatic metastases presented statistically significance in terms of survival [42]; similar results were also reported by Kolev et al., and Merideth et al. respectively, no significant difference being revealed between cases with solitary liver masses and multiple lesions [32, 49]. Oppositely to these studies, Niu et al. reported an improved survival for patients diagnosed with a single metastases versus those with multiple lesions (55.4 months versus 26.06 months, $p = 0.018$). However, this fact did not reach statistical significance in multivariate analysis ($p = 0.085$) [46]. The diameter of the largest liver metastasis was proven to have a significant importance in Gerard Abood's study, conducted at Loloya University Medical Center, in which 10 patients were included. According to this study, tumor size larger than 5 cm was associated with a significantly increased survival (with a reported median survival of 17.2 months versus 11.2 months in patients with smaller tumors, $p = 0.046$); the authors explained this surprising aspect by the fact that cases with larger tumors have in fact less hepatic tumor burden due to the smaller number of lesions [48].

## Other Prognostic Factors

When it comes to other possible prognostic factors such as the tumor histology and degree of differentiation, no significant influence in terms of survival has been demonstrated [32, 42, 46]. In the study conducted by Yoon et al. a favorable tumor biology (reflected in a slow growing pattern, limited to liver disease and long disease free interval) associated with a good biological status of the patient represents the ideal scenario for performing liver resection for ovarian cancer metachrnous hepatic metastases [30]. An interesting aspect was revealed by Roh's study which demonstrated that a higher upper abdominal burden is significantly associated with a decreased survival (patients with a higher pelvic tumor burden reported a median overall survival of 38 months while with those with a higher upper abdominal burden reported a median overall survival of 11 months, $p = 0.032$) [47].

### The Significance of Hematogenous Hepatic Metastases in the Setting of Relapsed Stage Ovarian Cancer

In order to determine if a difference in terms of survival is maintained at the moment of secondary cytoreduction for peritoneal versus hematogenous lesions, a study involving 15 patients was conducted in Fundeni Clinical Institute, Bucharest. Disease free interval between surgery for ovarian cancer and diagnosis of liver metastases was 30 months. An R0 resection (defined as no residual tumor) was achieved in 12 patients. The histopathological findings revealed the presence of peritoneal lesions in six patients while in the other nine patients entirely parenchimatous lesions have been found. When it came to the type of liver resection, minor hepatectomies (defined as liver resection of less than two segments) were performed in 14 cases while in the fifteenth case a major hepatectomy was performed. In order to maximize the cytoreductive effort, associated visceral resections were performed: splenectomy (in four cases), bowel resection (in four cases), diaphragmatic resections (in three cases) and subtotal gastrectomy (in a single case).

The postoperative morbidity arte was 27% while the liver surgery related complication rate was 13% and consisted of biliary leak and a hepatic abscess respectively. Although it did not present statistical significance, patients with liver metastases with peritoneal origin had a better outcome when compared to those with hematogenous lesions (14.51 months versus 6.16 months, $p = 0.197$). However, liver resection proved to be a safe and effective method as part of secondary cytoreduction [41].

In conclusion, hepatic resection for metachronous liver metastases from ovarian cancer can be safely performed at the time of secondary cytoreduction with acceptable rates of postoperative liver related complications and almost zero mortality. However, mixed surgical teams including hepato-bilio-pancreatic surgeons, visceral surgeons and gynecologic oncologist should be created in order to maximize the effects of this aggressive surgical approach and to minimize the postoperative complication rates [42-45].

## Liver Resection Beyond Secondary Cytoreduction for Relapsed Ovarian Carcinoma

Data regarding the place of liver resection beyond tertiary cytoreduction are even scarcer, limited number of cases being reported. In the same study conducted in Fundeni Clinical Hospital, liver resection was performed in three cases as part of tertiary cytoreduction and in two patients submitted to quaternary cytoreduction. Liver resection at the moment of tertiary cytoreduction was performed after a mean interval of 54 months after the initial diagnosis. In two cases minor hepatectomies (defined as resection of less than 2 segments) was performed while in the third cases a major hepatectomy was performed. Postoperatively death occurred in a single case due to the development of a urinary fistula after synchronous resection of a pelvic recurrence. The postoperative course uneventful in the other two cases; the long term outcomes revealed a survival of 63 months for one case and 70 months for the second patient, the latter being alive at the moment of ending the study. As for the patients submitted to liver resection as part of quaternary cytoreduction,, the interval between the primary and quaternary cytoreduction was 40 and 33 months respectively. None of the patients experienced postoperative complications while the reported survival after quaternary cytoreduction was 16 and 20 months, both patients being dead of disease by the end of the study [41].

In another similar study conducted by Mario Leitao in which 26 patients submitted to tertiary cytoreduction liver resection was necessary in three cases: in two cases wedge resections were performed while in the third case a segmentectomy was necessary to resect the hepatic lesions with negative margins. The postoperative morbidity rate was 27% while the overall mortality rate was zero. However liver surgery related complications were not reported [56].

In the study conducted by K.K. Shih et al. regarding the role of cytoreductive surgery beyond tertiary cytoreduction, a single patient submitted to quaternary cytoreduction had recurrent disease in the liver at the preoperative imagistic studies [57].

## Laparoscopic and Robotic Approach for Ovarian Cancer Liver Metastases

Once the safety and effectiveness of laparoscopic and robotic techniques have been widely demonstrated, these minimally invasive techniques became more frequently used in liver surgery too. The main advantages consist of implementing a minimally invasive procedure which assures a rapid postoperative rehabilitation without compromising the oncologic outcomes. The first robotic procedure performed in a patient with liver recurrence after ovarian cancer came from Robert Holloway and was performed in Florida in 2010. It was the case of a 60-year-old patient diagnosed with a 3.4 cm liver metastasis developed on the dome of the right liver, invading the diaphragm which was successfully resected robotically, after a console time of 82 minutes; the estimated blood loss was 100 ml. Postoperatively she developed a pleural effusion which was punctioned, the patient being discharged on the fifth postoperative day. She was submitted to adjuvant chemotherapy 4 weeks postoperatively [58].

### Utility of Radiofrequency Ablation in Association with Liver Resection for Ovarian Cancer Hepatic Metastases

In an attempt to increase the rate of complete cytoreduction and in the meantime to decrease even more the rate of postoperative liver surgery related complications some studies focused on the possibility of association of radiofrequency ablation in the setting of advanced stage and relapsed ovarian cancer with liver involvement [59-61]. However, the utility of radiofrequency ablation was initially proved in patients with liver metastases from colorectal cancer, data regarding the utility of the method in ovarian cancer liver metastases still being scarce [60-64]. Although in cases with liver metastases from colorectal cancer radiofrequency ablation seems to be unjustified in the presence of extrahepatic disease, when it comes to ovarian cancer, it is perfectly justified in order to maximize the cytoreductive effort [59-61].

The main benefit in radiofrequency ablation is the fact that it provides a rapid, bloodless destruction of the hepatic lesion; in the meantime this method creates a circumferential coagulative necrosis of the surrounding liver parenchyma decreasing in this way the blood loss in cases in which hepatectomy is intentioned as the second step procedure. However, the method is still limited in cases presenting centro-hilar lesions: in these cases the close proximity of the large blood vessels will induce a "heat sink" effect, decreasing in this way the likelihood of complete ablation and secondarily increasing the risk of recurrence. In the meantime it can increase the risk of biliary fistula [28,65]. Another limitative factor remains the dimension of the lesions, lesions larger than 5 cm being associated with a higher risk of recurrence; however this risk can be decreased if radiofrequency ablation is followed by liver resection [28]. The method of radiofrequency ablation of liver metastases seems to be especially effective in patients with disseminated, bilobar parenchimatous lesions, in an attempt to spare as much as possible the healthy parenchyma without compromising the oncological outcomes. In the meantime peritoneal lesions seem to be best treated by classic surgical approach. In this way combining the two methods might maximize the cytoreductive effort [60].

In one of the most recent published series, Petrou et al. included 145 consecutive patients diagnosed with liver metastases from various primaries submitted to radiofrequency ablation assite liver resection in order to decrease the blood lost during surgery. The standard technique in these cases consists of applying the radiofrequency ablation needle along the line of parenchymal transsection in order to create at this level an area of bloodless coagulative necrosis. By applying this principle, it is estimated that liver ischemia-reperfusion injury which usually develop after partial or total vascular occlusion could be safely minimized. Among the 145 patients submitted to radiofrequency ablation followed by liver resection, oavrain primaries were reported in two cases; in one case radiofrequency ablation was followed by a minor hepatic resection while in the latter case a major hepatectomy was associated. After performing these maneuvers, liver tests were slightly elevate during the early postoperative period and were normalized within seven days after surgery. When it comes to the completeness of resection, an R0 resection was achieved in 114 patients while in the other 13 cases an R1 resection was performed, the remnant 18 patients being submitted to liver resection for benign conditions. Regarding the postoperative outcomes, morbidity developed in 47 cases, no-one requiring re-operation. The most common complication remained transient liver insufficiency, which was completely recovered in all cases. Postoperative bile-leaks developed in ten patients, the mean duration of the leak being 17 days (range 5-32 days). However the postoperative complication rates were similar between cases submitted to major versus minor resections, demonstrating the safety and efficacy of the method [66].

In the case series reported by Mateo et al. three patients submitted to liver resection and radiofrequency ablation were included. The first reported case was a 59-year-old woman initially diagnosed with a stage IV ovarian cancer for which she was submitted to neoadjuvant chemotherapy followed by optimal debulking surgery. Five years later the patient was diagnosed with isolated hepatic recurrence (located in segment VI according to Couinaud's classification). Intraoperatively the lesions were successfully resected; however the intraoperative ultrasound revealed the presence of other two lesions located in the caudate lobe, each one measuring less than 2 cm which were successfully ablated. Several peritoneal nodules were also found and resected, achieving a complete resection. At 13 months follow up the patient had no recurrent disease. The second reported case was the one of a 51-year-old patient initially diagnosed with stage III ovarian cancer for which she was submitted to debulking surgery followed by other two cytoreductive procedures for relapsed disease. Seven years after the initial diagnosis the patient was diagnosed with two liver metastases: the first one was developed on the right hepatic dome invading the diaphragm which was successfully resected while the second one measuring 2.8 cm was located in the proximity of the right hepatic vein and of the anterior branch of the right portal vein and was treated by radiofrequency ablation. At nine months follow up there was no sign of recurrent disease. In the third case radiofrequency ablation was the treatment of choice for a late recurrence after a stage III ovarian granulosa cell tumor. The patient had been previously submitted to surgery 19 years before, followed by adjuvant chemotherapy. At the time of recurrence she was diagnosed with an 18 cm tumor developed in the right hemiliver associated with a 2.5 cm lesion located in segment IV. The largest lesion was resected by an extended hepatectomy was the segment IV lesion, which was ablated by radiofrequency. Although the patient refused any adjuvant chemotherapy, she was free of any recurrent disease at 39 months follow up [60].

All of these encouraging results come to underline the benefits of association between radiofrequency ablation and liver resection for advanced stage or relapsed ovarian cancer with liver involvement.

## References

[1] Jemal A, Bray F, Center MM, Ferlay J, Ward E, Forman D (2011), Global cancer statistics, *CA Cancer J. Clin.* 61: 69-90.

[2] Kim HS, Kim JW, Shouten LJ, Larsson SC, Chung HH, Kim YB, Ju W, Park NH, Song YS, Kim SC, Kang SB (2010), Wine drinking and epithelial ovarian cancer risk: a meta-analysis, *J. Gynecol Oncol* 21: 112-118.

[3] Shih KK, Chi DS (2010), Maximal cytoreductive effort in epithelial ovarian cancer surgery, *J. Gynecol Oncol* 21: 75-80.

[4] Ozols RF (2005), Treatment goals in ovarian cancer, *Int.J.Gynecol Cancer* 15 Suppl 1: 3-11.

[5] Chang SJ, Bristow RE (2012), Evolution of surgical treatment paradigms for advanced-stage ovarian cancer: redefining 'optimal' residual disease, *Gynecol Oncol* 125: 483-492.

[6] Bristow RE, Tomacruz RS, Armstrong DK, Trimble EL, Montz FJ (2002), Survival effect of maximal cytoreductive surgery for advanced ovarian carcinoma during the platinum era: a meta-analysis, *J. Clin. Oncol* 20: 1248-1259.

[7] Salani R, Zahurak ML, Santillan A, Giuntoli RL, Bristow RE (2007), Survival impact of multiple bowel resections in patients undergoing primary cytoreductive surgery for advanced ovarian cancer: a case-control study, *Gynecol Oncol* 107: 495-499.

[8] Houvenaeghel G, Gutowski M, Buttarelli M, Cuisenier J, Narducci F, Dalle C, Ferron G, Morice P, Meeus P, Stockle E, Bannier M, Lambaudie E, Rouanet P, Fraisse J,

Leblanc E, Dauplat J, Querleu D, Martel P, Castaigne D (2009), Modified posterior pelvic exenteration for ovarian cancer, *Int. J. Gynecol Cancer* 19: 968-973.
[9] Tixier H, Fraisse J, Chauffert B, Mayer F, Causeret S, Loustalot C, Deville C, Bonnetain F, Sagot P, Douvier S, Cuisenier J (2010), Evaluation of pelvic posterior exenteration in the management of advanced-stage ovarian cancer, *Arch. Gynecol Obstet.* 281: 505-510.
[10] Estes JM, Leath CA, III, Straughn JM, Jr., Rocconi RP, Kirby TO, Huh WK, Barnes MN, III (2006), Bowel resection at the time of primary debulking for epithelial ovarian carcinoma: outcomes in patients treated with platinum and taxane-based chemotherapy, *J. Am. Coll. Surg.* 203: 527-532.
[11] Kuhn W, Glorack G, Roder J, Schmalfeldt B, Pache L, Rust M, et al. (1998), The influence of upper abdominal surgery on perioperative morbidity and mortality in patients with advanced ovarian cancer FIGO III and IV. *Int J Gynecol Cancer.* 8:56–63.
[12] Eisenkop SM, Spirtos NM, Friedman RL, Lin WC, Pisani AL, Perticucci S (2003), Relative influences of tumor volume before surgery and the cytoreductive outcome on survival for patients with advanced ovarian cancer: a prospective study, *Gynecol Oncol* 90: 390-396.
[13] Aletti GD, Dowdy SC, Gostout BS, Jones MB, Stanhope CR, Wilson TO, Podratz KC, Cliby WA (2006), Aggressive surgical effort and improved survival in advanced-stage ovarian cancer, *Obstet. Gynecol* 107: 77-85.
[14] Chi DS, Eisenhauer EL, Zivanovic O, Sonoda Y, Abu-Rustum NR, Levine DA, Guile MW, Bristow RE, Aghajanian C, Barakat RR (2009), Improved progression-free and overall survival in advanced ovarian cancer as a result of a change in surgical paradigm, *Gynecol Oncol* 114: 26-31.
[15] Cormio G, Rossi C, Cazzolla A, Resta L, Loverro G, Greco P, Selvaggi L (2003), Distant metastases in ovarian carcinoma, *Int. J. Gynecol Cancer* 13: 125-129.
[16] Nakayama K, Nakayama N, Katagiri H, Miyazaki K (2012), Mechanisms of ovarian cancer metastasis: biochemical pathways, *Int.J.Mol.Sci.* 13: 11705-11717.
[17] Rose PG, Piver MS, Tsukada Y, Lau TS (1989), Metastatic patterns in histologic variants of ovarian cancer. An autopsy study, *Cancer* 64: 1508-1513.
[18] FIGO Cancer Committee (1986). Staging announcement, *Gynecol Oncol* 25: 5.
[19] Rees M, Tekkis PP, Welsh FK, O'Rourke T, John TG (2008), Evaluation of long-term survival after hepatic resection for metastatic colorectal cancer: a multifactorial model of 929 patients, *Ann. Surg.* 247: 125-135.
[20] Sutcliffe R, Maguire D, Ramage J, Rela M, Heaton N (2004), Management of neuroendocrine liver metastases, *Am. J. Surg.* 187: 39-46.
[21] Slotta JE, Schuld J, Distler S, Richter S, Schilling MK, Kollmar O (2014), Hepatic resection of non-colorectal and non-neuroendocrine liver metastases - survival benefit for patients with non-gastrointestinal primary cancers - a case-controlled study, *Int. J. Surg.* 12: 163-168.
[22] Reddy SK, Barbas AS, Marroquin CE, Morse MA, Kuo PC, Clary BM (2007), Resection of noncolorectal nonneuroendocrine liver metastases: a comparative analysis, *J. Am. Coll. Surg.* 204: 372-382.
[23] Earle SA, Perez EA, Gutierrez JC, Sleeman D, Livingstone AS, Franceschi D, Levi JU, Robbins C, Koniaris LG (2006), Hepatectomy enables prolonged survival in select patients with isolated noncolorectal liver metastasis, *J. Am. Coll. Surg.* 203: 436-446.

[24] Martel G, Hawel J, Rekman J, Croome KP, Bertens K, Balaa FK, Hernandez-Alejandro R (2015), Liver resection for non-colorectal, non-carcinoid, non-sarcoma metastases: a multicenter study, *PLoS. One.* 10: e0120569.

[25] Lendoire J, Moro M, Andriani O, Grondona J, Gil O, Raffin G, Silva J, Bracco R, Podesta G, Valenzuela C, Imventarza O, Pekolj J, De Santibanes E (2007), Liver resection for non-colorectal, non-neuroendocrine metastases: analysis of a multicenter study from Argentina, *HPB (Oxford)* 9: 435-439.

[26] Adam R, Chiche L, Aloia T, Elias D, Salmon R, Rivoire M, Jaeck D, Saric J, Le Treut YP, Belghiti J, Mantion G, Mentha G (2006), Hepatic resection for noncolorectal nonendocrine liver metastases: analysis of 1,452 patients and development of a prognostic model, *Ann. Surg.* 244: 524-535.

[27] Kamel SI, de Jong MC, Schulick RD, Diaz-Montes TP, Wolfgang CL, Hirose K, Edil BH, Choti MA, Anders RA, Pawlik TM (2011), The role of liver-directed surgery in patients with hepatic metastasis from a gynecologic primary carcinoma, *World J. Surg.* 35: 1345-1354.

[28] Chi DS, Fong Y, Venkatraman ES, Barakat RR (1997), Hepatic resection for metastatic gynecologic carcinomas, *Gynecol Oncol* 66: 45-51.

[29] Chalkiadakis GE, Lasithiotakis KG, Petrakis I, Kourousis C, Georgoulias V (2005), Major hepatectomy and right hemicolectomy at the time of primary cytoreductive surgery for advanced ovarian cancer: report of a case, *Int. J. Gynecol Cancer* 15: 1115-1119.

[30] Yoon SS, Jarnagin WR, Fong Y, DeMatteo RP, Barakat RR, Blumgart LH, Chi DS (2003), Resection of recurrent ovarian or fallopian tube carcinoma involving the liver, *Gynecol Oncol* 91: 383-388.

[31] Tangjitgamol S, Levenback CF, Beller U, Kavanagh JJ (2004), Role of surgical resection for lung, liver, and central nervous system metastases in patients with gynecological cancer: a literature review, *Int. J. Gynecol Cancer* 14: 399-422.

[32] Merideth MA, Cliby WA, Keeney GL, Lesnick TG, Nagorney DM, Podratz KC (2003), Hepatic resection for metachronous metastases from ovarian carcinoma, *Gynecol Oncol* 89: 16-21.

[33] Ramia JM, De La Plaza R, Quiñones J, Veguillas P, Adel F, García-Parreño J (2012), Liver Metastases from Gynecological Cancers: Time to Resection?. *Surgical Science* 3, 120-125.

[34] Eisenhauer EL, Abu-Rustum NR, Sonoda Y, Levine DA, Poynor EA, Aghajanian C, Jarnagin WR, DeMatteo RP, D'Angelica MI, Barakat RR, Chi DS (2006), The addition of extensive upper abdominal surgery to achieve optimal cytoreduction improves survival in patients with stages IIIC-IV epithelial ovarian cancer, *Gynecol Oncol* 103: 1083-1090.

[35] Raspagliesi F, Ditto A, Martinelli F, Haeusler E, Lorusso D (2013), Advanced ovarian cancer: omental bursa, lesser omentum, celiac, portal and triad nodes spread as cause of inaccurate evaluation of residual tumor, *Gynecol Oncol* 129: 92-96.

[36] Benedetti PP, Di D, V, Fischetti M, Casorelli A, Perniola G, Musella A, Marchetti C, Palaia I, Berloco P, Muzii L (2015), Predictors of postoperative morbidity after cytoreduction for advanced ovarian cancer: Analysis and management of complications in upper abdominal surgery, *Gynecol Oncol* 137: 406-411.

[37] Bristow RE, Montz FJ, Lagasse LD, Leuchter RS, Karlan BY (1999), Survival impact of surgical cytoreduction in stage IV epithelial ovarian cancer, *Gynecol Oncol* 72: 278-287.
[38] Scholz HS, Tasdemir H, Hunlich T, Turnwald W, Both A, Egger H (2007), Multivisceral cytoreductive surgery in FIGO stages IIIC and IV epithelial ovarian cancer: results and 5-year follow-up, *Gynecol Oncol* 106: 591-595.
[39] Neumann UP, Fotopoulou C, Schmeding M, Thelen A, Papanikolaou G, Braicu EI, Neuhaus P, Sehouli J (2012), Clinical outcome of patients with advanced ovarian cancer after resection of liver metastases, *Anticancer Res.* 32: 4517-4521.
[40] Lim MC, Kang S, Lee KS, Han SS, Park SJ, Seo SS, Park SY (2009), The clinical significance of hepatic parenchymal metastasis in patients with primary epithelial ovarian cancer, *Gynecol Oncol* 112: 28-34.
[41] Bacalbasa N, Dima S, Brasoveanu V, David L , Balescu I, Purnichescu-Purtan R, Popescu I. Liver resection for ovarian cancer liver metastases as part of cytoreductive surgery is safe and may bring survival benefit. Bacalbasa et al. World Journal of Surgical Oncology DOI 10.1186/s12957-015-0652-0, in press.
[42] Bosquet JG, Merideth MA, Podratz KC, Nagorney DM (2006), Hepatic resection for metachronous metastases from ovarian carcinoma, *HPB (Oxford)* 8: 93-96.
[43] Scarabelli C, Gallo A, Carbone A (2001), Secondary cytoreductive surgery for patients with recurrent epithelial ovarian carcinoma, *Gynecol Oncol* 83: 504-512.
[44] Zang RY, Li ZT, Tang J, Cheng X, Cai SM, Zhang ZY, Teng NN (2004), Secondary cytoreductive surgery for patients with relapsed epithelial ovarian carcinoma: who benefits?, *Cancer* 100: 1152-1161.
[45] Eisenkop SM, Friedman RL, Spirtos NM (2000), The role of secondary cytoreductive surgery in the treatment of patients with recurrent epithelial ovarian carcinoma, *Cancer* 88: 144-153.
[46] Niu GC, Shen CM, Cui W, Li Q (2012), Hepatic Resection is Safe for Metachronous Hepatic Metastases from Ovarian Cancer, *Cancer Biol. Med.* 9: 182-187.
[47] Roh HJ, Kim DY, Joo WD, Yoo HJ, Kim JH, Kim YM, Kim YT, Nam JH (2011), Hepatic resection as part of secondary cytoreductive surgery for recurrent ovarian cancer involving the liver, *Arch. Gynecol Obstet.* 284: 1223-1229.
[48] Abood G, Bowen M, Potkul R, Aranha G, Shoup M (2008), Hepatic resection for recurrent metastatic ovarian cancer, *Am. J. Surg.* 195: 370-373.
[49] Kolev V, Pereira EB, Schwartz M, Sarpel U, Roayaie S, Labow D, Momeni M, Chuang L, Dottino P, Rahaman J, Zakashansky K (2014), The role of liver resection at the time of secondary cytoreduction in patients with recurrent ovarian cancer, *Int. J. Gynecol Cancer* 24: 70-74.
[50] Pekmezci S, Saribeyoglu K, Aytac E, Arvas M, Demirkiran F, Ozguroglu M (2010), Surgery for isolated liver metastasis of ovarian cancer, *Asian J. Surg.* 33: 83-88.
[51] Gold JS, Are C, Kornprat P, Jarnagin WR, Gonen M, Fong Y, DeMatteo RP, Blumgart LH, D'Angelica M (2008), Increased use of parenchymal-sparing surgery for bilateral liver metastases from colorectal cancer is associated with improved mortality without change in oncologic outcome: trends in treatment over time in 440 patients, *Ann. Surg.* 247: 109-117.

acetylglaucarubinone, and molvizarin have $IC_{50}$s lower than 100 nM in ovarian cancer cells and might have different mechanisms of action from those of platinum derivatives/paclitaxel, therefore providing potential ways to attack multidrug resistance in ovarian cancer without jeopardising the patient's treatment.

# 1. INTRODUCTION

## Ovarian Cancer

Ovarian cancer is the ninth most prevalent cancer in the US and is the leading cause of death in gynaecologic cancers in the UK and US [1]. Ovarian cancer forms in tissues of the ovary and most of them are either ovarian epithelial carcinomas (cancer that begins in the cells on the surface of the ovary) or malignant germ cell tumours (cancer that begins in egg cells). The major cause of death in women from ovarian cancer is largely due to poor diagnosis because there is a lack of any clear early detection or screening test. About 70% of cases are not diagnosed until they have reached advanced stages [2].

A number of interventions are currently in use or in trials for the treatment of ovarian cancer. These include surgery, radiotherapy, hyperthermia, laser therapy, gene therapy and chemotherapy. Conventional treatment mainly involves a combination of these interventions with surgery, radiotherapy and chemotherapy. However these interventions are not without disadvantages and limitations, which has been recognised by the scientific community. Some chemotherapeutic drugs employed in the treatment of cancers are cisplatin and carboplatin (Figure 1). Cisplatin is one of the platinum-based drugs used in the treatment of several cancers, such as testicular, small cell lung and ovarian cancers.

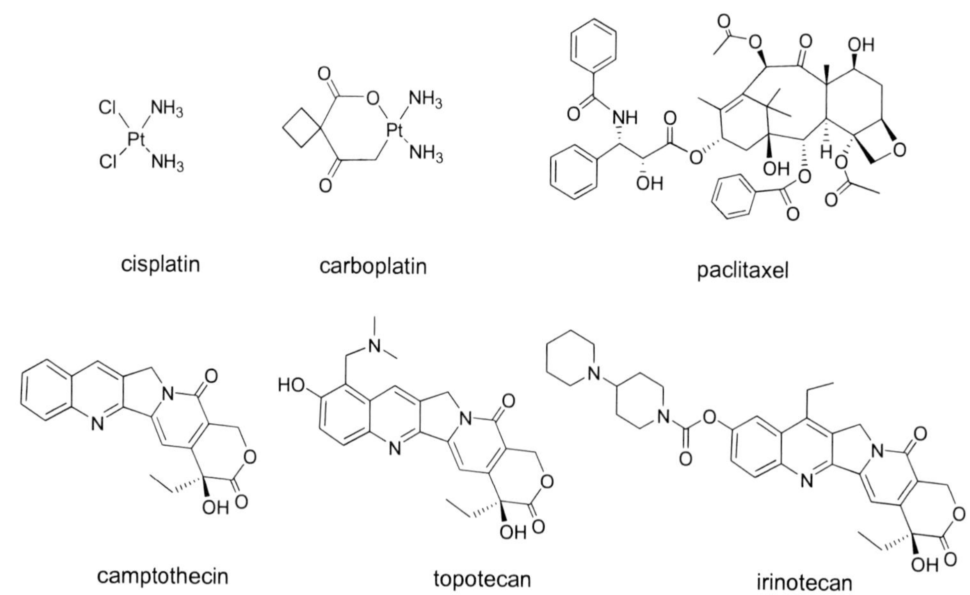


Figure 1. Structures of plant-derived natural products (drugs) and platinum-derived drugs used for the treatment of ovarian cancer.

The drug is very toxic and could cause damage to kidneys and nerves. Other adverse effects of cisplatin include loss of hearing, vomiting and bone marrow suppression resulting in anaemia. Due to these adverse side effects, cisplatin is used mainly in conjunction with other chemotherapeutic agents [3, 4]. Carboplatin is another platinum-based drug used in the treatment of lungs, head, neck and ovarian cancers. Unlike cisplatin, carboplatin is less toxic and thus has fewer side effects compared with cisplatin but the disadvantage is that it's less effective. Also, as with all platinum drugs, platinum resistance has been advancing which may cause the cancer to re-emerge [5, 6]. Thus, there is an urgent medical need for breakthrough drugs that have an effective therapeutic impact on ovarian cancer.

## Natural Products in Cancer Treatment

Since ancient times natural products (mainly plants) have been used for the treatment of various diseases. Natural products sources of drugs comprises of plants, marine/aquatic, terrestrial microbial/fungi, terrestrial animal and unspecified organism.

However, most drugs have been derived from plant sources from focused research, i.e., higher plants mainly because there is a great interest in investigating the medicinal plants across the continents [7]. According to the WHO survey, 80% of populations living in the developing countries rely almost exclusively on traditional medicine (mainly plants) for their primary health care needs [8]. It is estimated that there are about 250,000 known higher plant species in the world, of which only 5-15% have been studied for biological usefulness (bio-activity) [9]. About 200,000 secondary metabolites have been reported in plants [10]. Some of the important phytochemical constituents, found in plants, include alkaloids (atropine, quinine, etc.), flavonoids, tannins, terpenes, terpenoids, steroids, glycosides, saponins, phenolics, and quinones. The bio-activities of medicinal plants have been linked to the presence of one or more of the various classes of phytochemicals, with isoprenoids, phenolic compounds and alkaloids being the most commonly biosynthesised [7]. Investigations into the anticancer activity of plants have been for about 60 years and are fairly recent, with even fewer plants being screened [11].

The process of discovering anticancer drugs derived from plants includes preclinical and clinical studies. The preclinical study includes random or ethanopharmacology-based in vitro screening of plant extracts, isolation, structural elucidation of bioactive compounds, and toxicological and effectiveness tested on animals. If the compound passes all the testing, the results are submitted to the Food and Drug Administration (FDA) in US or a comparable agency in other countries before clinical studies. In the clinic, there are generally three phases of clinical trials. Phase I involves the evaluation of safety of a drug in healthy volunteers; Phase II includes the testing of efficacy and dose range in patients; while Phase III is to further validate the efficacy and safety in thousands of patients. If the tested compound passes all the evaluations and is approved by FDA after thorough review, the new drug can be offered for clinical use [12].

Within 1981-2010, about 50 natural products derived anti-cancer drugs were approved, either as un-modified compounds, or semi-synthesised analogues, or synthesised compounds based on natural product leads, with 5 drugs namely: romidepsin, cabazitaxel, eribulin, mifamurtide and vinflunine developed in 2010 alone. This underlines the importance of plants as sources of new cancer chemotherapeutic agents [13, 14].

The literature on five plant extracts and sixty-nine compounds isolated from higher plants and microorganisms before 2001 and with potential antitumor activity against ovarian neoplasia was reviewed [15]. In the current review, we will discuss plant-derived natural products and their derivatives, which have been approved in clinics, in clinical trials and in preclinical investigation for the treatment of ovarian cancer. In particular we list novel phytochemical structures with potent in vitro anti-cancer activity in ovarian cancer cell lines (Table 1), which were discovered from 2001 to 2014.

## 2. PHYTOCHEMICALS APPROVED FOR THE TREATMENT OF OVARIAN CANCER

### Camptothecin

Camptothecin (Figure 1) was isolated from the Chinese tree *Camptotheca acuminate* (family *Cornaceae*; www.theplantlist.org) by Dr. Monroe E. Wall and Dr. Mansukh C. Wani of Research Triangle Institute [16]. Camptothecin possesses a mechanism of action involving the inhibition of DNA relaxation by DNA topoisomerase I, more specifically the stabilization of a covalent binary complex formed between topoisomerase I and DNA [17]. It has been shown to have significant antitumor activity against: lung, ovarian, breast, pancreas and stomach cancers. To improve its water solubility and pharmacological properties, various semi-synthetic analogues of camptothecin have been made. Two of them, Hycamtin (topotecan) and Camptosar (irinotecan or CPT-11) (Figure 1) marketed by GlaxoSmithKline and Pfizer, respectively, are used for the treatment of ovarian and colon cancers [18].

### Paclitaxel

Paclitaxel (Figure 1) was originally discovered from the bark of the Pacific yew tree, *Taxus brevifolia* Nutt. (family *Taxaceae*) also by Dr. Monroe E. Wall and Dr. Mansukh C. Wani [19]. The mechanism of action of paclitaxel is to bind to beta-tubulin subunits of microtubule, therefore stabilizing the microtubule and protecting it from disassembly, which could cause defects in mitotic spindle assembly, chromosome segregation, and cell division [20]. The drug has been approved for use in the treatment of breast, lung, non-small cell lung and ovarian cancers. Paclitaxel is used in the first-line and second-line treatment of ovarian cancer. Cremophor EL is used as the vehicle in the delivery of paclitaxel due to its poor water solubility. However, this has led to increasing clinical toxicity of paclitaxel. Thus, paclitaxel in combination with other agents, such as carboplatin, which are less toxic, is often used. Furthermore, a number of its derivatives are explored for clinical trials. An albumin-paclitaxel called Abraxane is a water-soluble formulation where paclitaxel is covalently bound to albumin nano-particles. Abraxane was approved by FDA in 2005, which exhibited enhanced paclitaxel tissue distribution and tumour penetration with fewer side effects in multiple tumour types [21].

**Table 1. A list of novel and potent plant natural products against ovarian cancer cells discovered between 2001 and 2014 (the order of the compounds is arranged according to the year in which they were reported)**

| Compound name | Structure | Plant name (family) | $IC_{50}$ (A2780 ovarian cancer cell line) | Reference |
|---|---|---|---|---|
| trihydroxyalkylcyclohexenones | 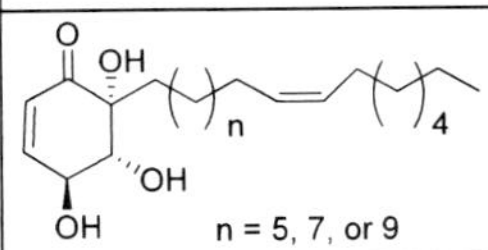  | *Pleiogynium timoriense* (A. DC.) Leenh. (*Anacardiaceae*) | 0.8, 0.7, and 0.8 μM, respectively. | [81] |
| securinine | 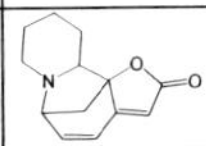 | *Margaritaria discoidea* (Baill.) G. L. Webster (*Euphorbiaceae*) | 3-16 μM (OVCAR-8, A2780 and A2780cis)[a] | [77] |
| 3-β-[(O-alpha-L-rhamnopyranosyl-(1-2)-α-L-arabinopyranosyl)oxy]-16-α-hydroxyolean-12-en-28-oic acid | 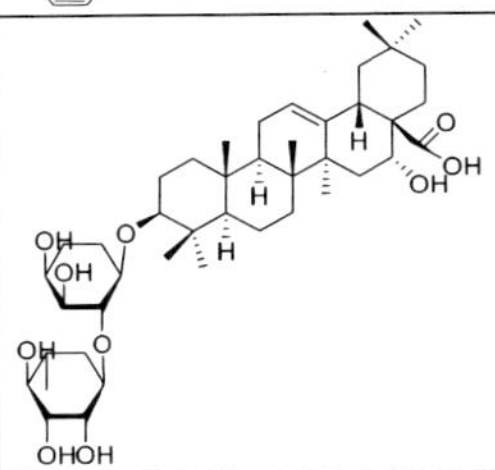 | *Polyscias duplicate* (Thouars ex Baill.) Lowry and G. M. Plunkett (*Araliaceae*) | 2.8 μM | [82] |
| (+)-1,2-dehydrotelobine and (+)-2'-norcocsuline | 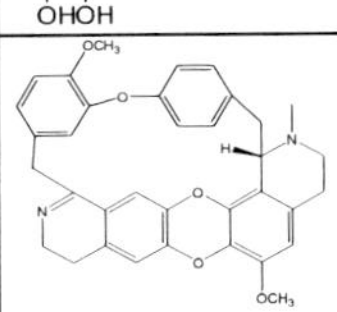 (+)-1,2-dehydrotelobine 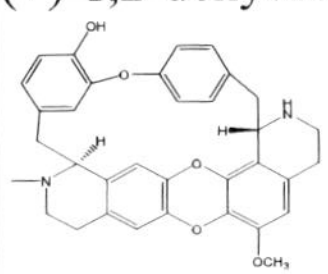 (+)-2'-norcocsuline | *Anisocycla grandidieri* Baill. (*Menispermaceae*) | 4.1 ± 0.3 and 2.7 ± 0.3 μM, respectively. | [83] |

**Table 1. (Continued)**

| Compound name | Structure | Plant name (family) | $IC_{50}$ (A2780 ovarian cancer cell line) | Reference |
|---|---|---|---|---|
| **bufatrienolides**[b] | 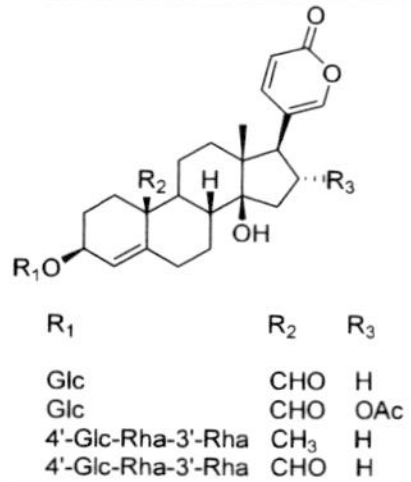  | *Urginea depressa* Baker (*Asparagaceae*) | 24.1, 11.2, 111, and 40.6 nM, respectively. | [84] |
| randianin, 2"-O-acetylrandianin and 6"-O-acetylrandianin | 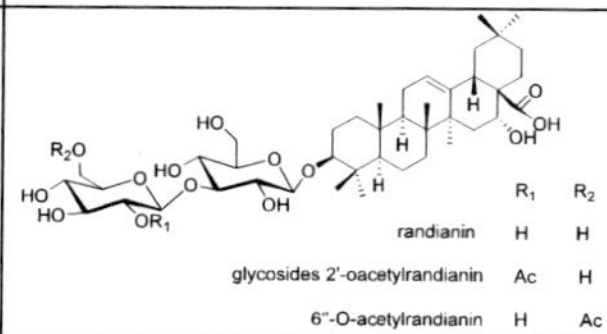  | *Nematostylis anthophylla* (A. Rich. ex DC.) Baill. (*Rubiaceae*) | 1.2, 1.7, and 2.2 μM, respectively. | [85] |
| 10-desoxygochnatiolide A | 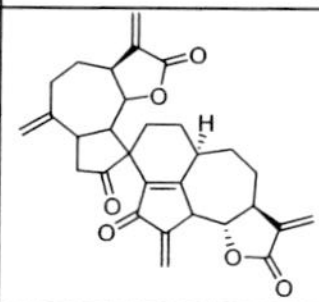 | *Gochnatia polymorpha* (Less) Cabr. ssp. floccosa Cabr. (*Compositae*) | 2.0 μM (OVCa3) | [86] |
| tavinin A and epi-tavinin A | 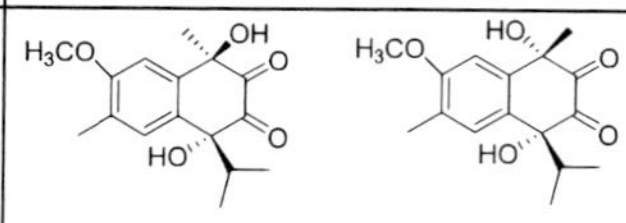  | *Sterculia taiva* Baill. (*Malvaceae*) | 5.5 and 6.7 μM, respectively. | [87] |
| madagascarensilide A and madagascarensilide B | 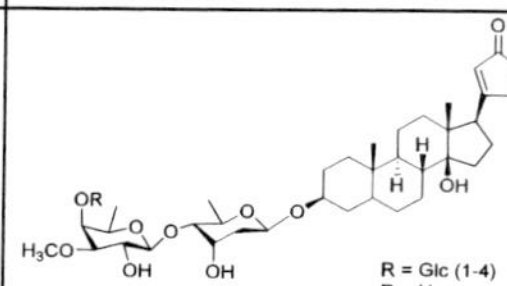  | *Leptadenia madagascariensis* Decne. (*Apocynaceae*) | 0.18 and 0.29 μM respectively. | [88] |

| Compound name | Structure | Plant name (family) | $IC_{50}$ (A2780 ovarian cancer cell line) | Reference |
|---|---|---|---|---|
| sampangine | 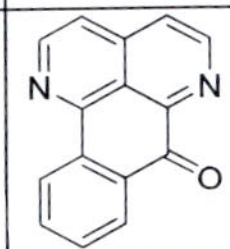 | *Ambavia gerrardii* (Baill.) Le Thomas (*Annonaceae*) | 0.58 μM | [89] |
| athrolide D | 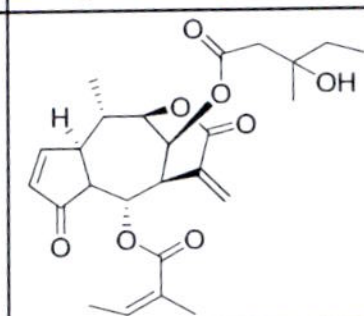 | *Athroisma proteiforme* (Humbert) Mattf. (*Compositae*) | 0.6 μM | [90] |
| 16,18-dihydroxykolavenic acid lactone | 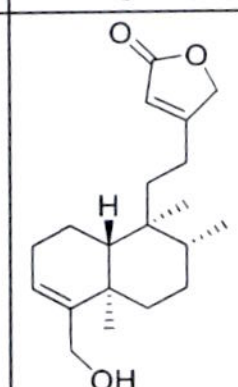 | *Cyphostemma greveana* Desc. (*Vitaceae*) | 0.44 μM | [91] |
| **2'-(R)-O-acetylglaucarubinone** | 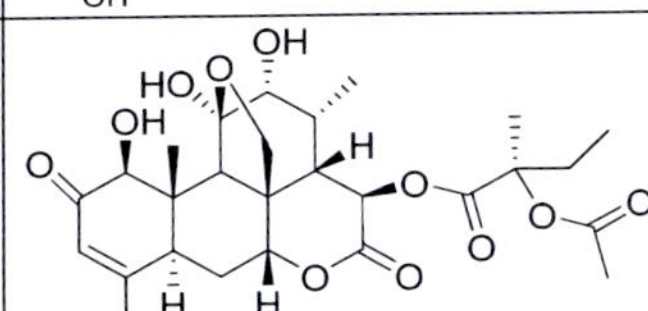 | *Quassia gabonensis* Pierre [Syn. *Odyendyea gabonensis* (Pierre) Engl.] (*Simaroubaceae*) | <18 nM (MSPC1, 2774-C10, HeyA8 Hoc7) | [92] |
| terminaliaside A | 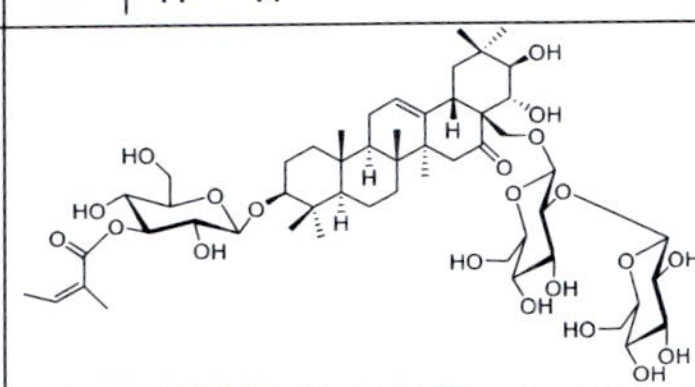 | *Terminalia tropophylla* H. Perrier (*Combretaceae*) | 1.2 μM | [93] |

**Table 1. (Continued)**

| Compound name | Structure | Plant name (family) | $IC_{50}$ (A2780 ovarian cancer cell line) | Reference |
|---|---|---|---|---|
| **cardenolide glycosides** | 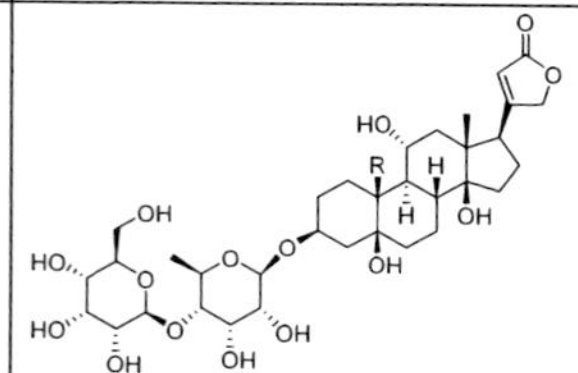 | *Elaeodendron alluaudianum* H. Perrier | 70 nM | [94] |
| isomahubannolide-23 | 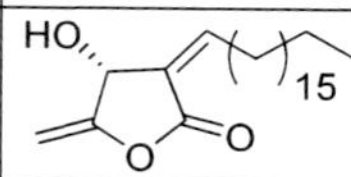 | *Machilus wangchiana* Chun (*Lauraceae*) | 2.66 μM | [95] |
| dodoneasides A and B | 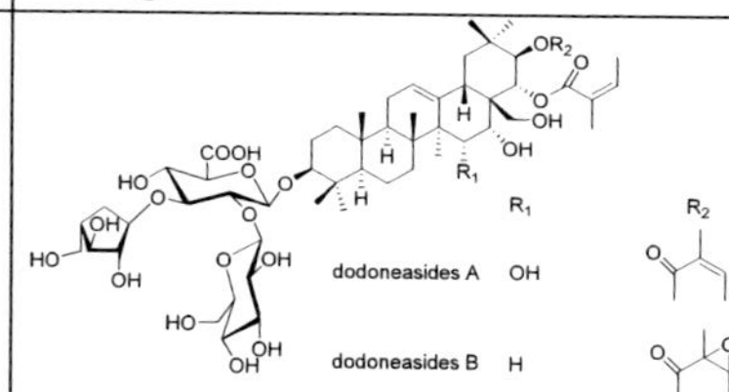 | *Dodonaea* wiscosa (L.) Jacq. (*Sapindaceae*) | 0.79 and 0.70 μM, respectively | [96] |
| parthenolide | 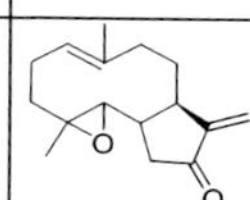 | *Magnolia kobus* DC. (*Magnoliaceae*) | 9.7 μM (SK-OV-3) | [97] |
| xanifolia-$Y_0$ | 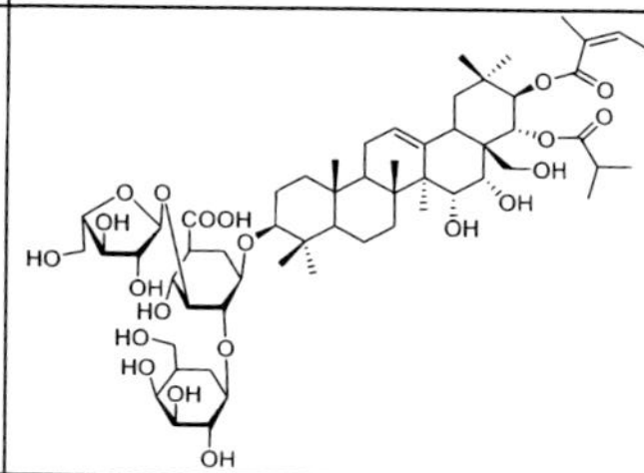 | *Xanthoceras sorbifolia* Bunge (*Sapindaceae*) | 4.2 ± 0.7 μM (OVCAR3) | [98] |

| Compound name | Structure | Plant name (family) | $IC_{50}$ (A2780 ovarian cancer cell line) | Reference |
|---|---|---|---|---|
| caseanigrescens A-D | 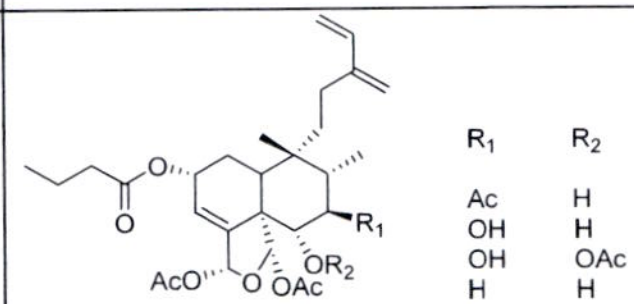 | *Casearia nigrescens* Tul. (*Salicaceae*) | 0.83-1.4 μM | [99] |
| atractyligenin 15 keto and atractyligenin 2,15-diketo | 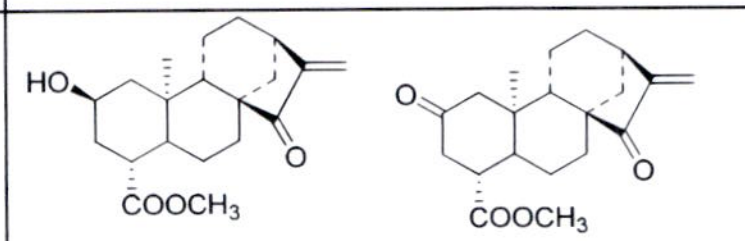 atractyligenin 15-keto atractyligenin 2,15-diketo | *Atractylis gummifera* L. (*Asteraceae*) | 0.3 and 0.2 μM (1A9), respectively. | [100] |
| boivinide A | 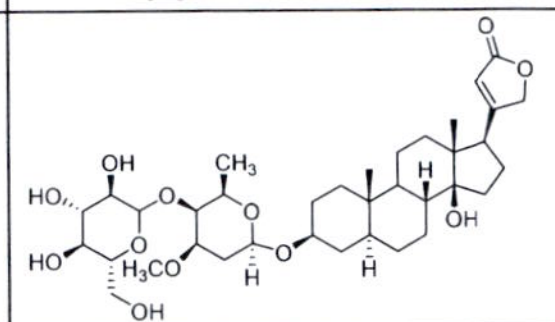 | *Roupellina (Strophanthus) boivinii* Baill. (*Apocynaceae*) | 0.17 μM | [101] |
| vedelianin, schweinfurthin E | 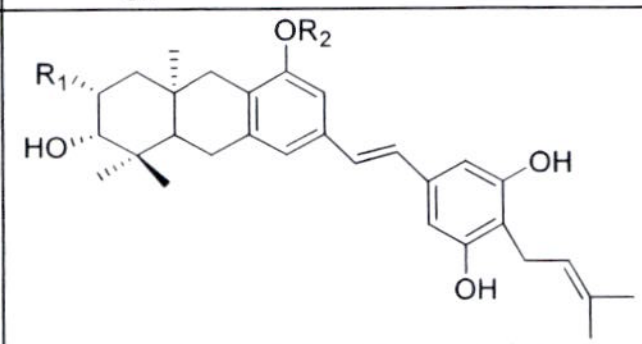 schweinfurthin E, $R_1$ = OH, $R_2$ = $CH_3$ vedelianin, $R_1$ = OH, $R_2$ = H | *Macaranga alnifolia* Baker (*Euphorbiaceae*) | 0.26 and 0.13 μM, respectively. | [102] |
| glaucolides M | 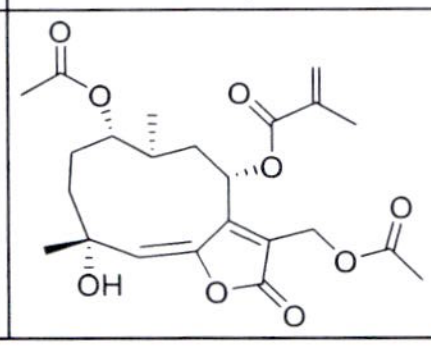 | *Vernonia pachyclada* Baker (*Compositae*) | 3.3 μM | [103] |

**Table 1. (Continued)**

| Compound name | Structure | Plant name (family) | $IC_{50}$ (A2780 ovarian cancer cell line) | Reference |
|---|---|---|---|---|
| **Ipomoeassin D** | 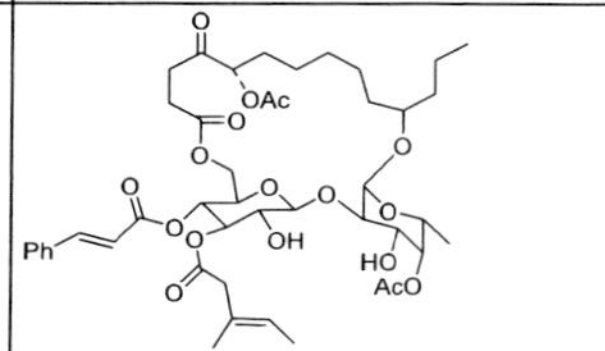 | *Ipomoea squamosal* Choisy (*Convolvulaceae*) | 35 nM | [104] |
| isomundulinol | 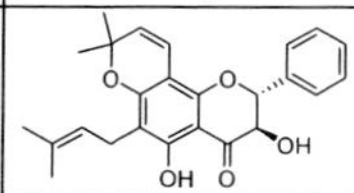 | *Mundulea chapelieri* (Baill.) Du Puy and Labat (*Leguminosae*) | 1.2 μM | [105] |
| **molvizarin** | 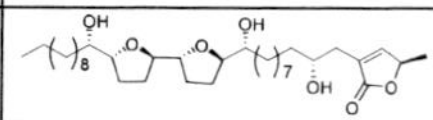 | Annonaceous plants | 12 pM (1A9 cell) | [106] |
| celastrol and pristimerin | 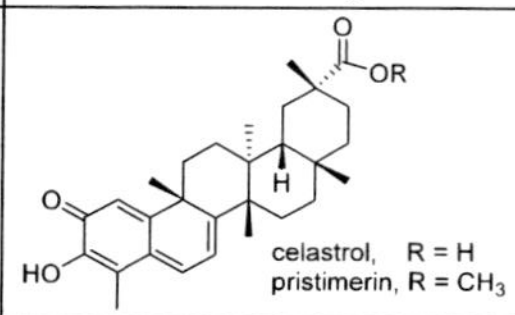 | *Reissantia buchananii* (Loes.) N. Hallé (*Celastraceae*) | 0.17 and 0.22 μM (1A9), respectively. | [107] |
| chlorojanerin | 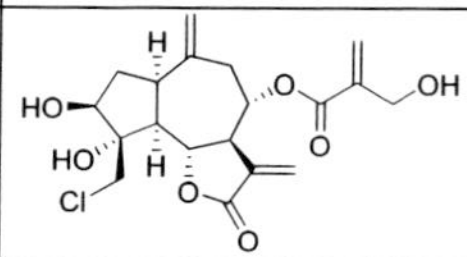 | *Centaurothamnus maximus* (Forssk.) Wagenitz and Dittrich (*Compositae*) | 15 μM (SK-OV-3) | [108] |
| cycloviolacin $O_2$ | Cyclic peptide | *Viola odorata* L. (Violaceae) | 1.32 μM (OVCA) | [78] |
| methyl (10S)-hydroxypheophorbide a | 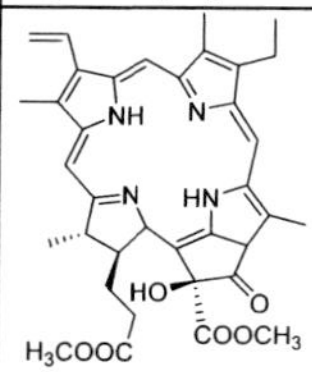 | *Clerodendrum calamitosum* L. (*Lamiaceae*) | 0.43 μM (1A9) | [109] |

[a]$IC_{50}$ in other ovarian cancer cell lines rather than A2780. [b]very potent compounds with $IC_{50}$ less than 100 nM are marked as bold.

Paclitaxel poliglumex is another water soluble conjugate of paclitaxel and poly(L-glutamic acid) which can reduce hypersensitivity reactions. Current pre-clinical pharmacokinetic studies and key phase I and II clinical trial in ovarian cancer indicates that this derivative is active in ovarian cancer, but has not been shown to possess significant benefit in terms of its side-effect profile over a standard taxane-based regimen [22].

## 3. PHYTOCHEMICALS IN CLINICAL STUDY FOR THE TREATMENT OF OVARIAN CANCER

Despite the advances in the treatment of ovarian cancer such as the developments of camptothecins and taxanes, FDA has approved no new drug for ovarian cancer since 2006 [23]. Currently, several plant-derived products are in clinical trials.

### Epipodophyllotoxin Derivatives Etoposide and Teniposide

Podophyllotoxin and epipodophyllotoxin (Figure 2) are lignans obtained from the roots of the North American May Apple, *Podophyllum peltatum* L. (family *Berberidaceae*). The compounds are used traditionally as a remedy for cough, skin diseases and have served as purgatives. The mechanism of action of podophyllotoxin lies in the formation of a complex with tubulin and prevention of the synthesis of microtubules.

Surprisingly, two glycosidic derivatives etoposide and teniposide are inhibitors of topoisomerase II. Etoposide is currently in clinical use as antineoplastic agents in the treatment of lung cancer, testicular cancer, kaposi sarcoma, lymphoma; while teniposide is used in the treatment of childhood acute lymphocytic leukaemia.

Clinical studies of etoposide for the treatment of ovarian cancer have been carried out. Single use of the compound showed activity in recurrent ovarian cancer after treatment with cisplatin, but response and survival periods are short [24].

A clinical trial that involved the use of alternating blotecan (a synthetic derivative of camptothecin) and oral etoposide in platinum-resistant ovarian cancer patients shows positive activity at the dose of 50 mg/day of etoptoside [25]. A clinical study suggested that the combination chemotherapy with irinotecan plus oral etoposide has provided clinical benefit to patients with recurrent ovarian cancer previously treated with platinum and taxane agents [26]. However, a more recent study of the same drugs combination based on 60 patients suggested a moderate response rate but did not meet the primary endpoint [27, 28]. More clinical studies are needed to confirm their efficacy and safety.

### Vinblastine Derivatives

The vinca alkaloids such as vinblastine and vincristine (Figure 2) were discovered from a Chinese medicinal plant *Catharanthus roseus* (L.) G. Don (family *Apocynaceae*) in the 1950s. They act on tubulin and prevent its formation of micriotubule in a similar way as podophyllotoxin [29].

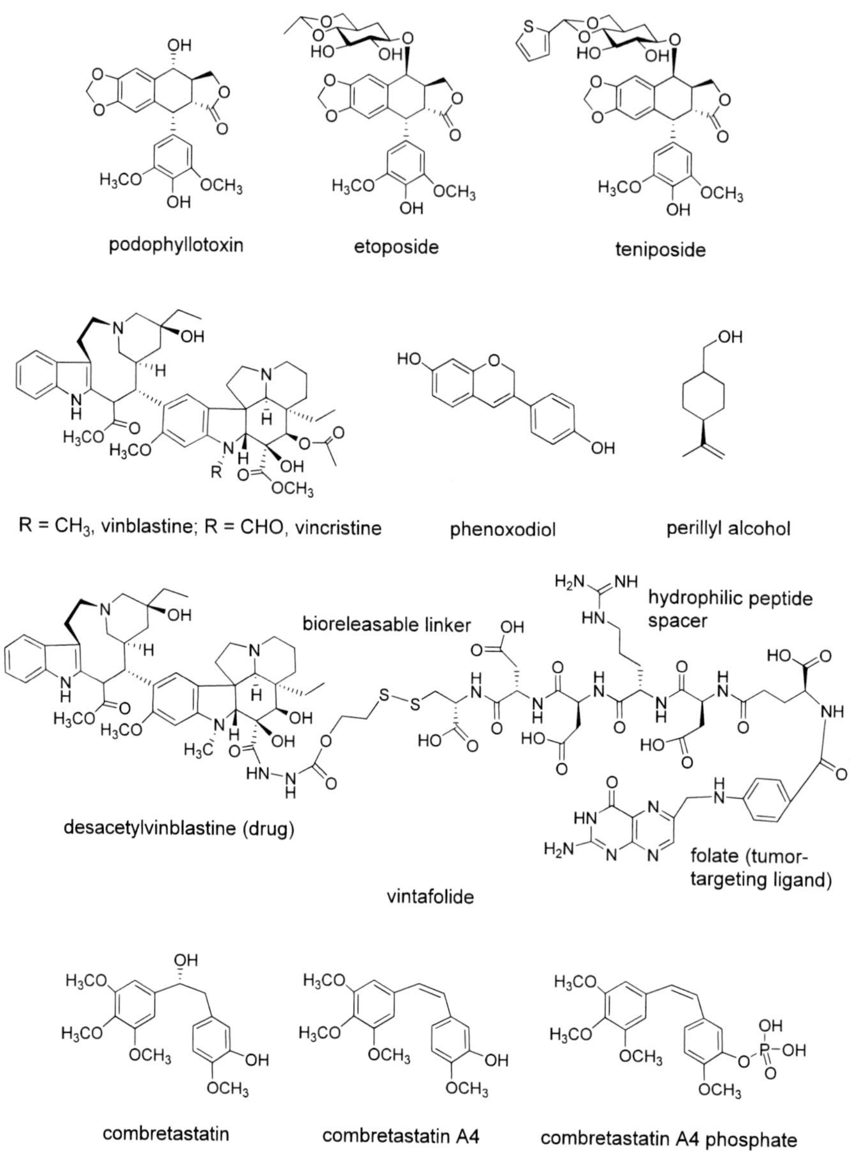


Figure 2. Phytochemicals and their derivatives currently in clinical trials for the treatment of ovarian cancer.

The vinca alkaloids were approved as antileukaemic agents. Vintafolide (EC145), a folic acid-desacetylvinblastine (folate receptor (FR)-targeted vinca alkaloid) conjugate is currently under development as a novel targeted agent for epithelial ovarian cancer [30]. The FR is overexpressed in ovarian cancer cells, which can be used as a target for anticancer agent as well as a diagnostic marker. The radiopharmaceutical, EC20, was therefore developed for non-invasive detection of functionally active FR. Vinofolate in companion with EC20 has shown promise in the trials in ovarian cancer [31]. In Phase I studies vintafolide demonstrated an acceptable safety profile. A Phase II study of vintafolide plus pegylated liposomal doxorubicin (PLD) versus PLD alone in patients with platinum-resistant ovarian cancer showed a statistically significant improvement in progression-free survival with combination therapy. A Phase III study is currently underway [32].

## Phenoxodiol

Phenoxodiol (2H-1-benzopyran-7-0,1,3-[4-hydroxyphenyl] is a derivative of plant isoflavone genistein (Figure 2) found in soybean [*Glycine* max (L.) Merr.; family *Fabaceae*].

Phenoxodiol is a multiple signal transduction regulator, enhancing mitotic arrest and apoptosis of tumour cells through multiple mechanisms that include decreasing the level of antiapoptotic proteins and inhibiting the activity of DNA topoisomerase II similar as etoposide and teniposide. Further research suggested that phenoxodiol may be an effective anticancer drug targeting the two drivers of tumour growth - the proliferation of the tumour cells themselves and the angiogenic and inflammatory stimulation of the vasculature [33]. Preclinical studies with this agent showed promising anticancer activity leading to a potential role in the treatment of a wide range of solid and hematologic cancers.

Early clinical studies, especially in chemotherapy-resistant ovarian cancer, showed minimal toxicity with minor antitumor activity. Hormone-refractory prostate cancer is another promising area in which phenoxodiol is being actively tested.

Studies are ongoing to define the optimal use of this novel anticancer agent [34]. The observation that an inverse relationship exists between dietary intake of isoflavones and cancer incidence has led to the evaluation of these compounds in cancer therapy. Phenoxodiol has been evaluated in advanced clinical trial for development as a "chemosensitizer" when combined with platinum drugs for the treatment of ovarian cancer [35] and as a monotherapy for cervical and prostate cancers [36].

A Phase II evaluation of phenoxodiol in combination with cisplatin or paclitaxel, within women with platinum/taxane-refractory/resistant epithelial ovarian, fallopian tube, or primary peritoneal cancers, in 2011 showed that a combination of phenoxodiol and cisplatin was active [37]. In contrast, a recent report indicated that orally delivered phenoxodiol showed no evidence of clinical activity, when combined with weekly AUC2-carboplatin in platinum-resistant ovarian cancer [38]. Thus, more clinical investigations on phenoxiodiol or its combination with other drugs are necessary.

## Combretastatins

Combretastatins (Figure 2) are stilbenoid phenols isolated from the South African bush willow tree, *Combretum caffrum* (Eckl. and Zeyh) Kuntze (family *Combretaceae*) [39]. The compounds were reported to be active against colon, lung and leukemia cancers. One of its analogues - combretastatin A-4 was suspected to be the most cytotoxic phytomolecule ($IC_{50}$ = 1 nM) among all isolated compounds [39, 40].

The mechanism of action of combretastatin A-4 is to bind to beta-tubulin at the colchicine-binding site and to inhibit tubulin polymerization [41]. Its poor solubility in water has necessitated the synthesis of several pro-drugs. Combretastatin A-4 phosphate, fosbretabulin (CA4P, Zybrestat) as a pro-drug has undergone phase 11 clinical trial for the treatment of relapsed ovarian cancer, NSCL and thyroid cancers [42]. A Phase II clinical trial of combretastatin A4 phosphate, carboplatin, and paclitaxel conducted in patients with platinum-resistant ovarian cancer, resulted in an improved response in the patients, with increased tolerance, than when the chemotherapeutic agents were administered without combretastatin A4 phosphate [43].

### Perillyl Alcohol

Perillyl alcohol (Figure 2) is a plant-derived monoterpene from lavendin, peppermint, spearmint, cherries, celery seed and other plants [44]. Its anticancer mechanism of action might involve blocking signal transduction by inhibition of post-translational isoprenylation of small G proteins [45]. In a phase II study of perillyl alcohol for the treatment of advanced ovarian cancer, orally administered perillyl alcohol with a dose 1200 to 1500 mg/m(2) did not exhibit signs of extending the time-to-progression in patients with advanced ovarian carcinoma [46]. Recent development of inhalation chemotherapy with perillyl alcohol for the treatment of recurrent malignant glioma seems to be effective and a safe strategy [47] and has been applied in clinical trials of patients with malignant brain tumours in Brazil [48].

## 4. Phytochemicals in Preclinical Study for the Treatment of Ovarian Cancer

### Quercetin

Quercetin (Figure 3) is a naturally occurring flavonoid found in foods like capers, dill, watercress, red onion and the leaves of fennel and radish. The compound has anti-allergic, anti-inflammatory and potentially anti-tumour activities. Quercetin exhibited a dose-dependent growth inhibition in the ovarian cancer cell line OVCA433 and also showed synergic antiproliferative activity with cisplatin [49]. A recent study on the anti-cancer activities of quercetin in A2780S ovarian cancer cells showed the induction of apoptosis and the activation of caspase 3 and 9.

The anticancer activities of quercetin on a xenograft A2780 ovarian tumour was studied by the administration of an intravenous solution of a nano-formulation of quercetin encapsulated in mono-methoxy poly(ethylene glycol)-poly(ε-caprolactone) particles. The researchers observed a significant retardation in tumour growth [50]. Studies have shown that quercetin has low toxicity and is able to enhance the therapeutic effects of cisplatin and paclitaxel in the treatment of ovarian cancer at low doses. The compound's ability to reverse multi-drug resistance of chemotherapeutic drugs has been established in *in vitro* experiments [51]. In a xenograft mouse model of ovarian cancer, quercetin has also been shown to enhance the antitumor effect of cisplatin recently [52].

## Baicalin and Baicalein

Baicalin and its aglycone, baicalein (Figure 3), are flavones found in several Chinese medicinal plants, such as *Scutellaria baicalensis* Georgi (family *Lamiaceae*) and *Scutellariae radix*. These compounds recently gained scientific focus and showed anti-inflammatory, neuroprotective and anti-cancer activities [53].

The study reported significant cytotoxic activities in OVCAR3 and CP-70 ovarian cancer cell lines, with minimized cytotoxicity in normal ovarian cells. Baicalein with $IC_{50}$ of 25-40 μM had a slightly better inhibitory effect than baicalin with $IC_{50}$ of 45-55 μM in ovarian cancer cells [54]. Recently, baicalein was shown to inhibit the matrix metalloproteinase-2 expression and possibly involve the p38 MAPK-dependent NF-kappaB signalling pathway [55].

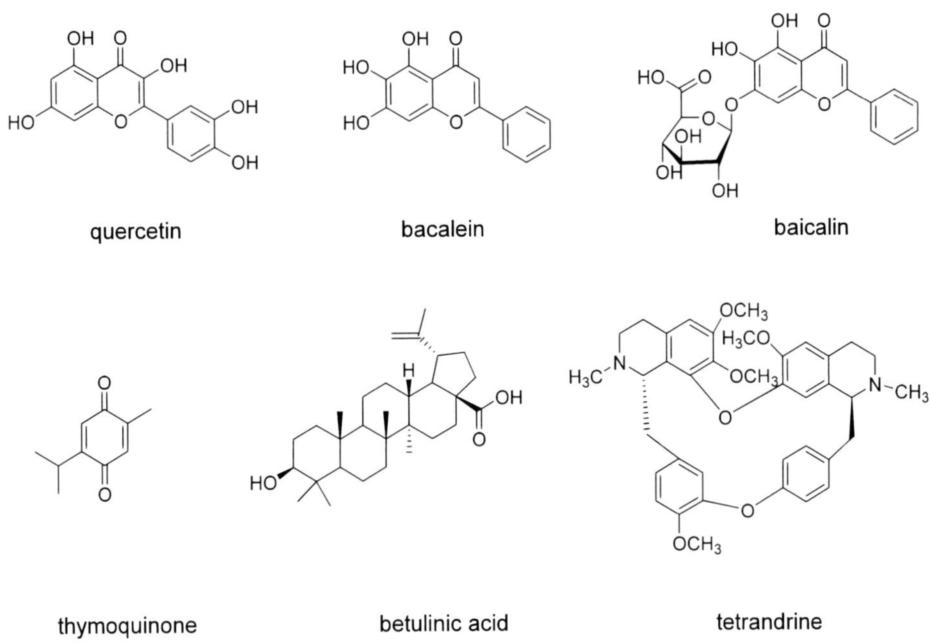


Figure 3. Structures of quercetin, baicalein, baicalin, thymoquinone, betulinic acid and tetrandrine.

## Thymoquinone

Thymoquinone (Figure 3), a promising anticancer agent is one of the compounds isolated from the volatile oil of *Nigella Sativa* L. (family *Ranunculaceae*) [56, 57]. Thymoquinone has demonstrated cytotoxicity against a wide range of cancers such as breast adenocarcinoma, colorectal cancer, leukaemia, lung cancer, pancreatic cancer, prostate cancer, osteosarcoma and ovarian cancer [57-59]. It has been shown to exhibit cytotoxicity to human ovarian adenocarcinoma cell line via induction of apoptosis but more resistance in non-cancerous cells [60]. Studies on the mechanism of action of thymoquinone in breast cancer cells showed that thymoquinone induced apoptosis, and activated caspases 8, 9 and 7 in a dose-dependent manner. It was found that progression of MDA-MB-231 cells was reduced in its presence.

Also thymoquinone increased peroxisome proliferator-activated receptor gamma (PPAR-γ) activity and down-regulated the expression of the genes for Bcl-2, Bcl-xL and survivin in breast cancer cells [61].

Thymoquinone not only killed pancreatic cancer cells but also prevented their occurrence in a study by Kimmel Cancer Centre in Philadelphia [62]. It prevented both cancer-causing histone deacetylases (HDAC) and several inflammation-causing cytokines from appearing more effectively than trichostatin A - a proven anticancer drug as a HDAC inhibitor. However, from a crystallographic study, it has been discovered that thymoquinone diplaces phosphopeptides in a non-covalent binding mode to bind to the phosphoserine/ phosphothreonine recognition site in the polo-box domain of polo-like kinase 1, a major mitotic regulator which is responsible for carcinogenesis when overexpressed [63]. An analogue of thymoquinone, poloxin also as an inhibitor of polo-like kinase is at the early clinical trial [64]. Thymoquinone showed synergic effect when used in combination with cisplatin and oxaliplatin in ovarian cancer cells [65-67].

Some synthetic analogues of thymoquinones have been made in our laboratory and tested their anti-ovarian cancer activity in vitro, as a result few of them such as a nitrogen-substituted thymoquinone showed more potent activity and higher water solubility [68].

## Betulinic Acid

Betulinic acid (Figure 3), a lupine-type pentacyclic triterpene is widely distributed in plants such as *Ziziphus mauritiana* Lam. (family *Rhamnaceae*), *Diospros Leucomelas* (family *Ebenaceae*), and *Crossopteryx febrifuga* (family *Rubiaceae*) [69, 70]. Betullinic acid has demonstrated cytotoxicity in neuroectodermal and malignant brain tumour cell lines. It also selectively inhibits the growth of human melanoma cell lines [69]. The cytotoxicity of betulinic acid in ovarian cancer cells has been reported and the compound demonstrated increased cytotoxic activities when administered with 5-fluorouracil in ovarian cancer cells [71].

## Tetrandrine

Tetrandrine, a bisbenzylisoquinoline alkaloid (Figure 3) isolated from the dried root of *Stephania tetrandra* S Moore (family *Menispermaceae*), exhibits very broad pharmacological actions, including anti-cancer activity [72].

In one study, tetrandine could reduce the paclitaxel concentration required to achieve 50% inhibition of cell growth to HCT15 (P-gp-positive) cells about 3100-fold, while they could not affect the accumulation and residual rate of rhodamine 123 in SK-OV-3 (P-gp-negative) cells. Therefore, tetrandrine was concluded to enhance the cytotoxicity of drugs via modulation of P-glycoprotein (P-gp) in the resistant cancer cells [73].

Tetrandrine could also increase growth suppression and apoptosis induced by cisplatin and cause redistribution of the cell cycle in ovarian cancer. *In vivo* tetrandrine and cisplatin exhibit the synergic and anti-cancer effect, which supports the application of tetrandrine as an adjunct to cisplatin in the chemotherapy of ovarian cancer [74].

Tetrandrine in combination with doxorubicin showed a significant synergistic effect in multidrug resistant Caco-2 and CEM/ADR5000 cancer cells. It could also reverse the multidrug resistance by reducing the expression of P-glycoprotein [75].

## Novel Phytochemicals Active against Ovarian Cancer

Searching for novel anti-ovarian cancer compounds from medicinal plants is on-going all over the world. A complete list of novel and potent plant natural products with $IC_{50}$s less than 10 μM in different ovarian cancer cell lines discovered from 2001-2014 has been compiled in Table 1.

In particular, Kingston's group at Virginia Polytechnic Institute, US has discovered a number of potent compounds including very promising and potent compounds such as bufatrienolides and ipomoeassin D from plants collected from Madagascar Rainforest (Table 1). Lee's group at University of North Carolina, US, also discovered many anti-ovarian cancer compounds such as 2'-(R)-O-acetylglaucarubinone and molvizarin (Table 1).

Bufatrienolides, ipomoeassin D, 2'-(R)-O-acetylglaucarubinone, and molvizarin showed very low $IC_{50}$s (less than 100 nM), which might possess different mechanisms of action from those of platinum/paclitaxel due to their unique and diverse chemical structures, and therefore providing a potential new therapy to attack multidrug resistance in ovarian cancer.

In our laboratory we are also focusing on the discovery of natural products from medicinal plants. Cycleanine, a bisbenzylisoquinoline alkaloid from *Triclisia subcordata* Oliv. (family *Menispermaceae*), was found to be an anti-ovarian cancer agent with $IC_{50}$ of 7.6 μM in A2780 cells [76]. Securinine and gallic acid have been identified from *M. discoidea*, which showed $IC_{50}$ ranging from 5 to16 μM in OVCAR8, A2780 and cisplatin resistant A2780cis ovarian cancer cell lines (Table 1) [77]. Semi-synthetic analogs of these compounds are being made to understand their structure-activity relationship and obtain more potent compounds for testing their toxicity in animals. Cyclotides as exceptionally stable disulphide–rich plant circular proteins have been reported to exert cytotoxic or lethal effects on ovarian cancer cell lines [78] which are probably due to its ability to target and bind to the cell membrane [79]. Varv A from *Viola yedeonsis* Makino (syn. *V. philippica* Cav.) (family *Violaceae*) showed $IC_{50}$s ranging from 4 to 10 μM in A2780, Igrov1 and OVCAR8 cells [80].

# 5. Prospects and Outlook

Plant-derived natural products continue to provide anti-cancer medicines for human health. In particular, paclitaxel and camptothecin have already been developed and widely used for ovarian cancer patients. During the last fifteen years a lot of phytochemicals with high potency have been discovered through *in vitro* bioassay-guided isolation and identification. Such approach should be continued for many untapped resources of medicinal plants. However, most of the ovarian cancer cell lines used in the previous bioassays were A2780 and/or SKOV3 cells (Table 1) which were categorized under being unlikely high-grade serious, therefore more serious and drug-resistant cell lines such as OVSAHO and SNU119 cell lines [110] should be used to evaluate the potency of plant extracts and pure compounds. Recently, plant endophytes that reside in the plant tissues have been found to produce phytochemicals including paclitaxel [111], camptothecin and vinblastine found in their host original plants, which provides an alternative production method for the minor components and a source of novel chemicals [11]. This is a promising area that needs more attention and intensive research. Furthermore, many natural products when isolated in pure form like camptothecin, paclitaxel and podophyllodoxin often have poor water solubility or high toxicity. Therefore the more water soluble and potent analogues must be found to overcome their shortcomings through semisynthesis and chemical modification of parent molecules. Following this approach, there have been plenty of successful examples, e.g., the making of topotecan and irinotecan based on podophyllodoxin.

In order to specifically target cancer cells without harming normal cells, drug (phytochemicals)-biologicals (antibody, biological agents, etc.) conjugates are promising candidates and are highly demanded for preclinical and clinical studies [112]. Therefore novel conjugates such as folate-paclitaxel and folate-camptothecin conjugates might be designed and prepared as vintafolide for targeting cancer cells. Metabolism of phytochemicals *in vivo* can also provide possible novel metabolites as potential drugs, which needs to be investigated. For example, SN-38 is an active metabolite of irinotecan via hydrolysis by carboxyesterase and metabolized through glucuronidation by UGT1A1, which is more bioactive and in current clinical trial [113].Another approach would be to investigate the combination of multiple drugs including the phytochemicals and approved drugs such as paclitaxel and platinum derivatives by targeting multiple targets and different pathways in order to inhibit the growth of cancer cells and to avoid drug resistance more effectively.

In summary, a multi-disciplinary and collaborative approach must be utilized by natural product chemists, synthetic chemists, chemical biologists, pharmacologist and clinicians in order to generate novel, safe and effective anti-ovarian cancer drugs based on the lead compounds discovered from plants. New drugs for the treatment of ovarian cancer can be expected and will emerge in future.

## Acknowledgments

Our work was supported by MRC and Keele University (W. W. Li), Nigerian ETF (A PhD studentship to O. R. Johnson-Ajinwo) and Nigerian ETF and NDDC (F. I. Uche). We also thank Jessica Li for editing the manuscript.

## References

[1] Siegel, R., Naishadham, D. and Jemal, A. (2013) Cancer statistics, 2013. *CA: a cancer journal for clinicians* 63(1):11-30.

[2] Xu, S. et al. (2012) Discovery of an orally active small-molecule irreversible inhibitor of protein disulfide isomerase for ovarian cancer treatment. *Proceedings of the National Academy of Sciences of the United States of America* 109(40):16348-16353.

[3] Loehrer, P. J. and Einhorn, L. H. (1984) Drugs five years later. Cisplatin. *Annals of internal medicine* 100(5):704-713.

[4] Milosavljevic, N. et al. (2010) Nongenomic effects of cisplatin: acute inhibition of mechanosensitive transporters and channels without actin remodeling. *Cancer Res.* 70 (19):7514-7522.

[5] Stordal, B., Pavlakis, N. and Davey, R. (2007) A systematic review of platinum and taxane resistance from bench to clinic: an inverse relationship. *Cancer treatment reviews* 33(8):688-703.

[6] Wheate, N. J., Walker, S., Craig, G. E. and Oun, R. (2010) The status of platinum anticancer drugs in the clinic and in clinical trials. *Dalton transactions* 39(35):8113-8127.

[7] Kinghorn, A. D., Pan, L., Fletcher, J. N. and Chai, H. (2011) The relevance of higher plants in lead compound discovery programs. *Journal of natural products* 74(6):1539-1555.

[8] Farnsworth, N. R., Akerele, O., Bingel, A. S., Soejarto, D. D. and Guo, Z. (1985) Medicinal plants in therapy. *Bulletin of the World Health Organization* 63(6):965-981.

[9] Cragg, G. M., Newman, D. J. and Snader, K. M. (1997) Natural products in drug discovery and development. *Journal of natural products* 60(1): 52-60.

[10] Tulp, M. and Bohlin, L. (2005) Rediscovery of known natural compounds: nuisance or goldmine? *Bioorganic and medicinal chemistry* 13(17):5274-5282.

[11] Cragg, G. M., Grothaus, P. G. and Newman, D. J. (2009) Impact of natural products on developing new anti-cancer agents. *Chemical reviews* 109(7):3012-3043.

[12] Lombardino, J. G. and Lowe, J. A. (2004) The role of the medicinal chemist in drug discovery-then and now. *Nature reviews Drug discovery* 3(10):853-862.

[13] Newman, D. J. and Cragg, G. M. (2007) Natural products as sources of new drugs over the last 25 years. *Journal of natural products* 70(3):461-477.

[14] Newman, D. J. and Cragg, G. M. (2012) Natural products as sources of new drugs over the 30 years from 1981 to 2010. *Journal of natural products* 75(3):311-335.

[15] Silva, J. S., Moura, M. D., Oliveira, R. A., Diniz, M. F. and Barbosa-Filho, J. M. (2003) Natural product inhibitors of ovarian neoplasia. *Phytomedicine: international journal of phytotherapy and phytopharmacology* 10(2-3):221-232.

[16] Wall, M. E. W., M. C.; Cook, C. E., Palmer, K. H., McPhail, A. T., Sim, G. A. (1966) Plant antitumor agents. I. Isolation and structure of camtothecin, a novel alkaloidal leukemia and tumor inhibitor from Camptotheca acuminata. *J. Am. Chem. Soc.* 88 (16):3888-3890.

[17] Thomas, C. J., Rahier, N. J. and Hecht, S. M. (2004) Camptothecin: current perspectives. *Bioorganic and medicinal chemistry* 12(7):1585-1604.

[18] Oberlies, N. H. and Kroll, D. J. (2004) Camptothecin and taxol: historic achievements in natural products research. *Journal of natural products* 67(2):129-135.

[19] Wani, M. C. T., H. L.; Wall, M. E., Coggin, P., McPhail, A. T. (1971) Plant antitumor agents. VI. Isolation and structure of taxol, a novel antileukemic and antitumor agent from Taxus brevifolia. *J. Am. Chem. Soc.* 93(9): 2325-2327.

[20] Lowe, J., Li, H., Downing, K. H. and Nogales, E. (2001) Refined structure of alpha beta-tubulin at 3.5 A resolution. *Journal of molecular biology* 313(5):1045-1057.

[21] Chen, N. et al. (2015) Albumin-bound nanoparticle (nab) paclitaxel exhibits enhanced paclitaxel tissue distribution and tumor penetration. *Cancer chemotherapy and pharmacology* 76(4):699-712.

[54] Chen, J. et al. (2013) Inhibitory effect of baicalin and baicalein on ovarian cancer cells. *International journal of molecular sciences* 14(3): 6012-6025.

[55] Yan, H. et al. (2015) Baicalein inhibits MMP-2 expression in human ovarian cancer cells by suppressing the p38 MAPK-dependent NF-kappaB signaling pathway. *Anti-cancer drugs* 26(6):649-656.

[56] El-Dakhakhany, M. (1963) Studies on the chemical constitution of Egyptian N. sativa L. seeds. *Planta Medica* (11):465-470.

[57] Schneider-Stock, R., Fakhoury, I. H., Zaki, A. M., El-Baba, C. O. and Gali-Muhtasib, H. U. (2014) Thymoquinone: fifty years of success in the battle against cancer models. *Drug discovery today* 19(1):18-30.

[58] Gali-Muhtasib, H., Roessner, A. and Schneider-Stock, R. (2006) Thymoquinone: a promising anti-cancer drug from natural sources. *The international journal of biochemistry and cell biology* 38(8):1249-1253.

[59] Woo, C. C., Kumar, A. P., Sethi, G. and Tan, K. H. (2012) Thymoquinone: potential cure for inflammatory disorders and cancer. *Biochemical pharmacology* 83(4):443-451.

[60] Shoieb, A. M., Elgayyar, M., Dudrick, P. S., Bell, J. L. and Tithof, P. K. (2003) In vitro inhibition of growth and induction of apoptosis in cancer cell lines by thymoquinone. *International journal of oncology* 22(1): 107-113.

[61] Woo, C. C. et al. (2011) Anticancer activity of thymoquinone in breast cancer cells: possible involvement of PPAR-gamma pathway. *Biochemical pharmacology* 82(5): 464-475.

[62] Chehl, N., Chipitsyna, G., Gong, Q., Yeo, C. J. and Arafat, H. A. (2009) Anti-inflammatory effects of the Nigella sativa seed extract, thymoquinone, in pancreatic cancer cells. *HPB: the official journal of the International Hepato Pancreato Biliary Association* 11(5):373-381.

[63] Yin, Z., Song, Y. and Rehse, P. H. (2013) Thymoquinone blocks pSer/pThr recognition by Plk1 Polo-box domain as a phosphate mimic. *ACS chemical biology* 8(2):303-308.

[64] Liu, X. (2015) Targeting Polo-Like Kinases: A Promising Therapeutic Approach for Cancer Treatment. *Translational oncology* 8(3):185-195.

[65] Nessa, M. U., Beale, P., Chan, C., Yu, J. Q. and Huq, F. (2011) Synergism from combinations of cisplatin and oxaliplatin with quercetin and thymoquinone in human ovarian tumour models. *Anticancer research* 31(11):3789-3797.

[66] Wilson, A. J., Saskowski, J., Barham, W., Yull, F. and Khabele, D. (2015) Thymoquinone enhances cisplatin-response through direct tumor effects in a syngeneic mouse model of ovarian cancer. *Journal of ovarian research* 8(1):46.

[67] Huq F. et al. (2014) Combinations of platinums and selected phytochemicals as a means of overcoming resistance in ovarian cancer. *Anticancer research* 34(1):541-545.

[68] Li, W. W. et al. (2013) Anti-cancer thymoquinone from Nigella sativa. *Planta Medica* 79:SL71.

[69] Cichewicz, R. H. and Kouzi, S. A. (2004) Chemistry, biological activity, and chemotherapeutic potential of betulinic acid for the prevention and treatment of cancer and HIV infection. *Medicinal research reviews* 24(1):90-114.

[70] Zhang, D. M. et al. (2015) Betulinic Acid and its Derivatives as Potential Antitumor Agents. *Medicinal research reviews* DOI: 10.1002/med.21353.

[71] Wang, Y. J., Liu, J. B. and Dou, Y. C. (2015) Sequential treatment with betulinic acid followed by 5-fluorouracil shows synergistic cytotoxic activity in ovarian cancer cells. *International journal of clinical and experimental pathology* 8(1):252-259.

[72] Chen, Y. J. (2002) Potential role of tetrandrine in cancer therapy. *Acta pharmacologica Sinica* 23(12):1102-1106.

[73] Choi, S. U. et al. (1998) The bisbenzylisoquinoline alkaloids, tetrandine and fangchinoline, enhance the cytotoxicity of multidrug resistance-related drugs via modulation of P-glycoprotein. *Anti-cancer drugs* 9(3): 255-261.

[74] Zhang, Y. et al. (2011) Combination of Tetrandrine with cisplatin enhances cytotoxicity through growth suppression and apoptosis in ovarian cancer in vitro and in vivo. *Cancer letters* 304(1):21-32.

[75] Sun, Y. F. and Wink, M. (2014) Tetrandrine and fangchinoline, bisbenzylisoquinoline alkaloids from Stephania tetrandra can reverse multidrug resistance by inhibiting P-glycoprotein activity in multidrug resistant human cancer cells. *Phytomedicine: international journal of phytotherapy and phytopharmacology* 21(8-9):1110-1119.

[76] Uche, F., Li, W. W., Richardson, A. and Greenhough, T. J. (2014) Anti-ovarian cancer activities of alkaloids from Triclisia subcordata olive (Menispermecaea). *Planta Medica* 80:PF7.

[77] Johnson-Ajinwo, O. R., Richardson, A. and Li, W. W. (2015) Cytotoxic effects of stem bark extracts and pure compounds from Margaritaria discoidea on human ovarian cancer cell lines. *Phytomedicine: international journal of phytotherapy and phytopharmacology* 22(1):1-4.

[78] Lindholm, P. et al. (2002) Cyclotides: a novel type of cytotoxic agents. *Molecular cancer therapeutics* 1(6):365-369.

[79] Troeira Henriques, S., Huang, Y. H., Chaousis, S., Wang, C. K. and Craik, D. J. (2014) Anticancer and toxic properties of cyclotides are dependent on phosphatidylethanolamine phospholipid targeting. *Chembiochem: a European journal of chemical biology* 15(13):1956-1965.

[80] Uche, F. I., Li, W. W., Richardson, A. and Greenhough, T. J. (2014) Anti-cancer activities of Cyclotides from Viola yedeonsis Makino (violaceae). *Planta Medica* 80: PG17.

[81] Eaton, A. L., Rakotondraibe, L. H., Brodie, P. J., Goetz, M. and Kingston, D. G. (2015) Antiproliferative Trihydroxyalkylcyclohexenones from Pleiogynium timoriense. *J. Nat. Prod.* 78 (7): 1752-1755.

[82] Eaton, A. L. et al. (2015) Bioactive oleanane glycosides from Polyscias duplicata from the Madagascar dry forest. *Natural product communications* 10(4):567-570.

[83] Liu, Y. et al. (2013) Structure elucidation of antiproliferative bisbenzylisoquinoline alkaloids from Anisocycla grandidieri from the Madagascar dry forest. *Magnetic resonance in chemistry: MRC* 51(9): 574-579.

[84] Dai, Y. et al. (2013) Antiproliferative Homoisoflavonoids and Bufatrienolides from Urginea depressa. *Journal of natural products* 76(5):865-872.

[85] Dai, Y. et al. (2013) Two antiproliferative triterpene saponins from Nematostylis anthophylla from the highlands of Central Madagascar. *Chemistry and biodiversity* 10 (2):233-240.

[86] Strapasson, R. L. et al. (2012) Bioactivity-guided isolation of cytotoxic sesquiterpene lactones of Gochnatia polymorpha ssp. floccosa. *Phytotherapy research: PTR* 26(7): 1053-1056.

[87] Dai, Y. et al. (2012) Isolation and synthesis of two antiproliferative calamenene-type sesquiterpenoids from Sterculia tavia from the Madagascar rain forest. *Bioorganic and medicinal chemistry* 20(24): 6940-6944.

[88] Pan, E. et al. (2011) Cardenolides of Leptadenia madagascariensis from the Madagascar dry forest. *Bioorganic and medicinal chemistry* 19(1): 422-428.

[89] Pan, E. et al. (2011) Isolation and synthesis of antiproliferative eupolauridine alkaloids of Ambavia gerrardii from the Madagascar Dry Forest. *Journal of natural products* 74 (5):1169-1174.

[90] Pan, E. et al. (2011) Antiplasmodial and antiproliferative pseudoguaianolides of Athroisma proteiforme from the Madagascar Dry Forest. *Journal of natural products* 74(10):2174-2180.

[91] Cao, S. et al. (2011) Antiproliferative compounds of Cyphostemma greveana from a Madagascar dry forest. *Chemistry and biodiversity* 8(4): 643-650.

[92] Usami, Y. et al. (2010) Antitumor Agents. 282. 2'-(R)-O-acetylglaucarubinone, a quassinoid from Odyendyea gabonensis as a potential anti-breast and anti-ovarian cancer agent. *Journal of natural products* 73(9):1553-1558.

[93] Cao, S. et al. (2010) Saponins and a lignan derivative of Terminalia tropophylla from the Madagascar Dry Forest. *Phytochemistry* 71(1):95-99.

[94] Hou, Y. et al. (2009) Antiproliferative cardenolide glycosides of Elaeodendron alluaudianum from the Madagascar Rainforest. *Bioorganic and medicinal chemistry* 17 (6):2215-2218.

[95] Cheng, W. et al. (2009) Chemical constituents of the bark of Machilus wangchiana and their biological activities. *Journal of natural products* 72(12):2145-2152.

[96] Cao, S. et al. (2009) Antiproliferative triterpenoid saponins of Dodonaea viscosa from the Madagascar dry forest. *Journal of natural products* 72(9):1705-1707.

[97] Park, H. W. et al. (2010) Cytotoxic germacranolide sesquiterpenes from the bark of Magnolia kobus. *Archives of pharmacal research* 33(1):71-74.

[98] Chan, P. K., Zhao, M., Che, C. T. and Mak, E. (2008) Cytotoxic acylated triterpene saponins from the husks of Xanthoceras sorbifolia. *Journal of natural products* 71(7): 1247-1250.

[99] Williams, R. B. et al. (2007) Cytotoxic clerodane diterpenoids and their hydrolysis products from Casearia nigrescens from the rainforest of Madagascar. *Journal of natural products* 70(2):206-209.

[100] Rosselli. S. et al. (2007) Cytotoxic activity of some natural and synthetic ent-kauranes. *Journal of natural products* 70(3):347-352.

[101] Karkare, S. et al. (2007) Cytotoxic cardenolide glycosides of Roupellina (Strophanthus) boivinii from the Madagascar rainforest. *Journal of natural products* 70(11):1766-1770.

[102] Yoder, B. J. et al. (2007) Antiproliferative prenylated stilbenes and flavonoids from Macaranga alnifolia from the Madagascar rainforest. *Journal of natural products* 70(3): 342-346.

[103] Williams, R. B. et al. (2005) Cytotoxic sesquiterpene lactones from Vernonia pachyclada from the Madagascar rainforest. *Journal of natural products* 68(9):1371-1374.

[104] Cao, S. et al. (2005) Ipomoeassins A-E, cytotoxic macrocyclic glycoresins from the leaves of Ipomoea squamosa from the Suriname rainforest. *Journal of natural products* 68(4):487-492.

[105] Cao, S. et al. (2004) Cytotoxic compounds from Mundulea chapelieri from the Madagascar Rainforest. *Journal of natural products* 67(3):454-456.

[106] Nakanishi, Y. et al. (2003) Acetogenins as selective inhibitors of the human ovarian 1A9 tumor cell line. *Journal of medicinal chemistry* 46(15):3185-3188.

[107] Chang, F. R. et al. (2003) Antitumor agents. 228. five new agarofurans, Reissantins A-E, and cytotoxic principles from Reissantia buchananii. *Journal of natural products* 66 (11):1416-1420.

[108] Muhammad, I. et al. (2003) Cytotoxic sesquiterpene lactones from Centaurothamnus maximus and Vicoa pentanema. *Phytotherapy research: PTR* 17(2):168-173.

[109] Cheng, H. H. et al. (2001) Cytotoxic pheophorbide-related compounds from Clerodendrum calamitosum and C. cyrtophyllum. *Journal of natural products* 64(7): 915-919.

[110] Domcke, S., Sinha, R., Levine, D. A., Sander, C. and Schultz, N. (2013) Evaluating cell lines as tumour models by comparison of genomic profiles. *Nat. Commun.* 4:2126.

[111] Stierle, A., Strobel, G. and Stierle, D. (1993) Taxol and taxane production by Taxomyces andreanae, an endophytic fungus of Pacific yew. *Science* 260(5105):214-216.

[112] Matsumoto, K., Onda, T. and Yaegashi, N. (2015) Pharmacotherapy for recurrent ovarian cancer: current status and future perspectives. *Japanese journal of clinical oncology* 45(5):408-410.

[113] Etienne-Grimaldi, M. C. et al. (2015) UGT1A1 genotype and irinotecan therapy: general review and implementation in routine practice. *Fundam. Clin. Pharmacol.* 29 (3):219-237.

In: Handbook on Ovarian Cancer
Editor: Bethany R. Collier

ISBN: 978-1-63483-874-0


*Chapter 11*

# MOLECULAR ALTERATIONS CHEMORESISTANCE-RELATED IN OVARIAN CANCER PATIENTS AND RELATED TARGET THERAPIES

***Lucrezia Amoroso, Francesca De Iuliis and Susanna Scarpa***
Experimental Medicine Department, Sapienza University of Rome, Italy

## ABSTRACT

**Introduction.** Ovarian cancer has the highest rate of mortality among gynecological malignancies and it is the fifth leading cause of cancer-related death in women of developed countries. It is often diagnosed at late stage, therefore, despite optimal cytoreduction by debulking surgery and adjuvant chemotherapy, recurrence is frequent.

New therapeutic strategies are needed to treat relapses and advanced stage chemoresistant ovarian cancer. Ovarian cancer is characterized by different molecular phenotypes, and it can be classified in five tumor types with different clinical, pathologic and prognostic properties, and with different chemosensitivity.

**Objective.** This review will focus on molecular alterations involved in ovarian cancer carcinogenesis, which may become new targets for therapy in the future. Biological therapies can impact on the prognosis, especially in advanced chemoresistant ovarian cancer patients.

**Discussion.** The most important pathways involved in ovarian cancer chemoresistance are PI3K/ AKT/ mTOR, KRAS/ MAPK/ ERK, BRCA1/BRCA2, Notch and Forkhead Box M1 pathways.

The amplification of PI3K is more frequent in high-grade ovarian tumors rather than in low grade ones, together with AKT phosphorylation, contributing to disease progression.

KRAS mutations are frequent in low-grade ovarian tumors, and their expression varies in different histopathological types. Loss of PTEN is frequently present in high-grade serous carcinomas and correlates with a poor prognosis.

Several protein kinases and other signaling molecules, such as KRAS, BRAF, PI3KCA and CTNNB1, have been evaluated and their mutations have been correlated with prognosis. Epigenetic modifications are promising targets for ovarian cancer treatment. Several studies on molecular alterations have been conducted on ovarian cancer tissue, but further studies are needed to tailor every therapy to the specific histotype of ovarian cancer.

Actually, the approved biological therapies currently used in ovarian cancer patients are only three: Bevacizumab (a monoclonal antibodies directed against VEGF, usually utilized in platinum-pretreated patients), Pazopanib (tyrosine) and Olaparib (PARP-inhibitor, utilized in BRCA1/2 mutated patients).

Further studies are needed to better evaluate different chemoresistance related pathways, and to find new targets on which to focus clinical research.

**Conclusions.** Among the analyzed studies, only molecular alterations of PI3KI seem to have the strongest correlation with prognosis. These mutations could be future targets of therapy for chemoresistant patients, but more studies are required.

**Keywords:** Ovarian cancer, chemoresistance, targeted-therapy, pathway

## INTRODUCTION

Ovarian cancer (OC) has the highest rate of mortality among gynecological malignancies, and it is the fifth leading cause of cancer-related death in women of developed countries, due to the lack of clear early symptoms and the lack of obvious risk genetic markers [1]. It may present either acute or sub-acute symptoms. Most common symptoms are abdominal fullness, bloating, vague pelvic or abdominal pain, and symptoms related to tumor infiltration or compression, such as pleural effusion, small bowel obstruction and venous thromboembolism [2].

Approximately 60–70% of ovarian cancers are diagnosed at advanced stage, or can present abdominal metastases at diagnosis. Only 17-36% of women have a life expectancy of 5 years. Considering that an early detection can increase the 5-year survival rate to 70–90%, it is important to investigate the molecular pathogenesis of ovarian cancer, with the aim to obtain an early diagnosis and to discover new targeted therapies [1, 3-4].

During the last 40 years, several trials have been conducted to establish the "gold standard" in ovarian cancer treatment. The most relevant trial is the pivotal Gynecologic Oncology Group (GOG)-111 study of 1996 conducted in women with advanced epithelial ovarian cancer: this trial focused on the use of paclitaxel, demonstrating that combination of cisplatin and paclitaxel conferred a substantial survival advantage over cisplatin and cyclophosphamide [5].

A recent Japanese Gynecologic Oncology Group phase III clinical trial in patients with advanced ovarian carcinoma compared the conventional regimen of paclitaxel and carboplatin every 3 weeks with weekly dose-dense paclitaxel and carboplatin every 3 weeks, demonstrating a large progression free survival (PFS) advantage for the dose-dense schedule [6].

Although the standard of care in the primary setting is the combination of debulking surgery and cytotoxic chemotherapy (carboplatin and paclitaxel based), approximately 80% of women with advanced OC experience relapsed disease, chemoresistance, and death due to cancer-associated morbidity [7]. Single agents as gemcitabine, doxorubicin and topotecan have been used in recurrent disease without any success in prolonging survival [8].

Chemoresistance has multifactorial origin, with different mechanisms involved. Ovarian cancer is a heterogeneous disease with different molecular characteristics. Histologically, OC can be classified in five tumor types: high-grade serous (70%), endometrioid (10%), clear cell (10%), mucinous (3%), and low-grade serous (< 5%) carcinomas. Every subtype is associated with different genetic risk factors, molecular events during carcinogenesis, and chemotherapy response [9]. The understanding of OC molecular pathogenesis is needed to demonstrate the impact of molecular alterations on clinical features of this tumor and to develop appropriate and effective therapies to overtake chemoresistance.

In this chapter review, we discuss the associations among hystotypes of ovarian cancers and the related molecular alterations. We will focus on the most important pathways involved in ovarian cancer chemoresistance such as PI3K/AKT/mTOR. Finally, we will discuss current therapies and potential target treatments to overcome chemoresistance in the different subtypes.

# 1. Serous Carcinomas

The most common subtype of OC is serous carcinoma, subdivided into high-grade (grade 2 and 3) and low grade (grade 1) [10]. Serous carcinoma has an epithelial phenotype arising from the mesothelium, either from cells lining the fallopian tube or the ovarian surface [11, 12].

## 1.1. High Grade Serous Carcinoma and Molecular Alterations

High-grade serous carcinomas (HGSCs) are the most frequent ovarian cancers characterized by poor prognosis and often presenting high-volume ascites [13].

Several mutations such as WT1 (Wilms tumor1) and loss of heterozygosity (LOH) of chromosomes 7q have been associated with better prognosis, and considered a valid prognostic marker for HGSCs [14]. Furthermore PI3K/AKT/mTOR (phosphatidylinositol 3-kinase/kinase B/ mammalian target of rapamycin) pathway is involved in HGSCs carcinogenesis. The most consistent data on molecular alterations are on TP53 and BRCA (breast cancer) mutations [12-9].

Aside from BRCA abnormalities, which are well known markers, we will focus our study on the mutation of p53 protein, which requires further studies in order to understand its peculiar function in HGSC.

TP53 gene mutations play a crucial role in HGSCs because ubiquitous in stage III or IV disease and very high in low stage of the disease [15-16]. An early somatic mutation in TP53 has been suggested to be the earliest event of carcinogenesis, followed by deletions or LOH of chromosomes carrying TP53, BRCA1 or BRCA2 [15]. TP53 mutation has been found also in tubal intraepithelial carcinomas (TICs), which are suggested to be the early invasive lesions of HGSCs, mutated in patients with and without BRCA1 /BRCA2 mutations.

Brachova et al. have analyzed TP53 mutation in patients who had undertaken primary platinum and taxane based chemotherapy: TP53 mutation analysis was performed through exon sequencing and TP53 was divided into four groups: known oncomorphic, known loss of function (LOF), unclassified, or wildtype (WT). Probably, WT p53 contributes to chemoresistance of drugs that act especially in mitosis, acting on cell cycle checkpoints.

Thus, it is important to investigate the status of both alleles of TP53, because this gene may be a potential therapeutic target for ovarian cancer with this type of mutation.

The same authors demonstrated also that tumors with TP53 mutation have increased expression of activated growth pathways, such as phosphorylation of EGFR (epidermal growth factor receptor), Her2 (human epidermal growth factor receptor 2), and retinoblastoma protein (Rb). Besides, mTOR (mammalian target of rapamycin) and β catenin proteins were significantly increased in tumors with TP53 mutation. They described that patients with unclassified mutations are significantly more chemosensitive and have lower rates of relapses, opposite to patients with the oncomorphic TP53 mutations, which are associated with a worse progression free survival (PFS) and higher rates of chemoresistance and recurrence [17].

Among the studies on TP53 mutations, there are discordances about the influence of TP53 on survival and recurrence in HGSCs. Considering the high incidence of TP53 mutations in sporadic and familial cases (a percentage of 60–80%), [12] and the high reliance of HGSCs on TP53 mutations, further studies are necessary to investigate the initial carcinogenic events that lead to inactivation of TP53 and to investigate the biological significance of the different types of TP53 mutations. This target could represent an evolution in the treatment of HGSC patients, with the aim to obtain better outcomes in terms of survival and response to chemotherapy [18].

## 1.2. Low Grade Serous Carcinoma and Molecular Alterations

Low grade serous carcinoma (LGSCs) account for <5% of ovarian cancer and, despite a more favorable prognosis than HGSC, it presents poor response rates to chemotherapy [9]. LGSC seems to originate from serous cystadenoma/adenofibroma which progress into ovarian serous borderline tumor (OSBT) that includes: atypical proliferative serous tumor (APST) and micropapillary serous carcinoma (MPSC). The epithelial inclusion glands seem to derive from the fallopian tube [19-20]. Several studies report the association of PTEN and CTNNB1 mutations with low-grade tumors [21]. LGSC carcinogenesis is associated with KRAS (*Kirsten* rat sarcoma), BRAF (B-Raf proto-oncogene, serine/threonine kinase) and PIK3CA (phosphoinositide-3-kinase, catalytic, alpha polypeptide) mutations, LOH on chromosome Xq, microsatellite instability and expression of amphiregulin, but the most common alterations involved are KRAS and BRAF mutations [12]. KRAS mutation is associated with a good prognosis in LGSCs FIGO Stage I-II, but not in FIGO Stage III-IV. This could be explained from the fact that KRAS mutation is more frequent in less advanced tumors than in advanced ones [22]. However, some studies suggest that chemoresistance in late stage ovarian cancer may be due to the earliest mutations in KRAS that can activate and lead the over-activation of NF-κB (Nuclear factor-κB) in cancer stem cells (CSCs) [23]. In addition, it has recently been demonstrated that OSBT, APST and MPSC are associated with BRAF and KRAS mutations and LOH. The same mutations have been found in peritoneal implants [9]. Recent studies showed the presence of a variant allele of KRAS at rs61764370, that breaks a micro RNA binding site in this oncogene. Ratner et al. demonstrated that KRAS-variant was largely present in patients with ovarian cancer and their relatives, focusing the attention on the research on KRAS-variant in families with ovarian cancer [24]. Singer et al. evaluated the role of BRAF and KRAS mutations in LGSC analyzing both genes for three common mutations (at codon 599 of BRAF and codons 12 and 13 of KRAS). They demonstrated that KRAS and its downstream mediator BRAF were frequently present in OSBT, supporting the data on the involvement of KRAS/MAPK/ERK pathway [25]. KRAS and BRAF mutations or their overexpression in the MAPK pathway induce mitogen-activated protein kinase (MAPK) activation [26].

More recent studies have shown that patients who underwent taxane-platinum based chemotherapy have a poor prognosis in relation with MAPK1 amplification. Opposite to this, KRAS amplification did not have effects on survival. So, MAPK1 amplification may be cause of chemoresistance and/or increase chemoresistance in recurrent cancers [27]. In 40-60% of OC, MAPK interacts with estrogen receptor alpha (ERa): several studies have demonstrated a relationship between MAPK signaling and ERa, but it is not clear whether expression of ERa can influence tumor growth dependency from estrogens and whether targeting ERa could modify cell growth or survival of OC.

Some clinical trials on recurrent OC suggest some efficacy of the inhibition of estrogen signaling; hence, anti-estrogen therapy may be advantageous in patients with ERα positive, also using a selective MEKi (*Mitogen*-activated protein/extracellular signal-regulated kinase kinase inhibitor) to down-regulate the estrogen pathway. In fact the signaling network of MAPK can interact with estrogen receptors [28]. Hou et al. have demonstrated that MEKi can enhance ERα over-expression and can sensitize ovarian cells to antiestrogens (such as fulvestrant) [28].

New therapeutic approaches for patients with recurrent ovarian cancer are represented by new target therapies as Selumetinib (AZD6244), an inhibitor of MEK-1/2, which demonstrated a disease stability rate of 65% with a major efficacy respect to conventional chemotherapy [29].

Further phase II clinical trials are ongoing to test other MEK inhibitors, which can be new valid options **in the treatment of LGSC.** Currently, an international randomized phase II/III study of another MEK inhibitor, trametinib, compared with standard therapy, is under development for women with recurrent low-grade serous carcinoma [30-31].

These findings propose KRAS and BRAF mutations as early events of the initiation of LGSC and underline the importance of MAPK amplification in and the role of MEK in LGSCs.

## 2. Endometrioid Carcinoma and Molecular Alterations

Endometrioid carcinomas (ECs) represent 10% of OC [9] and several studies consider endometriosis as a probable precursor of EC [32].

This association is supported from data which report that OC develops in 0.3–1.6% of women with endometriosis, while endometriosis is observed in 4–29% of patients with ovarian cancer [33]. Identification of genetic alterations in endometriotic lesions endorses this hypothesis. Endometrial cysts of the ovary could be precancerous form of EC: LOH at locus 10q23.3 and mutation of the PTEN tumor suppressor gene have high incidence in EC and in endometrial cysts of the ovary [34].

The most frequent abnormalities, apart KRAS and BRAF, that are no common alterations, are somatic mutations of beta-catenin (CTNNB1) and PTEN alterations [9].

PI3K/AKT/mTOR pathway is involved in the primordial follicle genesis and it is frequently altered in EC, but there are not clear data about these genetic alterations as critical drivers for EC. Anyway, PI3K/AKT activation is known to contribute to a decreased chemotherapy response [32].

A deregulation of Wnt/β-cat signaling pathway and/or PI3K/Pten signaling was found in EC. But there are no data that showed b-catenin mutations in human endometriotic lesions in the absence of endometrioid adenocarcinoma [35]. In EC, but also in OCCC, mutations in the gene encoding the AT-rich interacting domain containing protein 1A (ARID1A) have been found.

Most of these alterations induce a loss of expression of the ARID1A protein. Recent studies found a correlation between ARID1A mutations and PI3K/AKT pathway, which seems to be activated from ARID1A [32].

Loss of ARID1A expression may induce tumor cells to depend on PI3K/AKT-pathway activation, making cells more sensitive to PI3K/AKT inhibitors.

Eleftherios et al. demonstrated the sensitivity of ARID1A-deficient tumor cells to PI3K/AKT-inhibition. These cells presented a high rate of apoptosis in relation to PI3K- and AKT-inhibitors, supporting the importance of PI3K/AKT-pathway as a therapeutic target [36]. Activation of the PI3K-AKT signaling pathway can inhibit apoptosis, inactivating PTEN. PI3K can also be activated through PIK3CA mutations, which are associated with poor prognosis [37].

## 3. Clear Cell Carcinoma and Molecular Alterations

Clear cell carcinoma (CCC) is usually diagnosed at early stage and it is often associated with endometriosis and with a favorable prognosis, but they have a lower response to chemotherapy and a poorer prognosis than HGSCs. Rarely, it occurs at advanced stage with poor prognosis and with a lower response to chemotherapy.

Approximately, 46-57% of CCC presents ARID1A mutations and lack of BAF250 protein [9]; BAF250a is a protein involved in chromatin remodeling via the multi-protein SWI–SNF (SWItch/Sucrose non fermentable) complex, encoded by ARID1A. Loss or decreased expression of ARID1A, a gene involved in DNA repair, is associated to short disease free survival and chemoresistance. The effect of Paclitaxel consists in interrupting the function of microtubules and then blocking cell division. When ARID1A is decreased or lost, DNA cannot be repaired and the efficacy of Paclitaxel probably decreases because of lack of action site. Yokoyama et al. have demonstrated that ARID1A is less expressed in CCC stage III-IV, which usually relapse after complete clinical response after chemotherapy, suggesting that lack or decrease of ARID1A may be related to chemoresistance and recurrent disease [38].

ARID1A mutations have frequently been reported alongside mutations of PIK3CA and/or loss of PTEN expression, which both activate PI3K/AKT pathway [36]. This hypothesis is endorsed from several studies, as the study of Yamamoto who disclosed mutations of PIK3CA in 40% of CCCs, associated in more than 70% of cases with lack of ARID1A [39]. In agreement with the study of Yokoyama et al., further studies confirm the importance of the correlation between mutation of ARID1A and chemoresistance, suggesting that PI3K/AKT-inhibitors may become a target for therapies able to overtake chemoresistance in patients with loss or decrease of ARID1A [36].

## 4. Mucinous Carcinomas and Molecular Alterations

Mucinous carcinomas (MCs) represent 2 - 3% of ovarian tumors [40]. They are benign tumors in the 80% of cases and borderline tumors for the remaining 20%. The origin of MC is not known and most of them present gastrointestinal differentiation. In fact, MCs present genes that encode markers of intestinal differentiation, such as CDX2 and KRAS. KRAS is very common in low grade ovarian tumors and represents an early mutation in the carcinogenesis of MC [9, 41]. KRAS mutation is correlated to good prognosis and survival, but it hasn't been demonstrated a correlation between KRAS mutation and clinical stage, although its prevalence in well and moderately differentiated tumors at early stage of disease.

Considering the importance of KRAS in the prognosis of low grade tumors, Ras/Raf/MEK/ERK-pathway may be a target for therapies in this subtype of ovarian tumors [22].

## 5. A Brief Summary of Current Therapies

In the last three decades no remarkable changes have been reached in treatment and survival of patients with ovarian cancer. Patients at early stage have a 5-year survival rate of 50-90%, while it is of 25% in the late stage tumors. The deficiency in early detection is mainly due to the poor understanding of its pathogenesis, beyond the lack of symptoms in early stage. CA125 remains a good marker to monitor chemoresponse and recurrence during follow up; a new marker, HE4, is more sensitive to detect OC in premenopause patients [42]. Studies have shown that OC consists of dissimilar groups of malignancies, which have heterogeneous molecular alterations and different origin, arising from the distal fallopian tube or from the ovarian surface. This array can explain why the various subtypes of OCs respond in different ways to chemotherapy [43].

Over the past two decades, Carboplatin/paclitaxel has been the gold standard for primary epithelial OC [44-45]. For patients with recurrent OC, platinum-free interval (PFI) is important to choice the right chemotherapy. PFI is the interval between last platinum treatment and the diagnosis of recurrence. Patients are divided in "platinum sensitive", with a PFI of at least 6 months, and "platinum resistant", with a PFI less than 6 months. Platinum-based therapy is the principal treatment for patients with "platinum sensitive" recurrence, but combination chemotherapy has better PFS (progression free survival) and OS (overall survival). It has been showed that carboplatinum and pegylated liposomal doxorubicin (PLD) combination is more effective and less toxic than carboplatinum and paclitaxel combination. "Platinum resistant" recurrence includes different carcinomas that recur within 6 months of treatment or within 6 months of different lines of chemotherapy as dose-dense schedule of platinum, either cisplatin or carboplatin administred weekly in association with etoposide or paclitaxel, or platinum associated with gemcitabine. The most common drugs used in patients with "Platinum resistant" recurrence are PLD, paclitaxel, topotecan and gemcitabine [7].

At present, the only approved biological therapies currently used in ovarian cancer patients are identified in antiangiogenic agents (Bevacizumab), tyrosine (Pazopanib) and PARP inhibitors (Olaparib).

Bevacizumab, a humanized monoclonal antibody directed against vascular endothelial growth factor (VEGF), in combination with cytotoxic chemotherapy, improves response rate of both platinum sensitive and platinum resistant recurrences [12]. OCEANS and AURELIA trials have reported the efficacy of Bevacizumab in combination with cytotoxic chemotherapy in relapsed disease in terms of PFS and improved quality of life [46].

Pazopanib is a multifunctional tyrosine kinase inhibitor (TKI) that principally inhibits vascular endothelial growth factor receptors (VEGFR 1, 2, 3), platelet derived growth factor receptors (PDGFRα and β) and fibroblast growth factor receptor (FGFR). Additional targets include cell-factor receptor (c-kit), IL-2-inducible T-cell kinase, lymphocyte-specific protein tyrosine kinase, and colony-stimulating factor 1 receptor [47].

Du Bois et al. conducted an open-label, phase I/II study to evaluate safety and tolerability of Pazopanib in addition to a standard platinum-paclitaxel-based chemotherapy in patients with advanced gynecologic malignancies not previously treated. They demonstrated that Pazopanib 800 mg or 400 mg daily in association with standard paclitaxel and carboplatin chemotherapy was not appropriate in patients with recent diagnosis of gynecologic cancer, for an intolerable toxicity [48].

One of the most recent studies of Du Bois evaluated Pazopanib **as** maintenance therapy in patients with advanced stage OC with no evidence of disease progression after first-line chemotherapy. This study showed an improvement in progression-free survival but no benefits in terms of overall survival [49].

A phase I clinical trial of Fong PC et al. showed pharmacokinetic and pharmacodynamic characteristics of Olaparib, an oral inhibitor of the poly adenosine diphosphate [ADP]-ribose polymerases (PARPs), in patients with BRCA1/2 mutations, resistant to standard treatment or lacking of suitable therapies. In this study, Olaparib showed good tolerance with lower side effects along with valid pharmacokinetic and pharmacodynamic characteristics [50].

Another phase II study including ovarian cancer patients with BRCA1/2 mutations, showed efficacy of Olaparib 400 mg twice daily, demonstrating a clinical benefit rate of 66% and a median response duration of 9.5 months [51]. Actually, Olaparib has been approved as maintenance therapy in patients completely or partially responsive to platinum-based chemotherapy. It is addressed to platinum sensitive patients with BRCA germline and/or somatic mutations, in case of recurrence from high-grade serous epithelial ovarian cancer, fallopian tube or primary peritoneal carcinoma [52]. This therapy was based on a phase II trial, called Study 19, which recruited 265 patients with serous ovarian carcinoma who responded to platinum –based chemotherapy treated with Olaparib 400 mg twice daily or placebo.

This study described a median improvement of progression free survival of 6.9 months and an overall survival improvement of 3 months compared with placebo. Currently, phase III clinical studies are also evaluating maintenance therapy for advanced ovarian patients [53].

## 5.1. PI3K/AKT/mTOR Inhibitors

PI3K/AKT/mTOR pathway is prevalent in all histotypes of ovarian cancer [32, 54]; the inhibitors of PI3K/AKT/mTOR pathway consist of first-generation agent (rapamycin) and second-generation agents (everolimus and temsirolimus) that inhibit the mTORC1 complex by interacting with FK-binding protein 12 (FKBP12) [55-56].

PIK3CA mutation screening should be helpful for the use of PI3K/AKT/mTOR pathway inhibitors, although a single-agent is not sufficient because of concomitant escape mechanisms [32].

Sheppard et al. analyzed the response of 32 ovarian cancer cell lines to specific inhibitors of PI3K/mTOR (PF502) and RAS/ERK (PD901) signaling, which are currently used in clinical trials and they showed that PTEN loss or PIK3CA mutations did not relate with PF502 response [54]. In this study, concurrent inhibition of MEK and PI3K/mTOR pathways inhibited cell proliferation and induced cell death in PF502-resistant cells, furthermore inhibited tumor growth in vivo, suggesting that combination therapy with selective PI3K/mTOR and RAS/ERK pathway inhibitors can be an effective new treatment option for ovarian carcinoma [54].

KRAS and BRAF mutations confer sensitivity to MEK inhibition in several subtypes of ovarian cancer [57-59].

Inhibitors of mTOR are capable to limit proliferation and progression of the tumor. Patients with PIK3CA mutations are more responsive to PI3K/AKT/mTOR inhibitors than patients who not present these alterations [60]. Temsirolimus is an inhibitor of mammalian target of rapamycin (mTOR), a serine/threonine kinase involved in initiating mRNA translation. Behbakht et al. demonstrated that therapy with mTOR inhibitor, Temsirolimus, determined 9.3% response rate and 24.1% PFS at 6 months in patients with persistent/recurrent epithelial ovarian cancer and primary peritoneal cancer, but this response was insufficient to develop phase III studies in unselected patients with persistent cancer, recurrence or peritoneal carcinoma [61].

## 5.2. MEK Inhibitors and Other Potential Target Therapy

Selumetinib (AZD6244), an inhibitor of mitogen-activated protein kinase (MEK 1/2), has demonstrated a disease stability rate of 65%, with a major efficacy respect to conventional chemotherapy, in patients with recurrent LGSC [29].

Cossa et al. evaluated the role of MEK1/2 inhibitors in ovarian cancer cell lines containing platinum resistant variants expressing p53 mutations and ERK1/2 activation and showed that a MEK1/2 inhibitor can cooperate with platinum drugs in ovarian carcinoma cells by enhancing the induction of apoptosis [30].

Although the role of ERK1/2 in cell survival and induction of apoptosis is still discussed [62], it is important to highlight the role of ERK1/2 pathway by inhibiting MEK1/2 as a potential target therapy, principally in patients with activation of ERK1/2 pathway.

Mitogen-activated protein kinase (MAPK), also known as extracellular signal-regulated protein kinase (ERK), is activated from BRAF or KRAS mutations. These mutations led to overexpression of activated ERK1/2 in ovarian serous carcinomas. Phosphorylation of ERK1/2 activates a variety of cellular and nuclear proteins. Katagiri et al. demonstrated the importance of p-ERK1/2 expression, which depends on the activation of the MEK-ERK pathway, for cell migration and invasion of ovarian cancer. So, inactivating ERK1/2 through MEK inhibitor therapy, and using this therapy at the time of initial chemotherapy, can determine a decrease of any tumor residual and a prolongation of disease free interval. Furthermore, patients with primary tumors that express p-ERK1/2 may benefit from MEK inhibitors in combination with conventional chemotherapy [63].

## Conclusion

Ovarian cancer still remains the tumor with the highest incidence of death among gynecological tumors. Despite different subtypes have been described, it is still treated as a single disease, apart some new therapeutic approaches that include antiangiogenic therapies with Bevacizumab or PARP inhibitors, such as Pazopanib and Olaparib.

Different pathways have been analyzed but one of the most important pathways involved in both high and low-grade ovarian carcinomas is PI3K/Akt/mTOR.

In physiological conditions, PI3K/Akt/mTOR pathway protects the primordial follicles from destruction. Environmental toxins, as polycyclic aromatic hydrocarbons, cause atresia of primordial follicle leading to premature ovarian failure [64]. Follicles respond to this insult up-regulating PI3K/AKT/mTOR pathway that causes an increase of follicular proliferation [65]. PI3K/AKT/mTOR is implicated in the tumorigenesis of both high and low grade ovarian carcinomas. Low-grade ovarian carcinomas present a lower response to chemotherapy than high-grade ovarian tumors [66]. Certainly, PI3K/AKT/mTOR pathway plays a key role in ovarian cancer carcinogenesis, progression, and chemoresistance.

As previously discussed, low-grade cancers present cell signaling pathway mutations in KRAS, BRAF, CTNNB1, ARID1A and PTEN; numerous alterations in the tumor cell pathways are necessary to cause tumorigenesis [67].

Recently, new informations about ovarian carcinogenesis have been evaluated, recognizing that there are deep differences among several histotypes. Various OCs originate from the ovarian surface epithelium (mesothelium) and metaplastic changes lead to development of different histotypes. Each histotype (serous, endometrioid, clear cell, mucinous and transitional cell), correspond respectively to: fallopian tube, endometrium, gastrointestinal tract or endocervix and urinary bladder [68].

Deregulation of PI3K/AKT/mTOR can ensue from over-activation, alterations in the catalytic domains, in the regulatory domain, or aberrations to the downstream targets of PI3K. The most prevalent molecular alterations interest PIK3CA and PTEN [69].

We think that biological therapies will characterize the future of oncology and ovarian cancer treatment.

Several studies have been performed and other are in progress, but it is very important to focus attention on the importance of biological therapy which can be addressed to every singular type of ovarian cancer, overcoming resistances and overwhelming the most lethal gynecological carcinoma.

## REFERENCES

[1] Latha, TS; Panati, K; Gowd, DS; Reddy, MC; Lomada, D. Ovarian cancer biology and immunotherapy. *Int Rev Immunol.*, 2014, 33(5), 428-440.

[2] Argento, M; Hoffman, P; Gauchez, AS. Ovarian Cancer Detection and Treatment: Current Situation and Future Prospects. *Anticancer research*, 2008, 28, 3135-3138.

[3] Dong, X; Men, X1; Zhang, W; Lei, P. Advances in tumor markers of ovarian cancer for early Diagnosis. *Indian J Cancer*, 2014, 51 Suppl 3, e72-6.

[4] Hu, ZD; Wei, TT; Yang, M; Ma, N; Tang, QQ; Qin, BD; Fu, HT; Zhong, RQ. Diagnostic Value of Osteopontin in Ovarian Cancer: A Meta-Analysis and Systematic Review. *PLOS One.*, 2015, 10(5), e0126444

[5] McGuire, WP; Hoskins, WJ; Brady, MF; Kucera, PR; Partridge, EE; Look, KY; Clarke-Pearson, DL; Davidson, M. Cyclophosphamide and cisplatin compared with paclitaxel and cisplatin in patients with stage III and stage IV ovarian cancer. *N Engl J Med.*, 1996, 334(1), 1–6.

[6] Katsumata, N; Yasuda, M; Takahashi, F; Isonishi, S; Jobo, T; Aoki, D; Tsuda, H; Sugiyama, T; Kodama, S; Kimura, E; Ochiai, K; Noda, K. Dose-dense paclitaxel once a week in combination with carboplatin every 3 weeks for advanced ovarian cancer: a phase 3, open-label, randomised controlled trial. *Lancet.*, 2009, 374(9698), 1331-1338.

[7] Luvero, D; Milani, A; Ledermann, JA. Treatment options in recurrent ovarian cancer: latest evidence and clinical potential. *Ther Adv Med Oncol.*, 2014, 6(5), 229-239.

[8] Bookman, MA; Brady, MF; McGuire, WP; Harper, PG; Alberts, DS; Friedlander, M; Colombo, N; Fowler, JM; Argenta, PA; De Geest, K; Mutch, DG; Burger, RA; Swart, AM; Trimble, EL; Accario-Winslow, C; Roth, LM. Evaluation of new platinum-based treatment regimens in advanced-stage ovarian cancer: a Phase III Trial of the Gynecologic Cancer Intergroup. *J ClinOncol.*, 2009, 27(9), 1419–1425.

[9] Prat, J. Ovarian carcinomas: *five distinct diseases with different origins, genetic alterations, and clinicopathologicalfeatures. Virchows Arch.*, 2012, 460(3), 237-249.

[10] Tuna, M; Ju, Z; Smid, M; Amos, CI; Mills, GB. Prognostic relevance of acquired uniparental disomy in serous ovarian cancer. *Mol Cancer.*, 2015, 14(1), 29.

[11] Feeley, KM; Wells, M. Precursor lesions of ovarian epithelial malignancy. *Histopathology.*, 2001, 38(2), 87-95.

[12] Bast RC, Jr. Hennessy, B; Mills, GB. The biology of ovarian cancer: new opportunities for translation. *Nat Rev Cancer*, 2009, 9(6), 415–428.

[13] Feigenberg, T; Clarke, B; Virtanen, C; Plotkin, A; Letarte, M; Rosen, B; Bernardini, MQ; Kollara, A; Brown, TJ; Murphy, KJ. Molecular profiling and clinical outcome of high-grade serous ovarian cancer presenting with low- versus high-volume ascites. *Biomed Res Int.*, 2014, 2014, 367103.

[14] Köbel, M; Kalloger, SE; Boyd, N; McKinney, S; Mehl, E; Palmer, C; Leung, S; Bowen, NJ; Ionescu, DN; Rajput, A; Prentice, LM; Miller, D; Santos, J; Swenerton, K; Gilks, CB; Huntsman, D. Ovarian carcinoma subtypes are different diseases: implications for biomarker studies. *PLOS Med.*, 2008, 5(12), e232.

[15] Chien, J; Sicotte, H; Fan, JB; Humphray, S; Cunningham, JM; Kalli, KR; Oberg, AL; Hart, SN; Li, Y; Davila, JI; Baheti, S; Wang, C; Dietmann, S; Atkinson,

EJ; Asmann, YW; Bell, DA; Ota, T; Tarabishy, Y; Kuang, R; Bibikova, M; Cheetham, RK; Grocock, RJ; Swisher, EM; Peden, J; Bentley, D; Kocher, JP; Kaufmann, SH; Hartmann, LC; Shridhar, V; Goode, EL. TP53 mutations, tetraploidy and homologous recombination repair defects in early stage high-grade serousovarian cancer. *Nucleic Acids Res.*, 2015, pii: gkv111. [Epub ahead of print]

[16] Gursan, N; Sipal, S; Calik, M; Gundogdu, C. P53, bcl-2, ki-67 li (labeling index) status in benign, proliferative, and malignant ovarian surface epithelialneoplasms. *Eurasian J Med.*, 2009, 41(1), 10-14.

[17] Brachova, P; Mueting, SR; Carlson, MJ; Goodheart, MJ; Button, AM; Mott, SL; Dai, D; Thiel, KW; Devor, EJ; Leslie, KK. TP53 oncomorphic mutations predict resistance to platinum- and taxane-based standard chemotherapy in patients diagnosed with advanced serous ovarian carcinoma. *Int J Oncol.*, 2015, 46(2), 607-618.

[18] Ahmed, AA; Etemadmoghadam, D; Temple, J; Lynch, AG; Riad, M; Sharma, R; Stewart, C; Fereday, S; Caldas, C; Defazio, A; Bowtell, D; Brenton, JD. Driver mutations in TP53 are ubiquitous in high grade serous carcinoma of the ovary. *J Pathol.*, 2010, 221(1), 49-56.

[19] Tsang, YT; Deavers, MT; Sun, CC; Kwan, SY; Kuo, E; Malpica, A; Mok, SC; Gershenson, DM; Wong, KK. KRAS (but not BRAF) mutations in ovarian serous borderline tumor are associated with recurrent low-grade serous carcinoma. *J Pathol.*, 2013, 231(4), 449-456.

[20] Kurman, RJ; Shih, IeM. Molecular pathogenesis and extraovarian origin of epithelial ovarian cancer--shifting the paradigm. *Hum Pathol.*, 2011, 42(7), 918-931.

[21] Willner, J; Wurz, K; Allison, KH; Galic, V; Garcia, RL; Goff, BA; Swisher, EM. Alternate molecular genetic pathways in ovarian carcinomas of common histological types. *Hum Pathol.*, 2007, 38(4), 607-613

[22] Nodin, B; Zendehrokh, N; Sundström, M; Jirström, K. Clinicopathological correlates and prognostic significance of KRAS mutation status in a pooled prospective cohort of epithelial ovarian cancer. *Diagn Pathol.*, 2013, 8,106.

[23] Saldanha, SN; Tollefsbol TO. Pathway modulations and epigenetic alterations in ovarian tumorbiogenesis. *J Cell Physiol.*, 2014, 229(4), 393-406.

[24] Ratner, E; Lu, L; Boeke, M; Barnett, R; Nallur, S; Chin, LJ; Pelletier, C; Blitzblau, R; Tassi, R; Paranjape, T; Hui, P; Godwin, AK; Yu, H; Risch, H; Rutherford, T; Schwartz, P; Santin, A; Matloff, E; Zelterman, D; Slack, FJ; Weidhaas, JB. A KRAS-variant in ovarian cancer acts as a genetic marker of cancer risk. *Cancer Res.*, 2010, 70(16), 6509-6515.

[25] Singer, G; Oldt, R 3rd; Cohen,Y; Wang, BG; Sidransky, D; Kurman, RJ; Shih, IeM. Mutations in BRAF and KRAS characterize the development of low-grade ovarian serous carcinoma. *J Natl Cancer Inst.*, 2003, 95(6), 484-486.

[26] Rescigno, P; Cerillo, I; Ruocco, R; Condello, C; De Placido, S; Pensabene, M. New hypothesis on pathogenesis of ovarian cancer lead to future tailored approaches. *Biomed Res Int.*, 2013, 2013, 852839.

[27] Rahman, MT; Nakayama, K; Rahman, M; Katagiri, H; Katagiri, A; Ishibashi, T; Ishikawa, M; Sato, E; Iida, K; Nakayama, N; Ishikawa, N; Miyazaki K. KRAS and MAPK1 Gene Amplification in Type II Ovarian Carcinomas. *Int J Mol Sci.*, 2013, 14(7), 13748-13762.

[28] Hou, JY; Rodriguez Gubin, A; Samaweera, L; Hazan, R; Goldberg, GL; Horwitz, SB; McDaid HM. *Exploiting MEK inhibitor-mediated activation of ERα for therapeutic intervention in ER-positive ovarian carcinoma.*, 2013, 8(2), e54103.

[29] Farley, J; Brady, WE; Vathipadiekal, V; Lankes, HA; Coleman, R; Morgan, MA; Mannel, R; Yamada, SD; Mutch, D; Rodgers, WH; Birrer, M; Gershenson, DM. Selumetinib in women with recurrent low-grade serous carcinoma of the ovary or peritoneum: an open-label, single-arm, phase 2 study. *Lancet Oncol.*, 2013, 14(2), 134-140.

[30] Cossa, G; Lanzi, C; Cassinelli, G; Carenini, N; Arrighetti, N; Gatti, L; Corna, E; Zunino, F; Zaffaroni, N; Perego, P. Differential outcome of MEK1/2 inhibitor-platinum combinations in platinum-sensitive and -resistant ovariancarcinoma cells. *Cancer Lett.*, 2014, 347(2), 212-224.

[31] Bedard, PL; Tabernero, J; Janku, F; Wainberg, ZA; Paz-Ares, L; Vansteenkiste, J; Van Cutsem, E; Pérez-García, J; Stathis, A; Britten, CD; Le, N; Carter , K; Demanse, D; Csonka, D; Peters, M; Zubel, A; Nauwelaerts, H; Sessa, C. A phase Ib dose-escalation study of the oral pan-PI3K inhibitor buparlisib (BKM120) in combination with the oral MEK1/2 inhibitor trametinib (GSK1120212) in patients with selected advanced solid tumors. *Clin Cancer Res.*, 2015, 21(4), 730-738.

[32] Samartzis, EP; Noske, A; Dedes, KJ; Fink, D; Imesch, P. ARID1A mutations and PI3K /AKT pathway alterations in endometriosis and endometriosis-associated ovariancarcinomas. *Int J Mol Sci.*, 2013, 14(9), 18824-18849.

[33] Kim, HS; Kim, TH; Chung, HH; Song, YS. Risk and prognosis of ovarian cancer in women with endometriosis: a meta-analysis. *Br J Cancer.*, 2014, 110(7), 1878-1890.

[34] Sato, N; Tsunoda, H; Nishida, M; Morishita, Y; Takimoto, Y; Kubo, T; Noguchi, M. Loss of heterozygosity on 10q23.3 and mutation of the tumor suppressor gene PTEN in benign endometrial cyst of the ovary: possible sequence progression from benign endometrial cyst to endometrioid carcinoma and clearcell carcinoma of the ovary. *Cancer Res.*, 2000, 60(24), 7052-7056.

[35] Wu, R; Hendrix-Lucas, N; Kuick, R; Zhai, Y; Schwartz, DR; Akyol, A; Hanash, S; Misek, DE; Katabuchi, H; Williams, BO; Fearon, ER; Cho, KR. Mouse model of human ovarian endometrioid adenocarcinoma based on somatic defects in the Wnt/beta-catenin and PI3K/Pten signaling pathways. *Cancer Cell.*, 2007, 11(4), 321-333.

[36] Samartzis, EP; Gutsche, K; Dedes, KJ; Fink, D; Stucki, M; Imesch, P. *Loss of ARID1A expression sensitizes cancer cells to PI3K- and AKT-inhibition.*, 2014, 5(14), 5295-5303.

[37] Catasus, L; Gallardo, A; Cuatrecasas, M; Prat, J. PIK3CA mutations in the kinase domain (exon 20) of uterine endometrial adenocarcinomas are associated with adverse prognostic parameters. *Mod Pathol*, 2008, 21(2), 131–139.

[38] Yokoyama, Y; Matsushita, Y; Shigeto, T; Futagami, M; Mizunuma, H. Decreased ARID1A expression is correlated with chemoresistance in epithelial ovarian cancer. *J Gynecol Oncol.*, 2014, 25(1), 58-63.

[39] Yamamoto, S; Tsuda, H; Takano, M; Tamai, S; Matsubara, O. PIK3CA mutations and loss of ARID1A protein expression are early events in the development of cystic ovarianclear cell adenocarcinoma. *Virchows Arch.*, 2012, 460(1), 77-87.

[40] P, JG; R, VC; P, KM; Narasimhan, L. Primary ovarian mucinous carcinoma with signet ring cells - report of a rare case. *J Clin Diagn Res.*, 2014, 8(6), FD12-13.

[41] Garrett, AP; Lee, KR; Colitti, CR; Muto, MG; Berkowitz, RS; Mok, SC. K-ras mutation may be an early event in mucinous ovarian tumorigenesis. *Int J Gynecol Pathol.*, 2001, 20(3), 244-251.

[42] Biskup, K; Braicu, EI; Sehouli, J; Tauber, R; Blanchard, V. The serum glycome to discriminate between early-tage epithelial ovarian cancer and benign ovarian diseases. *Dis Markers.*, 2014, 2014, 238197.

[43] Grendys, EC Jr; Fiorica, JV; Orr, JW Jr; Holloway, R; Wang, D; Tian, C; Chan, JK; Herzog, TJ. Overview of a chemoresponse assay in ovarian cancer. *Clin Transl Oncol.*, 2014, 16(9), 761-769.

[44] Du Bois, A; Lück, HJ; Meier, W; Adams, HP; Möbus, V; Costa, S; Bauknecht, T; Richter, B; Warm, M; Schröder, W; Olbricht, S; Nitz, U; Jackisch, C; Emons, G; Wagner, U; Kuhn, W; Pfisterer, J. Arbeitsgemeinschaft Gynäkologische Onkologie Ovarian Cancer Study Group. A randomized clinical trial of cisplatin/paclitaxel versus carboplatin/paclitaxel as first-line treatment of ovarian cancer. *J Natl Cancer Inst.*, 2003, 95(17), 1320–1329.

[45] Bookman, MA; Brady, MF; McGuire, WP; Harper, PG; Alberts, DS; Friedlander, M; Colombo, N; Fowler, JM; Argenta, PA; De Geest, K; Mutch, DG; Burger, RA; Swart, AM; Trimble, EL; Accario-Winslow, C; Roth, LM. Evaluation of new platinum-based treatment regimens in advanced stage ovarian cancer: a Phase III Trial of the Gynecologic Cancer Intergroup. *J ClinOncol.*, 2009, 27(9), 1419–1425.

[46] Yoshida, H; Yabuno, A; Fujiwara, K. Critical appraisal of bevacizumab in the treatment of ovarian cancer. *Drug Des Devel Ther.*, 2015, 9, 2351-2358.

[47] Davidson, BA; Secord, AA. Profile of pazopanib and its potential in the treatment of epithelial ovarian cancer. *Int J Womens Health.*, 2014, 6, 289-300.

[48] Du Bois, A; Vergote, I; Wimberger, P; Ray-Coquard, I; Harter, P; Curtis, LB; Mitrica I. Open-label feasibility study of pazopanib, carboplatin, and paclitaxel in women with newly diagnosed, untreated, gynaecologic tumours: a phase I/II trial of the AGO study group. *Br J Cancer.*, 2012, 106(4), 629–632.

[49] Du Bois, A; Floquet, A; Kim, JW; Rau, J; Del Campo, JM; Friedlander, M; Pignata, S; Fujiwara, K; Vergote, I; Colombo, N; Mirza, MR; Monk, BJ; Kimmig, R; Ray-Coquard, I; Zang, R; Diaz-Padilla, I; Baumann, KH; Mouret-Reynier, MA; Kim, JH; Kurzeder, C; Lesoin, A; Vasey, P; Marth, C; Canzler, U; Scambia, G; Shimada, M; Calvert, P; Pujade-Lauraine, E; Kim; BG; Herzog, TJ; Mitrica, I; Schade-Brittinger, C; Wang, Q; Crescenzo, R; Harter, P. Incorporation of pazopanib in maintenance therapy of ovarian cancer. *J ClinOncol.*, 2014, 32(30), 3374-3382.

[50] Fong, PC; Boss, DS; Yap, TA; Tutt, A; Wu, P; Mergui-Roelvink, M; Mortimer, P; Swaisland, H; Lau, A; O'Connor, MJ; Ashworth, A; Carmichael, J; Kaye, SB; Schellens, JH; de Bono, JS. Inhibition of poly(ADP-ribose) polymerase in tumors from BRCA mutation carriers. *N Engl J Med*, 2009, 361(2), 123–134.

[51] Audeh, MW; Carmichael, J; Penson, RT; Friedlander, M; Powell, B; Bell-McGuinn, KM; Scott, C; Weitzel, JN; Oaknin, A; Loman, N; Lu, K; Schmutzler, RK; Matulonis, U; Wickens, M; Tutt, A. Oral poly(ADP-ribose) polymerase inhibitor olaparib in patients with BRCA1 or BRCA2 mutations and recurrent ovarian cancer: a proof-of-concept trial. *Lancet*, 2010, 376(9737), 245–251.

[52] Frampton, JE. Olaparib: a review of its use as maintenance therapy in patients with ovarian cancer. *BioDrugs.*, 2015, 29(2), 143-150.

[53] Ledermann, J; Harter, P; Gourley, C; Friedlander, M; Vergote, I; Rustin, G; Scott, CL; Meier, W; Shapira-Frommer, R; Safra, T; Matei, D; Fielding, A; Spencer, S; Dougherty, B; Orr, M; Hodgson, D; Barrett, JC; Matulonis, U. Olaparib maintenance therapy in patients with platinum-sensitive relapsed serous ovarian cancer: a preplanned retrospective analysis of outcomes by BRCA status in a randomised phase 2 trial. *Lancet Oncol.*, 2014, 15(8), 852-861.

[54] Sheppard, KE; Cullinane, C; Hannan, KM; Wall, M; Chan, J; Barber, F; Foo, J; Cameron, D; Neilsen, A; Ng, P; Ellul, J; Kleinschmidt, M; Kinross, KM; Bowtell, DD; Christensen, JG; Hicks, RJ; Johnstone, RW; McArthur, GA; Hannan, RD; Phillips, WA; Pearson, RB. Synergistic inhibition of ovarian cancer cell growth by combining selective PI3K/mTOR and RAS/ERK pathwayinhibitors. *Eur J Cancer.*, 2013, 49(18), 3936-3944.

[55] Liu, P; Cheng, H; Roberts, TM; Zhao, JJ. Targeting the phosphoinositide 3-kinase pathway in cancer. *Nat Rev DrugDiscov*, 2009, 8(8), 627–644.

[56] Markman, B; Dienstmann, R; Tabernero, J. *Targeting thePI3K/Akt/mTOR pathway—beyond rapalogs. Oncotarget*, 2010, 1(7), 530–543.

[57] Garon, EB; Finn, RS; Hosmer, W; Dering, J; Ginther, C; Adhami, S; Kamranpour, N; Pitts, S; Desai, A; Elashoff, D; French, T; Smith, P; Slamon, DJ. Identification of common predictive markers of in vitro response to the Mek inhibitor selumetinib (AZD6244; ARRY-142886) in human breast cancer and non-small cell lung cancer cell lines. *Mol Cancer Ther*, 2010, 9(7), 1985–1994.

[58] Yeh, JJ; Routh, ED; Rubinas, T; Peacock, J; Martin, TD; Shen, XJ; Sandler, RS; Kim, HJ; Keku, TO; Der, CJ. KRAS/BRAF mutation status and ERK1/2 activation as biomarkers for MEK1/2 inhibitor therapy in colorectal cancer. *Mol Cancer Ther*, 2009, 8(4), 834–843.

[59] Nakayama, N; Nakayama, K; Yeasmin, S; Ishibashi, M; Katagiri, A; Iida, K; Fukumoto, M; Miyazaki, K. KRAS or BRAF mutation status is a useful predictor of sensitivity to MEK inhibition in ovarian cancer. *Br J Cancer*, 2008, 99(12), 2020–2028.

[60] Husseinzadeh, N; Husseinzadeh, HD. mTOR inhibitors and their clinical application in cervical, endometrial and ovarian cancers: a critical review. *Gynecol Oncol.*, 2014, 133(2), 375-381.

[61] Behbakht, K; Sill, MW; Darcy, KM; Rubin, SC; Mannel, RS; Waggoner, S; Schilder, RJ; Cai, KQ; Godwin, AK; Alpaugh, RK. Phase II trial of the mTOR inhibitor, temsirolimus and evaluation of circulating tumor cells and tumor biomarkers in persistent and recurrent epithelial ovarian and primary peritoneal malignancies: a Gynecologic Oncology Group study. *Gynecol Oncol.*, 2011, 123(1), 19–26.

[62] Cagnol, S; Chambard, JC. ERK and cell death: mechanisms of ERK-induced cell death–apoptosis, autophagy and senescence. *FEBS J.*, 2010, 277(1), 2–21.

[63] Katagiri, A; Nakayama, K; Rahman, MT; Rahman, M; Yeasmin, S; Ishikawa, M; Iida, K; Nakayama, N; Miyazaki, K. MEK inhibition suppresses cell invasion and migration in ovarian cancers with activation of ERK1/2. *Exp Ther Med.*, 2010, 1(4), 591-596.

[64] Borman, SM; Christian, PJ; Sipes, IG; Hoyer, PB. Ovotoxicity in female fischer rats and b6 mice induced by low-dose exposure to three polycyclic aromatic hydrocarbons:

Comparison through calculation of an ovotoxic index. *Toxicol Appl Pharmacol.*, 2000, 167(3), 191–198.

[65] Sobinoff, AP; Nixon, B; Roman, SD; McLaughlin, EA. Staying alive: Pi3k pathway promotes primordial follicle activation and survival in response to 3mc-induced ovotoxicity. *Toxicol Sci*, 2012, 128(1), 258–271.

[66] Kurman, RJ; Shih, IeM. *The origin and pathogenesis of epithelial ovarian cancer: a proposed unifying theory.*, 2010, 34(3), 433-443.

[67] Wu, R; Hu, TC; Rehemtulla, A; Fearon, ER; Cho, KR. Preclinical testing of pi3k/akt/mtor signaling inhibitors in a mouse model of ovarian endometrioid adenocarcinoma. *Clin. Cancer Res.*, 2011, 17(23), 7359–7372.

[68] Kinross, KM; Montgomery, KG; Kleinschmidt, M; Waring, P; Ivetac, I; Tikoo, A; Saad, M; Hare, L; Roh, V; Mantamadiotis, T; Sheppard, KE; Ryland, GL; Campbell, IG; Gorringe, KL; Christensen, JG; Cullinane, C; Hicks, RJ; Pearson, RB; Johnstone, RW; McArthur, GA; Phillips, WA. An activating pik3ca mutation coupled with pten loss is sufficient to initiate ovarian tumorigenesis in mice. *J. Clin. Investig.*, 2012, 122(2), 553–557.

[69] Cancer Genome Atlas Research Network. Integrated genomic analyses of ovarian carcinoma. *Nature*, 2011, 474 (7353), 609–615.

In: Handbook on Ovarian Cancer
Editor: Bethany R. Collier
ISBN: 978-1-63483-874-0


*Chapter 12*

# PRIMARY CYTOREDUCTION IN EPHITELIAL OVARIAN CANCER

***E. Delgado, M. Martín-Cameán and I. Zapardiel****
Gynecologic Oncology Unit, La Paz University Hospital, Madrid, Spain

## ABSTRACT

Worldwide, ovarian cancer is the seventh cancer in frequency and the eighth cause of death from cancer in women. Epithelial ovarian cancer is also the leading cause of death among gynaecologic malignancies. Nowadays, the standard management of epithelial ovarian cancer is the correct surgical staging and optimal tumor cytoreduction followed by platinum plus taxane-based chemotherapy. Standard surgical treatment for early stages consists on peritoneal washings, total hysterectomy and bilateral anexectomy, inspection all organs and peritoneum surface, taking samples of suspicious areas, omentectomy and pelvic and para-aortic lymphadenectomy. Laparoscopic approach allows to do this surgical staging with less morbidity and mortality than a more aggressive laparotomy approach. After this complete surgical staging, the International Federation of Gynaecology and Obstetrics (FIGO) staging system for ovarian cancer ought to be applied to determine the management and prognosis of the patient. In advanced stages complete tumor cytoreduction has demonstrated survival advantage compared to incomplete debulking. The morbidity associated with the debulking surgery does not increase mortality. However, some patients with advanced epithelial ovarian cancer undergo debulking surgery but complete cytoreduction is not achieved, with an increase of the morbidity and no improvement in overall survival. There are some criteria to predict the cytoreduction outcomes, based on serum biomarkers levels, preoperative imaging techniques and laparoscopic based scores. Optimization of patient selection for primary cytoreduction would determine which patients could benefit from a complete cytoreduction or which ones might benefit from neoadjuvant chemotherapy and interval surgery.

* Corresponding author: Ignacio Zapardiel, Gynecologic Oncology Unit, La Paz University Hospital, Madrid, Spain, ignaciozapardiel@hotmail.com.

## INTRODUCTION

Worldwide, epithelial ovarian cancer (EOC) is the seventh most common cancer and the eight cause of death from cancer between women (3.6% of cases and 4.6% of deaths) [1]. In USA, ovarian cancer is the second most common gynecological malignancy and the most deadly with an estimated 21290 new cases and 14180 deaths in 2015 [2-4]. The incidence increases with age, so most of them are diagnosed in women between 40 and 65 years [5]. In Europe is the fourth most common gynecologic cancer with an incidence varying from 6 to 14 per 100,000 person-years [6]. This elevated death rate is due to its indolent course and screening methods which are ineffective. 60% of the EOC are diagnosed at an advanced stage (stages IIB to IV), with a median age at diagnosis of 63 years [4, 7-9]. The advanced-stage ovarian cancer has a 5-year survival rate of 30-55% compared to early stages where 5-year survival exceeds 80% [4]. In Europe, only a third of women are alive at five years from diagnosis [10]. In young patients, EOC seems to be associated with better prognosis: higher overall and progression-free survival, higher platinum sensitivity rate and a better clinical outcome [5].

There are several types of ovarian carcinoma, but the most frequent of all of them is the epithelial ovarian carcinoma, which represents the 95% of the ovarian neoplasias. The rest derive from other ovarian cells (germ cell tumors, sex cord-stromal tumors) [4]. EOC is also the most frequent cause of death from gynecological neoplasias [5, 6, 9-11].

It is described some risk factors associated with ovarian cancer. One established risk factor is nulliparity, with childless-women having between a two-three increased risk compared to parous women. Patients with endometriosis, history of pelvic inflammatory disease and ovulatory abnormalities such us polycystic ovarian syndrome also show high risk of EOC [12].

A woman risk's of developing ovarian cancer at the age of 75 varies by countries, between 0.5-1.6% [10]. Women with BRCA1 and BRCA2 mutation have higher risk of developing ovarian cancer (36-46% and 10-27% respectively) [4].

The origin and pathogenesis of EOC remains unclear. Several studies tried to identify precursors of the ovarian neoplasia, without success. This has led the proposal that ovarian cancer develops the novo [13]. Another pathological mechanisms suggested are the differentiation of ovarian surface epithelium or because of distal fallopian tube cells, which reach the ovary during ovulation [11].

We can distinguish to different types of ovarian neoplasia [13]: type I (low-grade serous, low-grade endometrioid, clear cell, and mucinous), which constitute the 25% of the ovarian cancers and 10% of the ovarian cancer deaths; and type II (high-grade serous and undifferentiated carcinomas, and malignant mixed mesodermal tumors) which represent the 75% of the ovarian cancers and are responsible of the 90% of ovarian cancer deaths.

The methods that are currently being used to screen women are pelvis examination, transvaginal ultrasound and measurement of serum CA 125 [13], but they are not effective in detecting all the different types of ovarian carcinoma. Type I are easily detected by pelvic examination or transvaginal ultrasound. They grow slowly and have a big size even when they are still confined to the ovary. Type II should be targeted for screening but they are confined to the ovary only the 0.5% of the cases at the moment of diagnosis [10]. A multiinstitutional prospective study showed the futility of the screening: despite annual screening with CA 125 and transvaginal ultrasound, 70% of the women presented advanced ovarian cancer, similar to the unscreened population [14].

To perform a correct staging procedure is important to know the spread pattern of ovarian carcinoma [14, 15]. Ovarian cancer arises within the ovarian surface epithelium, grows focally, and ultimately breaches the ovarian capsule and metastasizes by exfoliation or by the abdominal or pelvic lymphatic system. Cancer cells spread into the fluid initially implant throughout the pelvis and right paracolic gutters and across the right diaphragm and gastrointestinal organs.

## PREOPERATIVE EVALUATION

In specialized ovarian cancer centers, the surgeon precise preoperative evaluation of the tumor burden and metastatic disease in order to plan a multivisceral surgery and have an idea if it will be possible to achieve complete resection of the tumor [16].

There are strong recommendations to do a correct preoperative evaluation [17] with complete anamnesis (aiming to identify risk factors of ovarian cancer), physic and pelvic examination, transvaginal and abdominal sonography, serum tumor biomarkers, abdominopelvic CT or MRI (to evaluate pelvic and abdominal extension of the disease). Henrich et al. [16 demonstrated in a prospective study the predictive value of preoperative staging of transvaginal sonography (TVS), and they suggested that it should be done by routine. It is cost-effective, safe and easily available, compared to other imaging modalities. It decreases the number of unnecessary surgeries because it allows the differentiation between benign and malignant disease, and it makes the decision of doing laparoscopy or laparotomy easier and more accurate. It can assess precisely the size of the tumor, the presence of uterine or bladder invasion, peritoneal invasion and the presence of ascites. It is not reliable to prove intestinal invasion, but CT and MRI have similar limitations.

## CURRENT MANAGEMENT

Nowadays, the standard management of epithelial ovarian cancer is the complete surgical tumor cytoreduction followed by platinum and taxane-based chemotherapy in advanced stages [1, 10, 17-19].

For early stages standard surgical staging consists on peritoneal washings, total hysterectomy and bilateral anexectomy, inspection all organs and peritoneum surface, taking samples of suspicious areas, omentectomy and pelvic and para-aortic lymphadenectomy [17]. After this surgical staging, the International Federation of Gynecology and Obstetrics (FIGO) staging system for ovarian cancer ought to be applied to determine the management and prognosis of the patient. There is a new ovarian cancer staging approved since 1 January 2014, shown in table 1 [20]. Approximately, from 16% to 35% of the ovarian cancer, which were presumed to be an early stage, are later upstaged [21].

However, in advanced stages, if complete primary cytoreduction is impossible to achieve due to the extension of the disease or poor conditions, the treatment could be neoadjuvant chemotherapy followed by interval debulking surgery [2, 17-19, 22-24].

The group of Aletti et al. [1] identified a subgroup of patients who might benefit from neoadjuvant chemotherapy depending on the preoperative characteristics of the patients: high tumor dissemination or stage IV, poor performance status (ASA $\geq$ 3) or nutritional status (preoperative albumin levels $\geq$ 3.0 g/dL), and age $\geq$ 75 years. In this group the benefit of aggressive surgery does not appear to outweigh the risk. The consideration should be given to a primary neoadjuvant approach, in order to do a surgical procedure safer in those who respond to chemotherapy.

A randomized study carried out by Vergote et al. [24] showed no differences in mortality between the groups who underwent incomplete primary cytoreduction and the one with neoadjuvant treatment before surgery. The median overall survival was 29 months and 30 months respectively. The median progression free survival was 12 months for both groups. However, the overall survival was higher in the group who achieved complete primary surgery. The most frequent sites for residual disease after primary or interval surgery are the diaphragm, the abdominal peritoneum and the pelvis (pouch of Douglas, uterus, bladder, rectum and sigmoid).

## PRIMARY CYTOREDUCTION

There are three main types of advanced ovarian cancer surgery [17]: primary cytoreduction (its objective is to remove the higher tumor mass before any other treatment), interval surgery (used in patients who benefit from neoadjuvant chemotherapy before surgery), and secondary surgery (for tumor relapses).

Primary debulking surgery is performed to achieve complete cytoreduction, because the amount of residual tumor is the most important prognostic factor in overall survival [1, 2, 10, 18, 19, 22-24]. It consists on removing completely all visible tumor, including when necessary splenectomy, diaphragmatic resection, liver resection, intestinal resection or any other abdominal organ surgery affected [25, 26]. Intestinal resection is one of the most common procedures in advanced ovarian cancer and it is performed up to 50% of complete cytoreduction surgery, specially the rectosigmoid segment [2].

The definition of optimal and suboptimal cytoreduction change between different studies [10], which make comparisons difficult between them [19]. Zapardiel el al. [27] described a new terminology for cytoreduction in advanced ovarian cancer, and made three groups, according to relevant terms of survival: no macroscopic disease, macroscopic disease less than 1 cm, and macroscopic disease higher than 1 cm. the three groups could be referred to as complete resection, minimal residual and gross residual, respectively.

Complete cytoreduction is the most important prognostic factor. The amount of disease after the surgery is a strong predictor of survival [2, 10, 17, 19]. It is better as predictor of survival than the extent of metastatic disease before the surgery [1, 19]. Two studies [10] showed that each 10% increase in maximal cytoreduction was associated with a 5.5% increase in median survival. Several studies from the Gynecologic Oncology Group (GOG), GOG 52 and 97,showed that those patients with no residual disease had a 5-year survival rate of 60%, compared with 35% and < 20% of those with 0.1-1 or 1-2 cm residual disease, respectively [19]. Another GOG trials (111, 114, 132, 152, 158, 162 and 172) showed that complete resection (R0 resection) had the longest median overall survival (64 months versus

29 months for patients with < 1 cm disease) [19]. Another European prospective randomized studies [19] showed R0 resection was associated with 99.1 months of survival versus 36.2 months for < 1cm of residual disease. It is also correlated with the success of the chemotherapy applied after the surgery [10]. With debulking surgery, poorly vascularized tumor is removed, where the chemotherapeutic agents have poorly access. It also remove chemoresistant clones which are less susceptible to chemotherapy [2]. Radical surgery also reduces the risk of recurrence in a 30% [19].

Another factor related to survival is the surgeon's experience [1, 17]. Surgery performed by general surgeons or general gynecologist has lower survival outcomes than the one performed by gynecologist trained in gynecological oncology [2, 10]. Reported rates of complete cytoreduction vary widely in the literature, from 15 to 75% [18]. Several meta-analyses in USA have demonstrated an average complete cytoreduction rate of 42% [19].

The morbidity associated with complete debulking surgery does not increase the mortality [2]. Postoperative mortality of debulking surgery has been reported between 1% and 6% in several series [10]. Major surgical complications are: hemorrhage, thromboembolic disease, infection, myocardial infarction, bowel obstruction, visceral injuries, fistulae and wound breakdown [10]. However, the morbidity and mortality of primary surgery tends to be higher than in interval cytoreduction [24].

## PREDICTING INCOMPLETE DEBULKING

Some patients with advanced EOC undergo debulking surgery but complete cytoreduction is not achieved. Patients with incomplete resection will not experience the maximum advantage in survival and will have an increase of the morbidity [2, 22, 23].

Predicting which patients will have an incomplete cytoreduction could allow avoiding aggressive and unnecessary surgeries for patients who will benefit from neoadjuvant chemotherapy [2, 22, 23]. There are some criteria which help the surgeon to predict the results of debulking surgery, based on physical examination, preoperative imaging, serum biomarker levels and laparoscopic scores [2, 19].

CA-125 serum levels is one of the most studied parameters. They are elevated in more than 90% of the patients with advanced ovarian carcinoma [19]. Many studies identified the cut-off point of CA-125 in ≥ 500 to predict optimal cytoreduction [18, 19]. A follow up study showed that CA-125 was a predictor of upper abdominal disease and, if upper radical surgery is performed, it is not necessary associated with incomplete debulking [18]. However, other studies have shown conflicting results. A recent meta-analysis concluded that although a CA-125≥ 500 U/mL was a strong risk factor for incomplete debulking, it lacked the accuracy to independently predict surgical outcome, so it should be used in combination with other criteria to decide clinical management.

The group of Suidan et al. [18], in a prospective non-randomized study, found 3 clinical and 6 radiological criteria associated with suboptimal cytoreduction: age ≥ 60 years (OR 1.32), CA-125 ≥ 500 U/mL (OR 1.47), ASA 3-4 (OR 3.23), retroperitoneal lymph nodes above the renal hilum (including supradiaphragmatic) > 1cm (OR 1.59), diffuse small bowel adhesions/thickening (OR 1.87), periesplenic lesion > 1cm (OR 2.27), small bowel mesentery lesion > 1cm (OR 2.28), root of the superior mesenteric artery lesion > 1cm (OR 2.4), lesser sac lesion > 1cm (OR 4.61). Certain factors were more predictive than others, so they gave a predictive value score to each one. Age ≥ 60 years, CA-125 ≥ 500 U/mL, retroperitoneal lymph nodes above the renal hilum (including supradiaphragmatic) > 1cm and diffuse small bowel adhesions/thickening were each assigned a predictive value score of 1. Periesplenic lesion > 1cm, small bowel mesentery lesion > 1cm and root of the superior mesenteric artery lesion > 1cm had a predictive value score of 2. ASA 3-4 was assigned a value of 3, and lesser sac lesions > 1 cm a value of 4 (this suggests that in patients with disease that is extensive enough to involve the lesser sac, the disease has likely spread to several other anatomic locations as well.). Patients with a score of 0 (without criteria) had an incomplete resection rate of 5%. The incomplete resection rate of patients who had a score of 1–2, 3–4, 5–6, and 7–8 were 10%, 17%, 34%, and 52%, respectively. The highest incomplete resection rate, 74%, was found among patients who had a score of 9 or greater.

Fotopoulou et al. [28] identified that, in patients with advanced EOC, complete debulking surgery is more likely to be achieved if the tumor does not affect more than 4 abdominal fields. The fields more related to incomplete surgery are middle abdomen including radix mesentery and splenic (or left colic) flexure as well as the upper abdomen in the region of the porta hepatis. Moreover, this study did not show relation between the CA 125 levels, ascites or the FIGO stage with the resectability of the disease. Patients in whom R0 resection is unlikely to be achieved should be considered for neoadjuvant chemotherapy [17-19, 22-24], as explanied before.

## LAPAROSCOPY VS LAPAROTOMY

Minimally invasive surgery has improved over the last few years and is frequently used in gynecologic surgery. Many researchers have demonstrated that laparoscopic approach allows doing surgical staging with less morbidity and mortality than a more aggressive laparotomy approach [21, 29-33].

The patient treated with minimally invasive surgery can benefit from less adhesion formation, shorter hospitalization and minor postoperative complications compared to laparotomy [21, 29, 30, 32]. The volume of blood loss is decreased in laparoscopic and robotic surgery [29-32] so transfusion rates in both groups is lower [31]. Pain scores of the robotic and laparoscopic groups are also lower [31]. Laparoscopic approach is also advantageous when fertility preservation is desired because of the lower rate of adhesions compared to laparotomy [21], which is decreased until a 60% [33]. Patients treated with laparoscopy primary cytoreduction are able to undergo also laparoscopic secondary cytoreduction because of minimal postoperative adhesions (33). These benefits allow the patient to start the chemotherapy treatment earlier.

The overall survival, median survival and median progression-free survival is similar in patients treated with laparoscopic, robotic or laparotomic surgery [30, 32, 33].

It has been argued, related to laparoscopic surgery, the accuracy of surgical staging, the possibility of tumor spillage and port-site metastasis. However, many studies have solved these issues. Laparoscopy offers an excellent vision of the peritoneal surface, even better than direct vision during laparotomy. Certain areas are difficult to investigate for laparoscopy as well as at laparotomy [29, 32]. The risk of tumor spillage due to intraoperative mass rupture has not been supported by any prospective comparative study. Finally, the risk of port site implants is less than 1% in laparoscopy, and can be reduced by the use of laparoscopy bag [21, 29] and the initiation of chemotherapy in the early postoperative period [30].

The operative time is higher in laparoscopy than with the laparotomy approach in most of the studies [21, 29, 30, 33]. Although the higher is the surgeon's experience in laparoscopy the lower is the operative time. In fact, the group of Ching-Hui et al. [31] showed an operation time reduced in laparoscopic and roboctic surgery compared to laparotomy.

All these studies reveal that laparoscopy is feasible, safe and preferable for the staging and surgical treatment of early stage EOC compared to the gold standard laparotomic approach, with similar oncologic results.

## Conservative Treatment and Fertility Preservation

It is considered that 3-17% of all epithelial ovarian cancers occur in women under the age of 40 years [8] . As a result of late childbearing nowadays, there are cases of women in reproductive age with ovarian cancer who have not fulfilled their reproductive desires. In order to give a hope for conception to this patients, fertility-sparing surgery (FSS) have been successfully attempted in selected women with early ovarian cancer [34-39].

There are no unanimous consensus on which are the criteria for selecting this patients for a conservative surgery. According to the ESGO guidelines, patients should fulfill specific characteristics: patients younger than 40 years old, they should be referred to a tertiary center, patients should be compliant with a close follow-up during and after treatment in order to detect contralateral ovarian recurrence or uterine malignancy and should undergo an adequate staging, and pathology should be carried out by a designated gynecologic pathologist.

Many authors [34-37, 39, 40] agree that the optimal candidates to FSS are those with stage IA EOC with favorable histology (mucinous, serous, endometrioid or mixed histology) and grade 1 or 2. Patients with grade 3 or clear-cell histology of ovarian cancer should be excluded from a conservative surgery.

It is demonstrated [34, 36, 38, 39] that the recurrence rate in patients treated with EOC is similar to the one in patients who undergo radical comprehensive staging (RCS). In addition, the relapses in the FSS group occur in the residual ovary in 50% of the patients [34, 39], which can be managed successfully with surgery and chemotherapy. The type of surgery (FSS vs RCS) do not influence in DFS and OS [34, 36, 37].

Fertility sparing surgery includes unilateral salpingo-oophorectomy on the side of the ovarian tumor and complete staging including peritoneal sampling, pelvic and para-aortic lymph node disection and omentectomy [8]. A laparoscopic approach has been indicated for FSS due to reduced adhesion formation, which could also help for future fertility [8, 21, 38].

These patients are treated with carboplatin and paclitaxel, which are in less gonadotoxic compared to other cytostatics [8], under the concomitant ovarian protection with GnRH analogs (35). Several studies (8, 21) reflect the good obstetrical results after fertility sparing surgery with a pregnancy rate between 38 and 100% [8, 34, 39] and abortion rate under 30%.

We can conclude that fertility conservative treatment has oncological results comparable to radical surgery, so it is a safe option that can be offered in selected patients with EOC and reproductive desire [8, 34].

**Table 1. FIGO 2014 ovarian cancer staging [20]**

| | | |
|---|---|---|
| **STAGE I: Tumor confined to ovaries** | | |
| IA | Tumor limited to 1 ovary, capsule intact, no tumor on surface, negative washings | |
| IB | Tumor involves both ovaries otherwise like IA | |
| IC : Tumor limited to 1 or both ovaries | | |
| IC1 | Surgical spill | |
| IC2 | Capsule rupture before surgery or tumor on ovarian surface | |
| IC3 | Malignant cells in the ascites or peritoneal washings | |
| **STAGE II: Tumor involves 1 or both ovaries with pelvic extension (below the pelvic brim) or primary peritoneal cancer** | | |
| IIA | Extension and/or implant on uterus and/or Fallopian tubes | |
| IIB | Extension to other pelvic intraperitoneal tissues | |
| **STAGE III: Tumor involves 1 or both ovaries with cytologically or histologically confirmed spread to the peritoneum outside the pelvis and/or metastasis to the retroperitoneal lymph nodes** | | |
| IIIA: Positive retroperitoneal lymph nodes and/or microscopic metastasis beyond the pelvis) | | |
| IIIA1 | Positive retroperitoneal lymph nodes only | |
| | IIIA1(i) | Metastasis ≤ 10 mm |
| | IIIA1 (ii) | Metastasis > 10 mm |
| IIIA2 | Microscopic, extrapelvic (above the brim) peritoneal involvement ± positive retroperitoneal lymph nodes | |
| IIIB | Macroscopic, extrapelvic, peritoneal metastasis ≤ 2 cm ± positive retroperitoneal lymph nodes. Includes extension to capsule of liver/spleen | |
| IIIC | Macroscopic, extrapelvic, peritoneal metastasis > 2 cm ± positive retroperitoneal lymph nodes. Includes extension to capsule of liver/spleen | |
| **STAGE IV: Distant metastasis excluding peritoneal metastasis** | | |
| IVA | Pleural effusion with positive cytology | |
| IVB | Hepatic and/or splenic parenchymal metastasis, metastasis to extraabdominal organs (including inguinal lymph nodes and lymph nodes outside of the abdominal cavity) | |

## REFERENCES


[1] Aletti, GD; Eisenhauer, EL; Santillan, A; et al. Identification of patient groups at highest risk from traditional approach to ovarian cancer treatment. *Gynecol Oncol.*, 2011 Jan, 120(1), 23-8. doi: 10.1016/ j.ygy no.2010.09.010

[2] Narasimhulu, DM; Khoury-Collado, F; Chi, DS. Radical surgery in ovarian cancer. *Curr Oncol Rep.*, 2015 Apr, 17(4), 16. doi: 10.1007/ s 11912-015-0439-z.

[3] Siegel, RL; Miller, KD; Jemal, A. Cancer statistics, 2015. *See comment in PubMed Commons belowCA Cancer J Clin.* 2015 Jan-Feb, 65(1), 5-29. doi: 10.3322/caac.21254.

[4] Romanidis, K; Nagorni, EA; Halkia, E; et al. The role of cytoreductive surgery in advanced ovarian cancer: the general surgeon's perspective. *J BUON.*, 2014 Jul-Sep, 19(3), 598-604.

[5] Fotopoulou, C; Savvatis, K; Schumacher, G; et al. Surgical outcome and survival analysis of young patients with primary epithelial ovarian cancer. *Anticancer Res.*, 2009 Jul, 29(7), 2809-15.

[6] van Driel, WJ; Lok, CA; Verwaal, V; et al. The role of hyperthermic intraperitoneal intraoperative chemotherapy in ovarian cancer. *Curr Treat Options Oncol.*, 2015 Apr, 16(4), 14. doi: 10.1007/ s11864-015-0329-5.

[7] Horowitz, NS; Miller, A; Rungruang, B; et al. Does aggressive surgery improve outcomes? Interaction between preoperative disease burden and complex surgery in patients with advanced-stage ovarian cancer: an analysis of GOG 182. *See comment in PubMed Commons belowJ Clin Oncol.*, 2015 Mar 10, 33(8), 937-43. doi: 10.1200/JCO.2014.56.3106.

[8] Zapardiel, I; Diestro, MD; Aletti, G. Conservative treatment of early stage ovarian cancer: oncological and fertility outcomes. *Eur J Surg Oncol.*, 2014 Apr, 40(4), 387-93. doi: 10.1016/j.ejso.2013.11.028.

[9] Armstrong, DK; Bundy, B; Wenzel, L; et al. Intraperitoneal cisplatin and paclitaxel in ovarian cancer. *N Engl J Med.*, 2006 Jan 5, 354(1), 34-43.

[10] Elattar, A; Bryant, A; Winter-Roach, BA; et al. Optimal primary surgical treatment for advanced epithelial ovarian cáncer. *Cochrane Database Syst Rev.*, 2011 Aug 10, (8), CD007565. doi: 10.1002/14651858.

[11] Spiliotis, J; Halkia, E; Lianos, E; et al. Cytoreductive surgery and HIPEC in recurrent epithelial ovarian cancer: a prospective randomized phase III study. *Ann Surg Oncol.*, 2015 May, 22(5), 1570-5. doi: 10.1245/s10434-014-4157-9.

[12] Spiliotis, J; Halkia, E; Lianos, E; et al. Cytoreductive surgery and HIPEC in recurrent epithelial ovarian cancer: a prospective randomized phase III study. *Ann Surg Oncol.*, 2015 May, 22(5):1570-5. doi: 10.1245/s10434-014-4157-9.

[13] Kurman, RJ; Shih, IeM. The origin and pathogenesis of epithelial ovarian cancer: a proposed unifying theory. *Am J Surg Pathol.*, 2010 Mar, 34(3), 433-43. doi: 10.1097/PAS.

[14] Partridge, E; Kreimer, AR; Greenlee, RT; et al. Results from four rounds of ovarian cancer screening in a randomized trial. *Obstet Gynecol.*, 2009 Apr, 113(4), 775-82. doi: 10.1097/AOG.

[15] Fader, AN; Rose, PG. Role of surgery in ovarian carcinoma. *See comment in PubMed Commons belowJ Clin Oncol.*, 2007 Jul 10, 25(20), 2873-83.

[16] Henrich, W; Fotopoulou, C; Fuchs, I; Wolf, C; et al. Value of preoperative transvaginal sonography (TVS) in the description of tumor pattern in ovarian cancer patients: results of a prospective study. *Anticancer Res.*, 2007 Nov-Dec, 27(6C), 4289-94.

[17] Oncoguía SEGO: Cancer Epitelial de ovario, trompa y peritoneo 2014. Guías de práctica clínica en cáncer ginecológico y mamario. Publicaciones SEGO, Octubre 2014

[18] Suidan, RS; Ramirez, PT; Sarasohn, DM; et al. A multicenter prospective trial evaluating the ability of preoperative computed tomography scan and serum CA-125 to predict suboptimal cytoreduction at primary debulking surgery for advanced ovarian, fallopian tube, and peritoneal cáncer. *Gynecol Oncol.*, 2014 Sep, 134(3), 455-61. doi: 10.1016/j.ygyno.2014.07.002.

[19] Nick, AM; Coleman, RL; Ramirez, PT; et al. A framework for a personalized surgical approach to ovarian cancer. *Nat Rev Clin Oncol.*, 2015 Apr, 12(4), 239-45. doi: 10.1038/nrclinonc.2015.26.

[20] Mutch, DG; Prat, J. 2014 FIGO staging for ovarian, fallopian tube and peritoneal cáncer. *Gynecol Oncol.*, 2014 Jun, 133(3), 401-4. doi: 10.1016/j.ygyno.2014.04.013.

[21] Colomer, AT; Jiménez, AM; Bover Barceló, MI. Laparoscopic treatment and staging of early ovarian cancer. *J Minim Invasive Gynecol.*, 2008 Jul-Aug, 15(4), 414-9. doi: 10.1016/j.jmig.2008.04.002.

[22] Gómez-Hidalgo, NR; Martinez-Cannon, BA; Nick, AM; et al. Predictors of optimal cytoreduction in patients with newly diagnosed advanced-stage epithelial ovarian cancer: Time to incorporate laparoscopic assessment into the standard of care. *Gynecol Oncol.*, 2015 Jun, 137(3), 553-558. doi: 10.1016/j.ygyno.2015.03.049.

[23] Rutten, MJ; van de Vrie, R; Bruining, A; et al. Predicting surgical outcome in patients with International Federation of Gynecology and Obstetrics stage III or IV ovarian cancer using computed tomography: a systematic review of prediction models. *Int J Gynecol Cancer.*, 2015 Mar, 25(3), 407-15. doi: 10.1097/IGC.0000000000000368.

[24] Vergote, I; Tropé, CG; Amant, F; et al. Neoadjuvant chemotherapy or primary surgery in stage IIIC or IV ovarian cancer. *N Engl J Med.*, 2010 Sep 2, 363(10), 943-53. doi: 10.1056/NEJMoa0908806.

[25] Zapardiel, I; Peiretti, M; Zanagnolo, V; et al. Diaphragmatic surgery during primary cytoreduction for advanced ovarian cancer: peritoneal stripping versus diaphragmatic resection. *Int J Gynecol Cancer.*, 2011 Dec, 21(9), 1698-703. doi: 10.1097/IGC.

[26] Zapardiel, I; Peiretti, M; Zanagnolo, V; et al. Splenectomy as part of primary cytoreductive surgery for advanced ovarian cancer: a retrospective cohort study. *Int J Gynecol Cancer.*, 2012 Jul, 22(6), 968-73. doi: 10.1097/IGC.

[27] Zapardiel, I; Morrow, CP. New terminology for cytoreduction in advanced ovarian cancer. *Lancet Oncol.*, 2011 Mar, 12(3), 214. doi: 10.1016/S1470-2045(10)70292-8.

[28] Fotopoulou, C; Richter, R; Braicu, EI; et al. Can complete tumor resection be predicted in advanced primary epithelial ovarian cancer? A systematic evaluation of 360 consecutive patients. *Eur J Surg Oncol.*, 2010 Dec, 36(12), 1202-10. doi: 10.1016/j.ejso.2010.09.008.

[29] Ghezzi, F; Cromi, A; Uccella, S; et al. Laparoscopy versus laparotomy for the surgical management of apparent early stage ovarian cancer. *Gynecol Oncol.*, 2007 May, 105(2), 409-13.

[30] Magrina, JF; Zanagnolo, V; Noble, BN; et al. Robotic approach for ovarian cancer: perioperative and survival results and comparison with laparoscopy and laparotomy. *Gynecol Oncol.*, 2011 Apr, 121(1), 100-5. doi: 10.1016/j.ygyno.2010.11.045.

[31] Chen, CH; Chiu, LH; Chen, HH; et al. Comparison of robotic approach, laparoscopic approach and laparotomy in treating epithelial ovarian cáncer. *Int J Med Robot.*, 2015 Mar 25. doi: 10.1002/rcs.1655.

[32] Nezhat, FR; Pejovic, T; Finger, TN; et al. Role of minimally invasive surgery in ovarian cancer. *J Minim Invasive Gynecol.*, 2013 Nov-Dec, 20(6), 754-65. doi: 10.1016/j.jmig.2013.04.027.

[33] Fanning, J; Yacoub, E; Hojat, R. Laparoscopic-assisted cytoreduction for primary advanced ovarian cancer: success, morbidity and survival. *Gynecol Oncol.* 2011 Oct, 123(1), 47-9. doi: 10.1016/ j.ygyno. 2011. 06. 020.

[34] Ditto, A; Martinelli, F; Lorusso, D; et al. Fertility sparing surgery in early stage epithelial ovarian cancer. *J Gynecol Oncol.*, 2014 Oct, 25(4), 320-7. doi: 10.3802/jgo.2014.25.4.320.

[35] Fotopoulou, C; Braicu, I; Sehouli, J. Fertility-sparing surgery in early epithelial ovarian cancer: a viable option? *Obstet Gynecol Int.*, 2012, 2012, 238061. doi: 10.1155/2012/238061.

[36] Satoh, T; Hatae, M; Watanabe, Y; et al. Outcomes of fertility-sparing surgery for stage I epithelial ovarian cancer: a proposal for patient selection. *J Clin Oncol.*, 2010 Apr 1, 28(10), 1727-32. doi: 10.1200/ JCO.2009.24.8617.

[37] Ditto, A; Martinelli, F; Bogani, G; et al. Long-term safety of fertility sparing surgery in early stage ovarian cancer: Comparison to standard radical surgical procedures. *Gynecol Oncol.*, 2015 Jul, 138(1), 78-82. doi: 10.1016/j.ygyno.2015.05.004

[38] Cromi, A; Bogani, G; Uccella, S; et al. Laparoscopic fertility-sparing surgery for early stage ovarian cancer: a single-centre case series and systematic literature review. *J Ovarian Res.*, 2014 May 29, 7, 59. doi: 10.1186/1757-2215-7-59.

[39] Fruscio, R; Corso, S; Ceppi, L; et al. Conservative management of early-stage epithelial ovarian cancer: results of a large retrospective series. *Ann Oncol.*, 2013 Jan, 24(1), 138-44. doi: 10.1093/annonc/mds241.

[40] Liu, JH; Zanotti, KM. Management of the adnexal mass. *Obstet Gynecol.*, 2011 Jun, 117(6), 1413-28. doi: 10.1097/AOG.

In: Handbook on Ovarian Cancer
Editor: Bethany R. Collier

ISBN: 978-1-63483-874-0


*Chapter 13*

# Sensitizing Chemotherapy with Ultrasound

***Li Luo[1], Jinyan Li[1], Meijiao Wang[1], Lin Yu[2] and Tinghe Yu[1,*]***

[1]Key Medical Laboratory of Obstetrics and Gynecology,
The Second Affiliated Hospital, Chongqing Medical University, Chongqing, China
[2]Department of Otolaryngology, The First Affiliated Hospital,
Chongqing Medical University, Chongqing, China

## Abstract

Chemotherapy is limited by toxicity to noncancerous tissues and the development of chemoresistance. Here we discuss the use of low intensity ultrasound to modulate chemotherapy against ovarian cancer. Ultrasound can enhance the action of certain drugs, including circumvention of chemoresistance. Ultrasonic cavitation plays the leading role in sonochemotherapy, which permeabilizes the cell membrane favoring the influx of drugs. Recent trials suggest that ultrasound can modulate chemotherapy via multiple pathways, and synergize the sensitization due to a chemical modulator such as verapamil and cyclosporin A. Ultrasound can be efficiently delivered to the preselected volume within the body thus realizing a targeted therapy. This technique can be specifically developed as a non-drug technique to improve the therapeutic outcome of chemotherapy against ovarian cancer.

**Keywords:** Ultrasound, chemotherapy, chemoresistance, ovarian cancer, efficacy

## 1. Introduction

Chemotherapy-related toxicities and the formation of resistance remain the major obstacles to treatment of ovarian cancer [1]. It is urgently needed to develop effective

* Correspondence: Tinghe Yu, E-mail: yutinghe@hotmail.com

strategies that can potentiate anticancer agents (including reversal of chemoresistance), whilst decreasing adverse events. A chemical chemosensitizer such as cyclosporin A is limited by untoward events, and therefore a non-drug means may be an alternative.

Low intensity ultrasound has been preclinically employed to enhance the action of anticancer drugs since the late 1970s. Ultrasound has better tissue penetration, i.e., ultrasound can be focused on the preselected volume within the body without harming overlying/adjacent tissues. This results in structural and functional changes in exposed tissues, thereby realizing a targeted treatment [2-5].

Ultrasound induces thermal and non-thermal effects, depending on the intensity, frequency, insonation mode and acoustic property of the insonated medium. A higher intensity benefits the production of heat and of cavitation, and a lower frequency favors the occurrence of cavitation. The deposition of ultrasonic energy in tissues leads to temperature rise. A temperature of <56°C is termed ultrasonic hyperthermia, which can be applied for physiotherapy such as tissue healing and drug delivery. A temperature of >56°C results in immediate coagulative necrosis thus being a means to ablate tissues (i.e., high intensity focused ultrasound; HIFU). Cavitation is the most important non-thermal effect. Cavitation causes a localized high temperature ($10^4$–$10^6$ K) and high pressure ($10^4$ atmosperes), thus generating free radicals, microstreaming and microjetting [6-8]. These effects permeabilize the cell membrane including pore formation, thereby favoring the molecular influx. Ultrasonic hyperthermia can also impact on the cell membrane and has been employed for thermochemotherapy [4]. Indeed, ultrasonic chemotherapy is the utilization of membrane damage attributable to cavitation and hyperthermia, and cavitation is considered as the leading determinant. An increase of drug influx improves the intracellular drug level, thereby enhancing the action of drugs.

Here we summarize the data of using ultrasound to modulate chemotherapy for ovarian cancer. Ultrasound also can overcome chemotherapy resistance improving the therapeutic efficacy. These techniques should be developed to assist chemotherapy for ovarian cancer.

## 2. Biological Mechanisms of Ultrasonic Chemotherapy

Mechanisms of ultrasonic chemotherapy have not yet been understood thoroughly. Enhancement of the transmembrane drug delivery is usually considered as the leading determinant. Recent investigations demonstrate that ultrasound enhances the action of anticancer drugs via multiply pathways. Those factors are discussed below.

### 2.1. Increasing the Intracellular Drug Level

Insonation increases the intracellular drug accumulation mainly via cavitation [4, 6]. Cavitation causes damage to the cell membrane. Severely unrepairable damages will lead to cell rupture (i.e., cell lysis), and those repairable damages induce a transient increase in permeability. Ultrastructural examinations demonstrate the occurrence of pores and a reduction of microvilli and laminar ruffles on the plasma membrane of insonated cells [9]. The accumulation assay manifests that non-cytotoxic ultrasound can increase the intracellular drug level. In human ovarian cancer cells, ultrasound increased the intracellular adriamycin level in 3AO, A2780, A2780/ADR and SKOV3/ADR, and a higher level of active platinum was observed in COC1/DDP cells [10-14]. A2780/ADR, SKOV3/ADR and COC1/DDP are the chemoresistant subline. These findings suggest that ultrasound-increased drug influx is effective in resistant cancer cells. Therefore, sonochemotherapy may be a therapeutic modality for refractory ovarian cancer, considering the role of decreased intracellular drug level in chemotherapy resistance. Interestingly, an increase of intracellular adriamycin level was not confirmed in 3AO cells when using the mode of sonication prior to drug administration, but a lower percentage of survival cells was also detected [13]. The data indicate that other mechanisms play a role in ultrasonic chemotherapy.

Aforementioned details suggest that ultrasound only enhance the passive diffusion of drugs. The uptake of certain drugs is realized by both passive diffusion and active conveyance, and the role of each approach is dependent on cell type [15]. Additionally, plasma membrane of certain cells has a specific composition, protecting them against cavitation leading to a lack of permeabilization [16]. These need particular concerns in the development of sonochemotherapy.

## 2.2. Modulating Apoptosis

Most anticancer drugs deactivate cancer cells via inducing apoptosis. Ultrasound enhances adriamycin-induced apoptosis in SKOV3/ADR cells, and cisplatin-induced apoptosis in COC1/DDP cells, resulting in a higher percentage of apoptotic cells. The collapse of mitochondria membrane potential and activation of caspase-9 indicate that apoptosis is realized via the mitochondria pathway [14, 17].

Ultrasound-enhanced cell apoptosis can be understood from the perspective of intracellular pharmacokinetics–pharmacodynamics. Ultrasound favors transmembrane influx of drugs, improving the peak level and area under the concentration–time curve (AUC). The peak level and AUC are the determinant of efficacy of an antitumor drug. Therefore, ultrasound can modulate apoptosis attributable to a cytotoxic drug, and the apoptosis pathway depends on the drug itself. A chip assay indicates that ultrasound alone can affect the expression of genes related to apoptosis, e.g., up-regulating p53, p21/waf, Bip/GRP78, HSP, JUN, FOS and bid, and down-regulating Bcl-2, c-myb, prohibitin and mitofilin [18]. The gene expression pattern may play a part in apoptosis enhancement.

## 2.3. Enhancing Necrosis

Certain drugs (e.g., cisplatin) can induce both apoptotic and necrotic cell death, depending on cell type and the degree of damage [19]. In COC1/DDP cells subjected to cisplatin, a higher level of high mobility group box 1 (HMGB1) was detected when employing ultrasound [14]. HMGB1 is the biochemical marker of cell necrosis. The findings show that ultrasonic chemotherapy can induce cell necrosis directly. Directly inducing necrotic cell death may be a specific advantage, because the defect of apoptosis exists in certain cancer cells. The malfunction of apoptosis decreases the therapeutic efficacy, and can result in chemoresistance.

Usually, necrotic cell-death occurs only when the apoptosis pathway is blocked, or the damage is with the worst degree. The emergence of direct necrosis indicates that ultrasonic chemotherapy causes much severer DNA damage. This may be related to ultrasonic sensitization. Insonation decrease the threshold dose for inducing necrosis. Therefore, a dose that alone can only cause apoptosis, will induce cell necrosis. This effect has therapeutic implication, because inducing necrosis can be an alternative for cancers with apoptosis defect and with apoptosis-related chemoresistance [20, 21].

### 2.4. Modulating the Expression of Molecules Related to Chemoresistance

Mechanisms of chemoresistance in ovarian cancer are very complicated, and many molecules and pathways play a part [22]. Investigations reveal that some molecules can be modulated by insonation. Drug efflux decreases the drug level within cells, which is an active procedure mediated the efflux pumps such as multidrug resistance 1 (MDR1), lung resistance protein (LRP), multidrug resistance-related protein (MRP) and breast cancer resistance protein (BCRP) [22-24]. A lower level of LRP mRNA and protein was detected in COC1/DDP cells after insonation [14]. The suppression of MDR1 or MRP was reported in liver cancer cells HepG2/ADM [25]. Drug inactivation can decrease the anticancer effect, and glutathione S-transferase (GST) and glutathione (GSH) are the antidote for platinum [22, 26]. GSH, particularly the reduced form, was decreased in insonated COC1/DDP cells [14]. This suggest that the active form of a drug can be preserved, favoring the anticancer effect.

Resistant cells have an improved repair capacity, which can alleviate drug-induced harms leading to survival. For cisplatin, a higher capacity of DNA repair is related to resistance, where excision repair cross-complementing group 1 (ERCC1) plays the leading role [22]. The level of ERCC1 was decreased in sonicated COC1/DDP cells. This will cause severer DNA insult, which is supported with the findings in comet assay – a higher percentage of comet-formed cells occurred in the mode of cisplatin followed by ultrasound [14, 27].

Of aforementioned factors that lead to chemotherapy sensitization, the increase of intracellular drug level is the direct effect of ultrasound. Other factors indirectly enhance the action of anticancer drugs.

## 3. Strategies to Enhance the Efficacy of Ultrasonic Chemotherapy

The efficacy of ultrasonic chemotherapy is unsatisfactory in certain cells. Scientists hope to develop modalities that can enhance sonochemotherapy, thereby improving the therapeutic outcome.

### 3.1. Cavitation Modulators

Cavitation is the determinant of ultrasonic chemotherapy. Therefore, cavitation modulators have been used to enhance sonochemotherapy. The use of microbubbles is a popular area of research. Micobubbles can be the cavitation nuclei, thereby lowering the cavitation threshold. Further, the rupture of microbubbles under insonation leads to the formation smaller bubbles that can also favor the occurrence of cavitation (i.e., cavitation cascade) [6, 28].

Coadministration of microbubbles and anticancer drugs: Microbubbles enhance cavitation, thus enhancing membrane permeabilization. This improves the drug influx, leading to a higher level of anticancer drugs within cells. Microbubble-enhanced cavitation may destruct endothelium of tumor vessels thus favoring the extravasation of drugs. Under the image guidance, rupture of microbubbles can be triggered near the lesion, improving the therapeutic precision.

Encapsulation of drugs: Drugs are encapsulated into microbubbles or conjugated to the surface of microbubbles. Insonation is performed to destruct microbubbles when reaching the lesion, thereby releasing drugs from bubbles and enhancing the influx. These theoretically can realize a localized high concentration, i.e., targeted treatment. Antibodies or ligands can be linked to the surface of microbubbles to improve the treatment precision.

Sonosensitizers: Sonosensitizers engender free radicals under insonation, and are frequently used for sonodynamic therapy (SDT). A sonosensitizer is usually with a small molecular mass, indicating that it can enter into cells. Therefore, sonosensitizers can be used to assist the drugs (e.g., adriamycin) whose cytotoxicity is mediated by reactive radicals.

Dual/multiple frequency sonication: Biological tissues contain gases. A specific frequency of insonation is performed to trigger cavitation within the desired tissues producing massive microbubbles. Insonaiton with another specific frequency is then employed to rupture those newly formed bubbles thus amplifying the cavitation level.

## 3.2. Drug Form

Micelles adriamaycin is used for sonochemotherapy against A2780/ADR cells, and miceclles lead to a stronger anticancer effect compared with free drugs. This drug form is more effective than free drugs in vivo, resulting in a smaller tumor volume and longer survival time [10, 11].

Micelles can stabilize drugs, protecting them from the elimination from blood and ultrasonic cavitation. Micelles impact on the biodistribution of adriamycin. A higher concentration is detected within the tumor, and the heterogenous distribution of drugs within the tumor is decreased. The intratumoral drug level is increased when using insonation. Further, the adriamycin level in the heart when using micelles is much less than the level when using free adriamcyin. This will diminish the cardiotoxicity due to adriamycin [10, 11].

These stirring findings have been leading to the development of microparticles and nanoparticles containing antitumor drugs for ultrasonic chemotherapy. Scientists hope these forms can improve the therapeutic targeting.

## 3.3. Chemical Chemotherapy Modulators

Several chemical chemotherapy sensitizers (e.g., verapamil and cyclosporin) have been clinically tested. These modifiers are effective in preclinical investigations, but the dose required for sensitization is not available in vivo limiting clinical application. Ultrasound can enhance the sensitization attributable to verapamil in SKOV3/ADR cells, and that due to cyclosporin A in COC1/DDP cells [13, 14]. A combination of insonation and verapamil/cyclosporin enhanced adriamycin/cisplatin, leading to the smallest tumor size in transplanted tumors and the longest mean survival time in the orthotopic ovarian cancer model [14, 29]. Interesting, the mode of drug administration affected the sensitization effect. Verapmail pretreatment caused synergism; however, the synchronous use of verapmial and adriamycin produced no chemosensitization, and insonation cannot be an adjunct under the circumstances [13]. A chemical modifier usually takes effects via blocking specific molecules within cells and modulating the expression of specific genes [22, 24, 30, 31]. The down-regulation of genes due to cyclosporin A can be synergized by insonation – the lowest level of LRP and ERCC1 was detected in COC1/DDP cells [14]. Theoretically, the use of ultrasound can decrease the dose of a chemical modulator to a safe level. The alteration of gene expression using a chemical drug has a longer virtual time. Therefore, the combination of a chemical modulator with insonation will cause stronger and longer sensitization effect. These suggest that the combination may be a strategy when insonation or chemical modifier alone cannot produce satisfactory sensitization, and that the interaction between a chemical modulator and ultrasound need to be explored.

## 4. Implications from Available Clinical Trials

HIFU has been clinically used to manage solid tumors. Chemotherapy is performed to deactivate the residual and metastatic lesions. HIFU has been employed to treat recurrent and metastatic ovarian cancer that has no opportunity to receive other strategies [32].

HIFU ablates tissues via heat (>56°C) and cavitation. The intensity drastically attenuates outside the center of the focus (i.e., temperature is <56°C within a definite region outside the focus). Cavitation occurs in a wider region, including the pre- and post-focus area [33]. Thus, HIFU-chemotherapy provides a window to understanding the efficacy of ultrasonic chemotherapy [34].

Controlled trials (chemotherapy vs. chemotherapy + HIFU) are available in cancers of the liver, pancreas, breast, esophagus, stomach, intestine and colorectum. The combined modality increased the response rate in 35.0% (7/20) of trials [35]. The findings showed that ultrasonic chemotherapy may not improve the therapeutic outcome (even in a specific cancer type), and that chemotherapy should be curtailed in certain cases. The exact efficacy of ultrasonic chemotherapy on ovarian cancer remains unclear for lacking direct clinical data.

Unfortunately, factors that lead to a lack of chemosensitization are only limitedly understood. The efficacy of ultrasonic chemotherapy depends on cancer type and the drugs applied [36]. Pathologic type of ovarian cancer is very complicated. Reasonably, certain cancer types respond to sonochemotherapy poorly.

These data demonstrate a gap between the preclinical and clinical investigations – the present preclinical trials only partly reflect the clinical status leading to biases. In our opinion, following aspects need particular concerns in translational researches.

Sequence effect: Single drug regimen is usually adopted in the preclinical trials, but the combined regimen is the standard clinical strategy. The difference may play a part in the lack of sensitization in certain cases. There has a sequence effect when using multiple agents. The sequence of drug administration determines not only the anticancer effect but also untoward events. As an example, cisplatin followed by paclitaxel results in a reduced antitumor action and aggravates neutropenia, and the opposite sequence improves the anticancer effect [37]. Therefore, interactions between drugs, and between ultrasound and each drug should be explored. Representativeness of tumor models: Heterotopic xenograft (i.e., subcutaneous and intraperitoneal) is the mostly adopted model for ovarian cancer. Microenvironment in those sites differs from that in the ovary, making against the growth of cancer cells. Therefore, it is easy to treat a heterotopic tumor. Orthotopic transplantation provides appropriate microenvironment, so cancer cells can display their biological behavior thoroughly [38, 39]. Indeed, we found that sonochemotherpay led to a smaller tumor size in heterotopic tumors in mice, but not prolong the survival time in the orthotopic tumors in mice [14, 29].

Chemoresistant cancer model: A chemoresistant subline is obtained by exposing the parent line to anticancer drugs with gradually elevating concentration in the present study. The capacity of resistance decreases without the drug pressure, and ultimately decays completely [40]. The attenuation rate is much higher in vivo. The formation of a transplanted tumor need several weeks, suggesting that the formed tumor may not actually be chemoresistant. This will lead to an overestimation of the efficacy of a therapeutic modality. This can be solved by using intrinsic chemoresistant cells.

## CONCLUSION

Ultrasound can enhance the action of antitumor drugs for ovarian cancer including chemoresistant lesions, where cavitation plays the leading role. Ultrasound sensitizes drugs via multiple mechanisms, including the increase of drug influx and modulation the expression of molecules involving in drug efflux, detoxification and damage repair. Ultrasound can synergize the sensitization due to a chemical chemotherapy modulator in vitro and in vivo. The clinical data in certain solid cancers manifest that ultrasound cannot enhance anticancer drugs in certain cases, and demonstrate a gap between the preclinical and clinical trials. These need particular concerns in the translational studies. Insonation may be a non-drug technique to modulate chemotherapy against ovarian cancer.

## ACKNOWLEDGMENTS

The work in our laboratory was supported with grants from the Natural Science Foundation of China (34170822, 81300535) and the Sate Ministry of Education (SRFDP 20135503130002).

## REFERENCES

[1] Bookman MA. First-line chemotherapy in epithelial ovarian cancer. *Clin. Obstet. Gynecol.* 2012, 55, 96-113.

[2] Wood AKW, Sehgal CM. A review of low-intensity ultrasound for cancer therapy. *Ultrasound Med. Biol.* 2015, 41: 905-28.

[3] Tang J, Guha C, Tomé W. Biological effects induced by non-thermal ultrasound and implications for cancer therapy: A review of the current literature. *Technol. Cancer Res. Treat.* 2015, 14: 221-35.

[4] Yu T, Li S, Zhao J, et al. Ultrasound: A chemotherapy sensitizer. *Technol. Cancer Res. Treat.* 2006, 6: 51-60.

[5] Lakshmanan S, Gupta GK, Avci P, et al. Physical energy for drug delivery: Poration, concentration and activation. *Adv. Drug Deliv. Rev.* 2014, 71: 98-114.

[6] Pitt WG, Husseini GA, Staples BJ. Ultrasonic drug delivery – a general review. *Expert Opin. Drug Deliv.* 2004, 1, 37-56.

[7] Paliwal S, Mitragotri S. Ultrasound-induced cavitation: Applications in drug and gene delivery. *Expert Opin. Drug Deliv.* 2006, 3, 713-726.

[8] Mo S, Coussios CC, Seymour L, et al. Ultrasound-enhanced drug delivery for cancer. *Expert Opin. Drug Deliv.* 2012, 9: 1525-1538.

[9] Tachibana K, Uchida T, Ogawa K, et al. Induction of cell-membrane porosity by ultrasound. *Lancet* 1999, 353, 1409.

[10] Rapoport N. Combined cancer therapy by micellar-encapsulated drug and ultrasound. *Int. J. Pharm.* 2004, 277, 155-162.

[11] Rapoport NY, Christensen DA, Fain HD, et al. Ultrasound-triggered drug targeting of tumors in vitro and in vivo. *Ultrasonics* 2004, 42, 943-950.

[12] Yu T, Wang Z, Jiang S. Potentiation of cytotoxicity of adriamycin on human ovarian carcinoma cell line 3AO by low-level ultrasound. *Ultrasonics* 2001, 39, 307-309.

[13] Yu T, Hu K, Bai J, et al. Reversal of adriamycin resistance in ovarian carcinoma cell line by combination of verapamil and low-level ultrasound. *Ultrason. Sonochem.* 2003, 10, 37-40.

[14] Yu T, Yang Y, Zhang J, et al. Circumvention of cisplatin resistance in ovarian cancer by combination of cyclosporin A and low-intensity ultrasound. *Eur. J. Pharm. Biopharm.* 2015, 91, 103-110.

[15] Köberle B, Tomicic MT, Usanova SU, et al. Cisplatin resistance: Preclinical findings and clinical implications. *Biochim. Biophys. Acta* 2010, 1806, 172-182.

[16] Escoffre JM, Piron J, Novell A, et al. Doxorubicin delivery into tumor cells with ultrasound and microbubbles. *Mol. Pharm.* 2011, 8, 799-806.

[17] Yu T, Huang X, Hu K, et al. Mechanisms of reversal of adriamycin resistance in human ovarian cancer line by ultrasound. *Int. J. Gynecol. Cancer* 2004, 14, 76-81.

[18] Yu T, Wu M, Huang P, et al. Modulating apoptosis in cancer therapy with ultrasound and high intensity nanosecond electric pulses. In: Rodrigo R, Henning U. Eds. Trends in Stem Cell Proliferation and Cancer Research, Dordrecht: Springer Science, 2013, pp. 573-590.

[19] Cepeda V, Fuertes MA, Castilla J, et al. Biochemical mechanisms of cisplatin cytotoxicity. *Anticancer Agents Med. Chem.* 2007, 7, 3-18.

[20] Finkle E. Does cancer therapy trigger cell suicide? *Science* 1999, 286, 2256-2258.

[21] Kim R, Emi M, Tanabe K, et al. The role of apoptotic or nonapoptotic cell death in determining cellular response to anticancer treatment. *Eur. J. Surg. Oncol.* 2006, 32, 269-277.

[22] Agarwal R, Kaye SB. Ovarian cancers: Strategies for overcoming resistance to chemotherapy. *Nat. Rev. Cancer* 2003, 3, 502-516.
[23] Lage H, Denkert C. Resistance to chemotherapy in ovarian carcinoma. *Recent Results Cancer Res.* 2007, 176, 51-60.
[24] Xia CQ, Smith PG. Drug efflux transporters and multidrug resistance in acute leukemia: Therapeutic impact and novel approaches to mediation. *Mol. Pharmacol.* 2012, 82, 1008-1021.
[25] Xia W, Ma X, Li X, et al. Reversal effect of low-intensity ultrasound on adriamycin-resistant human hepatoma cells in vitro and in vivo. *Int. J. Imaging Syst. Technol.* 2014, 24, 23-28.
[26] Backos DS, Franklin CC, Reigan P. The role of glutathione in brain tumor drug resistance. *Biochem. Pharmacol.* 2012, 83, 1005-1012.
[27] He H, Huang H, Yu T. Detection of DNA damage in sonochemotherapy against cisplatin-resistant human ovarian cancer cells using the modified comet assay. *Int. J. Radiat. Biol.* 2014, 90, 897-902.
[28] May DJ, Allen JS, Ferrara KW. Dynamics and fragmentation of thick-shelled microbubbles. *IEEE Trans. Ultrason. Ferroelectr. Freq. Control* 2002, 49, 1400-1410.
[29] Yu T, Huang X, Hu K, et al. Treatment of transplanted adriamycin-resistent ovarian cancers in mice by combination of adriamycin and ultrasound exposure. *Ultrason. Sonochem.* 2004, 11, 287-291.
[30] Morjani H, Madoulet C. Immunosuppressors as multidrug resistance reversal agents. *Methods Mol. Biol.* 2010, 59, 433-446.
[31] Aouali N, Eddabra L, Macadré J, et al. Immunosuppressors and reversion of multidrug-resistance. *Crit. Rev. Oncol. Hematol.* 2005, 56, 61-70.
[32] Yu T, Fu X. Extracorporeal ultrasound-guided high intensity focused ultrasound: Implications from the present clinical trials. *Sci. World J.* 2014, 2014, 537260.
[33] Yin H, Qiao Y, Cao H, et al. Cavitation mapping by sonochemiluminescence with less bubble displacement induced by acoustic radiation force in a 1.2 MHz HIFU. *Ultrason. Sonochem.* 2014, 21, 559-565.
[34] Yu T, Zhang Y. Sonochemotherapy against cancers. In: Nowak FM. Eds. Sonochemistry: Theory, Reactions, Syntheses, and Applications. New York: Nova Science Publishers, 2010, pp. 189-200.
[35] Luo J, Ren X, Yu T. Efficacy of extracorporeal ultrasound-guided high intensity focused ultrasound: An evaluation based on controlled trials in China. *Int. J. Radiat. Biol.* 2015, 91, 480-485.
[36] He H, Yu T, Zhang Y. The interaction between a drug and ultrasound in sonochemotherapy against ovarian cancers. *Ultraschall. Med.* 2012, 33, 275-282.
[37] Vigano L, Locatelli A, Grasselli G, et al. Drug interactions of paclitaxel and docetaxel and their relevance for the design of combination therapy. *Invest. New Drugs* 2001, 19, 179-196.
[38] Ruggeri BA, Camp F, Miknyoczki S. Animal models of disease: Pre-clinical animal models of cancer and their applications and utility in drug discovery. *Biochem. Pharmacol.* 2014, 87, 150-161.
[39] KahnJ, Tofilon PJ, Camphausen K. Preclinical models in radiation oncology. *Radiat. Oncol.* 2012, 7, 223.

[40] Duesberg P, Li R, Sachs R, et al. Cancer drug resistance: The central role of the karyotype. *Drug Resist. Updat.* 2007, 10: 51-58.

In: Handbook on Ovarian Cancer
Editor: Bethany R. Collier
ISBN: 978-1-63483-874-0


*Chapter 14*

# ELDERLY OVARIAN CANCER PATIENTS: TREATMENT OPTIONS

***Francesca De Iuliis, Lucrezia Amoroso and Susanna Scarpa***
Experimental Medicine Department, Sapienza University of Rome, Italy

## ABSTRACT

**Introduction**. Ovarian cancer, the main cause of death among gynaecological malignancies, affects half of women in postmenopausal age. With the increase in older population, this tumor will be more frequent in elderly women, but not all the elderly patients can undertake standard treatments, due to comorbidities and less functional organ reserves.

New therapeutic approaches are needed to obtain an amendable overall survival and quality of life in this kind of patients.

**Objective**. Our aim is to propose the best management of elderly ovarian cancer patients, taking account of biological age over chronologic age, with the aim to assure suitable treatments with a better overall survival.

**Discussion**. Carboplatin-paclitaxel doublet is the standard treatment in patients with ovarian cancer; elderly patients are less treated with this therapy, due both to comorbidities and to the major toxicity. When the standard schedule every 21 days is administered in elderly patients, dose delay or previous stop for toxicity is frequent.

Furthermore, elderly are not candidate for intraperitoneal chemotherapy and HIPEC (hyperthermic intraperitoneal chemotherapy), due to highest toxicity. Chemotherapy is often the only possible choice for these patients, because a surgical debulking can be too much aggressive and associated with several morbidities.

Elderly have the same chemosensitivity than younger: geriatric assessment is fundamental to screen elderly population fitting for chemotherapy, and new strategies with less toxicity have to be investigated. Older patients with ovarian cancer have been underrepresented in clinical trials, so the few clinical studies with this kind of population must be evaluated.

It's not clear whether doublets or single agents are better in the treatment of elderly ovarian cancer patients. Single agent options for elderly patients include liposomal doxorubicin, topotecan, gemcitabine and vinorelbine. Doublet combinations every 21 days have been largerly investigated, but only small clinical trials have been conducted on weekly schedule. Weekly carboplatin and paclitaxel have demonstrated an optimal compliance among elderly patients.

For what concern targeted therapies, there are no elderly-specific data on PARP inhibitors, but they appear to be well tolerated, on the opposite to antiangiogenic agents, which require more caution in the older population.

Metronomic chemotherapy and weekly schedules are the best solutions for elderly patients, for their efficacy and tolerability, contributing to quality of life.

**Conclusions.** Metronomic therapy, comprising weekly schedules, can be an optimal option for elderly ovarian cancer patients. Prospective studies are needed to develop further strategies for these women.

**Keywords:** Elderly, ovarian cancer, metronomic therapy, targeted therapy

## INTRODUCTION

Ovarian cancer is the leading cause of mortality among gynecologic cancers in Western countries and more than 50% of diagnosed ovarian cancers is found in postmenopausal women. Indipendently from the initial management, more than 80% of patients experience relapse [1].

Older ovarian cancer patients have often the poorest outcome and decreased survival respect to the young patients, due to intrinsic factors such as comorbidity, which don't permit to utilize standard/aggressive treatments, beyond to molecular charachteristics of the neoplasia [2].

This major aggressivity in advanced age (higher grade, more advanced stage of disease) has not still an explanation; probably in older women intrinsic mechanisms of chemoresistance are involved, and together with malnutrition and medical illness, all translate in a sub optimal management.

Age is surely an independent prognostic factor of decreased overall survival. Elderly are not always enrolled in clinical trials, bringing to a lack of clinical data on this kind of patients [3-4].

Cytoreduction surgery is often associated with higher risk of perioperative mortality and morbidity within 30 days in elderly patients, as recently demonstrated. For this reason, neoadjuvant chemotherapy should always be proposed to advanced elderly patients, instead of surgery as first treatment [5]. In fact, relapsed women with more of 70 years are often excluded from surgery, but this point of view is still debated.

The standard chemotherapy for every ovarian cancer patient, including the elderly patients, is the doublet combination of carboplatin and paclitaxel every 21 days, a schedule that has largely demonstrated an improvement in progression-free and overall survival respect to best supportive care [6]. This schedule is recommended both in adjuvant and in first line, although an optimal dosage is still uncertain in elderly. Unfortunately, this schedule is associated to a discrete toxicity, and not all elderly patients can receive this doublet treatment [7].

Elderly often experience delays in platinum/paclitaxel administration and reduction of the dose intensity, which affect efficacy of the treatment and can impact on outcome [8-10]. The reasons of delay is commonly the hematologic toxicity.

Several trials by the Gynecology Oncology Group and Group d'Investigateurs Nationaux pour l'Etude des Cancers Ovariens (GINECO) have evaluated hematologic support during the chemotherapy in elderly patients.

MITO-7 trial (Multicentre Italian Trial in Ovarian Cancer) has recently demonstrated the efficacy and non inferiority of weekly schedule of carboplatin and paclitaxel in elderly women, respect to the standard every 3 weeks schedule [11].

In the last years, also intraperitoneal chemotherapy (HIPEC), in combination with standard intravenous chemoteraphy, have been considered in optimally advanced cytoreduced patients, although high toxicity rate reported.

The use of geriatric assessment tools can be useful to stratify elderly patients before the treatment, considering that baseline performance status is not a valid predictor of toxicity from chemotherapy.

All these results suggest that new strategies must be conducted on elderly ovarian cancer patients, respecting their chronological but also biological age, proposing therapies that do not affect quality of life.

## CURRENT STRATEGIES OF TREATMENT

Although ovarian cancer treatment is ruled by official guidelines, the onco-geriatric management is still object of discussion for what concern surgery, chemotherapy and HIPEC; elderly patients are frequently suboptimally treated, first of all for the risk of side effects determined by the treatments [12].

### Geriatric Assessment

Geriatric assessment (GA) can be a useful instrument to provide information about comorbidity, cognition, functional, psychological, social and nutritional status of elderly patients. In older cancer patients GA can estimate the risk of toxicity from chemotherapy and probably the future outcome.

Many authors suggested its use as an important evaluation before all kind of treatments [13]. The Preoperative Assessment of Cancer in the Elderly (PACE) tool utilizes the data of geriatric assessment from some tests (IADL: Instrumental Activities of Daily Living, ADL: Activities of Daily Living), from the PS (performance status) and from the surgical risk assessment tool, to predict the time of hospitalization; bad scores are associated with prolonged hospitalization [14].

A recent elder-specific study, (GOG273: Gynecologic Oncology Group) with 70 years and older ovarian cancer patients receiving first-line platinum-based chemotherapy, has evaluated two different regimens: every three weeks carboplatin AUC 5 and paclitaxel 135 mg/m$^2$ plus pegfilgrastim support, or every three weeks single agent carboplatin AUC 5 (in this latter arm, very older women, unlike to receive the combination therapy were enrolled). The ability of IADL score to predict the tolerability of chemotherapy (dose reduction and/or delay) was the primary end-point, but it was not reached [15].

The Vulnerable Elders Survey (VES-13) and the Cancer and Aging Research Group-GA (CARG-GA) are feasible tools that can predict toxicity and estimate survival. GINECO group has developed a Geriatric Vulnerability Score (GVS) to be utilized in very elderly ovarian cancer patients, built from a sery of up-front trials in older women with ovarian cancer. A score $\geq 3$ is associated with high risk of severe toxicity, hospitalization and early discontinuation of treatment [16].

All these instruments can be utilized for a better evaluation of elderly ovarian cancer patients, to choose the best treatment modality.

## Surgery

Ovarian cancer patients over the age of 70 years are less likely to receive surgery, and to have an optimal cytoreduction, so this contributes to the poor outcome of this category of patients.

There is clearly substantial toxicity associated with aggressive primary surgical cytoreduction in older patients, particularly those over 75 years of age.

Actually, primary debulking surgery (PDS), by removing as much tumor as possible, followed by chemotherapy platinum/taxane based, is the first line therapy and offers the greatest survival advantage in advanced stage.

Optimal tumor surgical eradication can remove drug resistant cells, helping chemotherapy to destroy the remaining cells. Resection of gross tumor burden greater than 1 cm is associated with an increased overall survival [17-18].

Two trials have evaluated PDS in a large number of patients: the first, European Organization for Research and Treatment of Cancer (EORTC) trial, has demonstrated that PDS without optimal tumor resection is not associated with a survival advantage. In patients with significant comorbidities, and contraindications for PDS, neo-adjuvant chemotherapy (NACT) is a valid approach. This trial demonstrated that NACT was associated with lower mortality, morbidity and with equivalent PFS and overall survival such as PDS [19]. The second trial, CHORUS trial, has confirmed a survival advantage in women undergoing PDS, therefore, in ovarian cancer women, survival with primary chemotherapy is non-inferior to primary surgery [20]. All these two trials concluded that morbidity is increased with surgery respect to chemotherapy [21].

Wright et al. recently published a survival analysis of 17 years using SEER-Medicare data and concluded that survival for PDS and NACT is equivalent [22].

## Chemotherapy

Several trials have been conducted on geriatric ovarian cancer women, especially utilizing weekly regimen of chemotherapy (as metronomic schedules), carboplatin as single agent, or with different kind of chemotherapeutic agents, with the aim to assure efficacy with less toxicity.

A recent survey on the standard treatments of elderly patients (with platinum and taxanes) has demonstrated that 29% of ovarian cancer women > 65 years received no chemotherapy and 25% received delayed or reduced doses [23]. In fact, the most important platinum and taxanes side effects, dose-limiting for elderly, are neutropenia and pheripheral neuropathy, which can hardly affect quality of life and survival of these patients.

GINECO group conducted trials with women affected by ovarian cancer > 80 years, previously evaluated with GVC to exclude patients not eligible for chemotherapy, treating the selected women with carboplatin/cyclophosphamide or carboplatin/paclitaxel or carboplatin single agent [24-25]. The results showed an evident superiority of carboplatin/paclitaxel in overall survival (25, 9 months), and a poor survival for the patients who underwent only carboplatin (17 months). Furthermore, in the same trial peripheral blood lymphocytes were collected from treated patients and telomere length analyzed. An association was found between shorter and median telomere length with shorter survival and higher risk of severe adverse events with chemotherapy [26].

Other possible biomarkers in aged patients have been evaluated, such as telomere length, p16INK4a expression in T lymphocytes and inflammatory cytokine expression. The European Organization for Research and Treatment of Cancer (EORTC) Elderly Task force is recently studying aging biomarkers in older cancer patients [27].

In the recent trial of Sabatier, 109 elderly ovarian cancer patients were retrospectively analyzed to find specific outcome prognostic factors. Multivariate analyses confirmed only age as an independent prognostic factor, while no correlation was observed between geriatric characteristics and type of chemotherapy or surgery [28].

MITO-7 trial has recently compared standard carbo/paclitaxel for 6 cycles every 21 days (carboplatin AUC 6, area under the curve 6 mg/mL/min, and paclitaxel 175 $mg/m^2$) to carboplatin AUC 2 mg/mL/min and paclitaxel 60 $mg/m^2$ weekly for 18 cycles. This trial has demonstrated a better toxicity profile of weekly schedule, preserving quality of life, and with no difference in PFS respect to standard chemotherapy (18.3 months with the weekly versus 17.3 months). Furthermore, the subanalysis of very elderly patients (> 70 years) has demonstrated an improvement in overall survival [11].

## Neoadjuvant Chemotherapy

NACT (Neoadjuvant chemotherapy), administered before cytoreduction, represents the standard approach both in Europe and in USA for elderly patients, assuring a similar overall survival respect to surgery. A large randomized study of neoadjuvant chemotherapy from the European Organization for Research and Treatment of Cancer (EORTC) evaluated 632 locally advanced patients, a group treated with surgery and following chemotherapy, and a group treated with NACT and then surgery. Complications linked to surgery as first approach were higher (first group) respect to side effects linked to chemotherapy [29].

Furthermore, a deep analysis of the older patients hasn't found differences in terms of responses respect to the younger counterpart [30].

The benefit of neoadjuvant therapy is strongly demonstrated in largest tumor burden, respect to small tumors. For these latters, surgery as first approach can be a considerable option.

## Intraperitoneal Chemotherapy

Severla trials demonstrated that HIPEC has a good efficacy and acceptable morbidity in cases of peritoneal involvement from metastasis of different origin, such as in recurrent ovarian cancer, impacting on survival [31].

The median overall survival after HIPEC was 22-64 months in the reported experiences, with a median DFS of 10-57 months [32].

However, a low number of patients, among those enrolled in these studies, were elderly. All these trials have been conducted with intraperitoneal cisplatin [33-35].

A trial of Fagotti compared a group of ovarian cancer patients treated with HIPEC and a group treated with surgery alone or chemotherapy alone, and morbidity and survival were then evaluated: HIPEC group showed better overall survival and time to relapse respect to the others [36]. The efficacy of HIPEC (after cytoreductive surgery) was also confirmed by Bakrin, in a trial with 566 ovarian cancer patients [37], as well as by Delotte, in a very recent experience only in elderly ovarian cancer women [38].

Despite the considerable morbidity reported in these trials [39], HIPEC can be a feasible option in elderly patients, which can be considered after a careful clinical evaluation.

## Other Agents

Elderly patients treated with first line platinum/paclitaxel chemotherapy can have longer DFS, but inevitably platinum resistance will occur. Other agents beyond platinum are needed, especially in frail (but suitable) elderly patients still curable.

Patients over 70 years have a median overall survival of only 23.6 months from recurrence versus 30.7 months of younger women, and are often treated in second line with a single chemotherapeutic agent [40].

In several trials, platinum sensitive patients have been randomized to continue platinum, adding a different agent at the place of paclitaxel, such as vinorelbine, gemcitabine [41] or liposomal doxorubicin [42].

ICON-4 trial is the only experience with a real benefit in terms of survival, with carboplatin and paclitaxel, but also with single agent carboplatin as valid option for frailer patients [43].

Kurtz has evaluated elderly patients treated with carboplatin/paclitaxel versus carboplatin/liposomal doxorubicin, demonstrated the same tolerability respect to younger patients, and similar rates of hematologic toxicity (only neuropathy was greater in older, while carboplatin hypersensitivity reactions were less common in older respect to younger patients) [44].

For platinum-resistant patients, a single agent is frequently preferred, with a overall respons rate of 10–25% and a duration of the response of 4-8 months. More commonly used agents are liposomal doxorubicin, topotecan, gemcitabine, weekly paclitaxel and vinorelbine [45].

Topotecan was utilized by Gronlund in 57 elderly patients, founding no differences in terms of toxicity and responses with younger patients [46].

Liposomal doxorubicin or gemcitabine can be other safety choices for older patients, but only lower responses and benefits in survival have been reported [45].

Beyond the second line, elderly patients should be only palliated, stopping chemotherapy [47]. Earlier hospice enrollment is beneficial, especially in older frail patients [48].

## Targeted Therapies

Ovarian cancer biological therapies are the poly(ADP-ribose) polymerase (PARP) inhibitors, the antiangiogenic agents and the antiangiogenic tyrosine kinase inhibitors.

PARP inhibitors are generally well tolerated, and also in the absence of specific data on elderly population, this therapy can be proposed to the eligible patients (only women with BRAC mutation). The described toxicities are mainly gastrointestinal and hematological disorders and fatigue, but all of low grade [49-50].

Antiangiogenic therapies are more toxic than PARP inhibitors; women treated with Bevacizumab can experience vascular and thromboembolic events, and although the reported responses are similar between younger and older patients, side effects are more conspicuous in older ones (8, 5% vs 2, 9%) [51].

Recently, anti-vascular endothelial growth factor (VEGF) tyrosine kinase inhibitors (TKIs) have been evaluated in ovarian cancer patients, showing an increase in DFS: pazopanib [52] and cediranib [53-54]; their most common toxicities are fatigue, diarrhea, and hypertension, but of low grade. Cediranib has been tested in elderly ovarian cancer, showing an increase in systolic blood pressure respect to younger women (15.9 vs 7.0 mm Hg)

Other anti VEGF TKIs drugs are sorafenib and sunitinib, but the results of the trials show too much toxicities (neutropenia, fatigue, and gastrointestinal symptoms) making them not safe for older [55-57].

# Conclusion

To improve the outcome of elderly patients affected by ovarian cancer, further trials are expected, to better understand molecular mechanisms at the basis of chemo resistance in aged patients and the differences with the younger, to better define schedule, dosing, timing of chemotherapy reducing toxicity and preserving efficacy at tyhe same time, to better discriminate which patients are eligible for the treatments and which are not. All the described approaches have proved efficacy, but every treatment has to fit the single patient, taking account of biologic age (better than chronologic age) and the willingness of the patient. Metronomic chemotherapy with weekly schedule carboplatin/paclitaxel based and PARP inhibitors is the only treatment that has shown proved efficacy in specific trials. HIPEC and surgery can be proposed only to suitable elderly patients, while single agent chemotherapies can be administered to every elderly population, due to the low toxicity, but with small benefits in terms of survival.

Every treatment choice should be previously based on objective geriatric assessment in order to improve the outcome in this population. Furthermore, new geriatric trials are needed to satisfy different unanswered questions.

## REFERENCES


[1] Oberaigner, W; Minicozzi, P; Bielska-Lasota, M; Allemani, C; De Angelis, R; Mangone, L; Sant, M. Eurocare Working Group; Survival for ovarian cancer in Europe: the across-country variation did not shrink in the past decade. *Acta Oncol.*, 2012, 51(4), 441–453.

[2] Langstraat, C; Aletti, GD; Cliby, WA. Morbidity, mortality and overall survival in elderly women undergoing primary surgical debulking for ovarian cancer: a delicate balance requiring individualization. *Gynecol Oncol.*, 2011, 123(2), 187–191.

[3] Cloven, NG; Manetta, A; Berman, ML; Kohler, MF; DiSaia, PJ. Management of ovarian cancer in patients older than 80 years of age. *Gynecol Oncol.*, 1999, 73(1), 137–139.

[4] Sundararajan, V; Hershman, D; Gann, VR; Jacobson, JS; Neugut, AI. Variations in the use of chemotherapy for elderly patients with advanced ovarian cancer: a populationbased study. *J Clin Oncol.*, 2002, 20(1), 173–178.

[5] Mandi, H; Wiechert, A; Lockhart, D; Rose, PG. Impact of Age on 30-Day Mortality and Morbidity in Patients Undergoing Surgery for Ovarian Cancer. *Int J Gynecol Cancer.*, Epub ahead of print, 2015.

[6] Eisenhauer, EL; Tew, WP; Levine, DA; Lichtman, SM; Brown, CL; Aghajanian, C; Huh, J; Barakat, RR; Chi, DS. Response and outcomes in elderly patients with stages IIIC–IVovarian cancer receiving platinum-taxane chemotherapy. *Gynecol Oncol.*, 2007, 106(2), 381–387.

[7] Pignata, S; Vermorken, JB. Ovarian cancer in the elderly. *Crit Rev Oncol Hematol.*, 2004, 49(1), 77–86.

[8] Joseph, N; Clark, RM; Dizon, DS; Lee, MS; Goodman, A; Boruta, D; Schorge, JO; Del Carmen, MG; Growdon, WB. Delay in chemotherapy administration impacts survival in elderly patients with epithelial ovarian cancer. *Gynecol Oncol Epub* ahead of print 2015 http://dx.doi.org /10.1016/j.ygyno.2015.03.052

[9] Chiara, S; Lionetto, R; Vincenti, M; Bruzzone, M; Nobile, MT; Gadducci, A; Carnino, F; Rosso, R; Conte, PF. Advanced ovarian cancer in the elderly: results of consecutive trials with cisplatin-based chemotherapy. Crit Rev Oncol Hematol., 2001, 37(1), 27–34.

[10] Hanna, RK; Poniewierski, MS; Laskey, RA; Lopez, MA; Shafer, A; Van Le, L; Crawford, J; Dale, DC; Gehrig, PA; Secord, AA; Havrilesky, LJ; Lyman, GH. Predictors of reduced relative dose intensity and its relationship to mortality in women receiving multi-agent chemotherapy for epithelial ovarian cancer. *Gynecol Oncol.*, 2013, 129(1), 74–80.

[11] Pignata, S; Scambia, G; Katsaros, D; MITO, GINECO, MaNGO, GCIG Investigators. Carboplatin plus paclitaxel once a week versus every 3 weeks in patients with advanced

ovarian cancer (MITO-7): a randomized, multicentre, open-label, phase 3 trial. *Lancet Oncol*, 2014, 15(4), 396–405.

[12] Pignata, S; Ferreandina, G; Scarfone, G; Scollo, P; Odicino, F; Cormio, G; Katsaros, D; Frigerio, L; Mereu, L; Ghezzi, F; Manzione, L; Lauria, R; Breda, E; Alletti, DG; Ballardini, M; Vernaglia, A; Sorio, R; Tumolo, S; Musso, P; Magni, G; Pisano, C; Morabito, A. Poor outcome of elderly patients with platinum-sensitive recurrent ovarian cancer: results from the SOCRATES retrospective study. *Crit Rev Oncol Hematol*, 2009, 71(3), 233–241.

[13] Kanesvaran, R; Li, H; Koo, HN; Poon, D. Analysis of prognostic factors of comprehensive geriatric assessment and development of a clinical scoring system in elderly Asian patients with cancer. *J Clin Oncol*, 2011, 29(27), 3620–3627.

[14] PACE participants; Audisio, RA; Pope, D; Ramesh, HS; Gennari, R; van Leeuwen, BL; West, C; Corsini, G; Maffezzini, M; Hoekstra, HJ; Mobarak, D; Bozzetti, F; Colledan, M; Wildiers, H; Stotter, A; Capewell, A; Marshall, E. Shall we operate? Preoperative assessment in elderly cancer patients (PACE) can help. A SIOG surgical task force prospective study. *Crit Rev Oncol Hematol*, 2008, 65(2), 156–163.

[15] Tewari, KS; Java, JJ; Gatcliffe, TA; Bookman, MA; Monk, BJ. Chemotherapy-induced neutropenia as a biomarker of survival in advanced ovarian carcinoma: an exploratory study of the gynecologic oncology group. *Gynecol Oncol*, 2014, 133(3), 439-435.

[16] Falandry, C; Weber, B; Savoye, AM; Tinquaut, F; Tredan, O; Sevin, E; Stefani, L; Savinelli, F; Atlassi, M; Salvat, J; Ujade-Lauraine, E; Freyer, G. Development of a geriatric vulnerability score in elderly patients with advanced ovarian cancer treated with first line carboplatin; a GINECO prospective trial. *Ann Oncol*, 2013, 24(11), 2808–2813.

[17] Morgan, RJ; Jr. Alvarez, RD; Armstrong, DK; Burger, RA; Chen, LM; Copeland, L; Crispens, MA; Gershenson, DM; Gray, HJ; Hakam, A; Havrilesky, LJ; Johnston, C; Lele, S; Martin, L; Matulonis, UA; O'Malley, DM; Penson, RT; Powell, MA; Remmenga, SW; Sabbatini, P; Santoso, JT; Schink, JC; Teng, N; Werner, TL; Dwyer, MA; Hughes, M. National comprehensive cancer networks; Ovarian cancer, version 2.2013. *J Natl Compr Canc Netw.*, 2013, 11(10), 1199-1209.

[18] Chang, S; Bristow, RE. Evolution of surgical treatment paradigms for advanced-stage ovarian cancer: redefining optimal residual disease. *Gynecol Oncol*, 2012, 125(2), 483–492.

[19] Vergote, CG; Trope, F; Amant, F; Kristensen, GB; Ehlen, T; Johnson, N; Verheijen, RHM; Van der Burg, MEL; Lacave, AJ; Panici, PB; Kenter, GG; Casado, A; Mendiola, C; Coens, C; Verleye, L; Stuart, GCE; Pecorelli, S; Reed, NS. European Org Res Treatment and N. C. T. Grp 2010; Neoadjuvant chemotherapy or primary surgery in stage IIIC or IV ovarian cancer. *N Engl J Med*, 2010, 363(10), 943–993.

[20] Kehoe, S; Hook, J; Nankivell, M; Jayson, GC; Kitchener, H; Lopes, T; Luesley, D; Perren, T; Bannoo, S; Mascarenhas, M; Dobbs, S; Essapen, S; Twigg, J; Herod, J; McCluggage, G; Parmar, M; Swart, AM. Primary chemotherapy versus primary surgery for newly diagnosed advanced ovarian cancer (CHORUS): an open-label, randomised, controlled, non-inferiority trial. Lancet, Epub ahead of print 2015, pii: S0140-6736(14)62223-6.

[21] Forde, GK; Chang, J; Ziogas, A; Tewari, K; Bristow, RE. Costs of treatment for elderly women with advanced ovarian cancer in a Medicare population. *Gynecol Oncol.*, 2015, 137(3), 479-484.

[22] Wright, JD; Cande, AV; Tsui, J; Glied, SA; Burke, WM; Yu-Shiang, I; Neugut, AI; Herzog, TJ; Hershman, DL. Comparative effectiveness of upfront treatment strategies in elderly women with ovarian cancer. *Cancer*, 2014, 120(8), 1246–1254.

[23] Fairfield, K.M; Murray, K; Lucas, FL; Wierman, HR; Earle, CC; Trimble, EL; Small, L; Warren, JL. Completion of adjuvant chemotherapy and use of health services for older women with epithelial ovarian cancer. *J Clin Oncol.*, 2011, 29(29), 3921–3926.

[24] Tredan, O; Geay, JF; Touzet, S; Delva, R; Weber, B; Cretin, J; Provencal, J; Martin, J; Stefani, L; Pujade-Lauraine, E; Freyer, G. Groupe d'Investigateurs Nationaux pour l'Etude des Cancers Ovariens; Carboplatin/cyclophosphamide or carboplatin/paclitaxel in elderly patients with advanced ovarian cancer? Analysis of two consecutive trials from the Groupe d'Investigateurs Nationaux pour l'Etude des Cancers Ovariens. *Ann Oncol.*, 2007, 18(2) 256–262.

[25] Freyer, G; Geay JF; Touzet S; Provencal, J; Weber, B; Jacquin; JP; Ganem, G; Tubiana-Mathieu, N; Gisserot, O; Pujade-Lauraine, E. Comprehensive geriatric assessment predicts tolerance to chemotherapy and survival in elderly patients with advanced ovarian carcinoma: a GINECO study. *Ann Oncol*, 2005, 16(11), 1795–1800.

[26] Falandry, C; Weber, B; Savoye, AM; Tinquaut, F; Tredan, O; Sevin, E; Stefani, L; Savinelli, F; Atlassi, M; Salvat, J; Pujade-Lauraine, E; Freyer, G. Development of a geriatric vulnerability score in elderly patients with advanced ovarian cancer treated with first-line carboplatin: a GINECO prospective trial. *Ann Oncol.*, 2013, 24(11), 2808-2813.

[27] Pallis, AG; Hatse, S; Brouwers, B; Pawelec, G; Falandry, C; Wedding, U; Lago, LD; Repetto, L; Ring, A; Wildiers, H. Evaluating the physiological reserves of older patients with cancer: the value of potential biomarkers of aging? *J Geriatr Oncol.*, 2014, 5(2), 204-218.

[28] Sabatier, R; Calderon, B; Lambaudie, E; Chereau, E; Provansal, M; Cappiello, MA; Viens, P; Rousseau, F. Prognostic factors for ovarian epithelial cancer in the elderly: a case-control study. *Int J Gynecol Cancer.*, 2015, 25(5), 815-822.

[29] Vergote, CG; Trope, F; Amant, F; Kristensen, GB; Ehlen, T; Johnson, N; Verheijen, RH; van der Burg, ME; Lacave, AJ; Panici, PB; Kenter, GG; Casado, A; Mendiola, C; Coens, C; Verleye, L; Stuart, GC; Pecorelli, S; Reed, NS. European Organization for Research and Treatment of Cancer-Gynaecological Cancer Group; NCIC Clinical Trials Group; Neoadjuvant chemotherapy or primary surgery in stage IIIC or IV ovarian cancer. *N Engl J Med.*, 2010, 363(10), 943-953.

[30] Van Meurs, H.S; Tajik, P; Hof, MH; Vergote, I; Kenter, GG; Mol, BW; Buist, MR; Bossuyt, PM. Which patients benefit most from primary surgery or neoadjuvant chemotherapy in stage IIIC or IV ovarian cancer? An exploratory analysis of the European Organisation for Research and Treatment of Cancer 55971 randomised trial. *Eur J Cancer.*, 2013, 49(15), 3191–3201.

[31] Cascales Campos, P. Morbidity and mortality outcomes of cytoreductive surgery and hyperthermic intraperitoneal chemotherapy in patients with primary and recurrent advanced ovarian cancer. *Eur J Surg Oncol.*, 2014, 40(8), 970–975.

[32] Chua, TC; Robertson, G; Liauw, W; Farrell, R; Yan, TD; Morris, DL. Intraoperative hyperthermic intraperitoneal chemotherapy after cytoreductive surgery in ovarian cancer peritoneal carcinomatosis: systematic review of current results. *J Cancer Res Clin Oncol.*, 2009, 135(12) 1637–1645.

[33] Markman, M; Bundy, BN; Alberts, DS; Fowler, JM; Clark-Pearson, DL; Carson, LF; Wadler, S; Sickel, J. Phase III trial of standard-dose intravenous cisplatin plus paclitaxel versus moderately high-dose carboplatin followed by intravenous paclitaxel and intraperitoneal cisplatin in small-volume stage III ovarian carcinoma: an intergroup study of the Gynecologic Oncology Group, Southwestern Oncology Group, and Eastern Cooperative Oncology Group *J Clin Oncol*, 2001, 19(4), 1001–1007.

[34] Armstrong, DK; Bundy, B; Wenzel, L; Huang, HQ; Baergen, R; Lele, S; Copeland, LJ; Walker, JL; Burger, RA. Gynecologic Oncology Group; Intraperitoneal cisplatin and paclitaxel in ovarian cancer. *N Engl J Med*, 2006, 354(1), 34–43.

[35] Alberts, DS; Liu, PY; Hannigan, EV; O'Toole, R; Williams, SD; Young, JA; Franklin, EW; Clarke-Pearson, DL; Malviya, VK; DuBeshter, B. Intraperitoneal cisplatin plus intravenous cyclophosphamide versus intravenous cisplatin plus intravenous cyclophosphamide for stage III ovarian cancer. *N Engl J Med.*, 1996, 335(26), 1950.

[36] Fagotti, A; Costantini, B; Petrillo, M; Vizzielli, G; Fanfani, F; Margariti, PA; Turco, LC; Piovano, E; Scambia, G. Cytoreductive surgery plus HIPEC in platinum-sensitive recurrent ovarian cancer patients: a case–control study on survival in patients with two year follow-up. *Gynecol Oncol.*, 2012, 127(3), 502–505.

[37] Bakrin, N; Bereder, JM; Decullier, E; Classe, JM; Msika, S; Lorimier, G; Abboud, K; Meeus, P; Ferron, G; Quenet, F; Marchal, F; Gouy, S; Morice, P; Pomel, C; Pocard, M; Guyon, F; Porcheron, J; Glehen, O. FROGHI (FRench Oncologic and Gynecologic HIPEC) Group; Peritoneal carcinomatosis treated with cytoreductive surgery and Hyperthermic Intraperitoneal Chemotherapy (HIPEC) for advanced ovarian carcinoma: a French multicentre retrospective cohort study of 566 patients. *Eur J Surg Oncol.*, 2013, 39(12), 1435–1443.

[38] Delotte, J; Arias, T; Guerin, O; Boulahssass, R; Bereder, I; Bongain, A; Benchimol, D; Bereder, JM. Hyperthermic intraperitoneal chemotherapy for the treatment of recurrent ovarian cancer in elderly women. *Acta Obstetricia et Gynecologica Scandinavica.*, 2015, 94(4), 435–439.

[39] Cascales-Campos, P; Gil, J; Gil, E; Feliciangeli, E; López, V; Gonzalez, AG; Ruiz-Pardo, J; Nieto, A; Parrilla, P. Cytoreduction and HIPEC after neoadjuvant chemotherapy in stage IIIC–IV ovarian cancer. Critical analysis in elderly patients. *Eur J Obstet Gynecol Reprod Biol.*, 2014, 179(1), 88–93.

[40] Pignata, S; Ferrandina, G; Scarfone, G; Feliciangeli, E; López, V; Gonzalez, AG; Ruiz-Pardo, J; Nieto, A; Parrilla, P. Poor outcome of elderly patients with platinum-sensitive recurrent ovarian cancer: results from the SOCRATES retrospective study *Crit Rev Oncol Hematol.*, 2009, 71(3), 233–234.

[41] Pfisterer, J; Plante, M; Vergote, I; du Bois, A; Hirte, H; Lacave, AJ; Wagner, U; Stähle, A; Stuart, G; Kimmig, R; Olbricht, S; Le, T; Emerich, J; Kuhn, W; Bentley, J; Jackisch, C; Lück, HJ; Rochon, J; Zimmermann, AH; Eisenhauer, E; AGO-OVAR; NCIC CTG; EORTC GCG. Gemcitabine plus carboplatin compared with carboplatin in patients with platinum-sensitive recurrent ovarian cancer: an intergroup trial of the AGO-OVAR, the NCIC CTG, and the EORTC GCG. *J Clin Oncol*, 2006, 24(29), 4699–4707.

[42] Pujade-Lauraine, E; Wagner, U; Aavall-Lundqvist, E; Gebski, V; Heywood, M; Vasey, PA; Volgger, B; Vergote, I; Pignata, S; Ferrero, A; Sehouli, J; Lortholary, A; Kristensen, G; Jackisch, C; Joly, F; Brown, C; Le Fur, N; du Bois, A. Pegylated liposomal Doxorubicin and Carboplatin compared with Paclitaxel and Carboplatin for patients with platinum-sensitive ovarian cancer in late relapse. *J Clin Oncol*, 2010, 28(20), 3323–3329.

[43] Parmar, MK; Ledermann, JA; Colombo, N; du Bois, A; Delaloye, JF; Kristensen, GB; Wheeler, S; Swart, AM; Qian, W; Torri, V; Floriani, I; Jayson, G; Lamont, A; Tropé, C. ICON and AGO Collaborators; Paclitaxel plus platinum-based chemotherapy versus conventional platinum-based chemotherapy in women with relapsed ovarian cancer: the ICON4/AGO-OVAR-2.2 trial. *Lancet*, 2003, 361(9375), 2099–2106.

[44] Kurtz, JE; Kaminsky, MC; Floquet, A;Veillard, AS; Kimmig, R; Dorum, A; Elit, L; Buck, M; Petru, E; Reed, N; Scambia, G; Varsellona, N; Brown, C; Pujade-Lauraine, E. Gynecologic Cancer Intergroup; Ovarian cancer in elderly patients: carboplatin and pegylated liposomal doxorubicin versus carboplatin and paclitaxel in late relapse: a Gynecologic Cancer Intergroup (GCIG) CALYPSO sub-study. *Ann Oncol*, 2011, 22(11), 2417–2423.

[45] Tew, WP; Lichtman SM; Ovarian cancer in older women. *Semin Oncol.*, 2008, 35(6), 582–589.

[46] Gronlund, B; Hogdall, C; Hansen, HH; Engelholm SA. Performance status rather than age is the key prognostic factor in second-line treatment of elderly patients with epithelial ovarian carcinoma. *Cancer.*, 2002, 94(7), 1961–1967.

[47] Griffiths, RW; Zee, YJ; Evans, S; Mitchell, CL; Kumaran, GC; Welch, RS; Jayson, GC; Clamp, AR; Hasan, J. Outcomes after multiple lines of chemotherapy for platinum-resistant epithelial cancers of the ovary, peritoneum, and fallopian tube. *Int J Gynecol Cancer.*, 2011, 21(1), 58–65.

[48] Lewin, SN; Buttin, BN; Powell, MA; Gibb, RK; Rader, JS; Mutch, DG; Herzog, TJ. Resource utilization for ovarian cancer patients at the end of life: how much is too much? *Gynecol Oncol*, 2005, 99(2), 261–266.

[49] Kaye, SB; Lubinski, J; Matulonis, U; Ang, JE; Gourley, C; Karlan, BY; Amnon, A; Bell-McGuinn, KM; Chen, LM; Friedlander, M; Safra, T; Vergote, I; Wickens, M; Lowe, ES; Carmichael, J; Kaufman, B. Phase II, open-label, randomized, multicenter study comparing the efficacy and safety of olaparib, a poly (ADP-ribose) polymerase inhibitor, and pegylated liposomal doxorubicin in patients with BRCA1 or BRCA2 mutations and recurrent ovarian cancer. *J Clin Oncol*, 2012, 30(4), 372–379.

[50] Boyd, J; Sonoda, J; Federici, M; Bogomolniy, F; Rhei, E; Maresco, DL; Saigo, PE; Almadrones, LA; Barakat, RR; Brown, CL; Chi, DS; Curtin, JP; Poynor, EA; Hoskins, WJ; Clinicopathologic features of BRCA-linked and sporadic ovarian cancer. *JAMA.*, 2000, 283(17), 2260–2265.

[51] Burger, RA; Brady, MF; Bookman, MA; Fleming, GF; Monk, BJ; Huang, H; Mannel, RS; Homesley, HD; Fowler, J; Greer, BE; Boente, M; Birrer, MJ; Liang, SX. Gynecologic Oncology Group; Incorporation of bevacizumab in the primary treatment of ovarian cancer, *N Engl J Med*, 2011, 365(26), 2473–2483.

[52] Du Bois, A; Floquet, A; Kim, JW; Rau, J; del Campo, JM; Friedlander, M; Pignata, S; Fujiwara, K; Vergote, I; Colombo, N; Mirza, MR; Monk, BJ; Kimmig, R; Ray-Coquard, I; Zang, R; Diaz-Padilla, I; Baumann, KH; Mouret-Reynier, MA; Kim, JH;

Kurzeder, C; Lesoin, A; Vasey, P; Marth, C; Canzler, U; Scambia, G; Shimada, M; Calvert, P; Pujade-Lauraine, E; Kim, BG; Herzog, TJ; Mitrica, I; Schade-Brittinger, C; Wang, Q; Crescenzo, R; Harter, P. Incorporation of pazopanib in maintenance therapy of ovarian cancer. *J Clin Oncol*, 2014, 32(30), 3374-3382.

[53] Raja, FA; Griffin, CL; Qian, W; Hirte, H; Parmar, MK; Swart, AM; Ledermann, JA. Initial toxicity assessment of ICON6: a randomised trial of cediranib plus chemotherapy in platinum-sensitive relapsed ovarian cancer. *Br J Cancer.*, 2011, 105(7), 884-889.

[54] Liu, JF; Tolaney, SM; Birrer, M; Fleming, GF; Buss, MK; Dahlberg, SE; Lee, H; Whalen, C; Tyburski, K; Winer, E; Ivy, P; Matulonis, UA. A Phase 1 trial of the poly(ADP-ribose) polymerase inhibitor olaparib (AZD2281) in combination with the anti-angiogenic cediranib (AZD2171) in recurrent epithelial ovarian or triple-negative breast cancer. *Eur J Cancer.*, 2013, 49(14), 2972-2978.

[55] Wong, H; Tang, YF; Yao TJ; Chiu, J; Leung, R; Chan, P; Cheung, TT; Chan, AC; Pang, RW; Poon, R; Fan, ST; Yau, T. The outcomes and safety of single-agent sorafenib in the treatment of elderly patients with advanced hepatocellular carcinoma (HCC). *Oncologist.*, 2011; 16(12),1721–1728.

[56] Gonsalves, W; Ganti, AK. Targeted anti-cancer therapy in the elderly. *Crit Rev Oncol Hematol.*, 2011, 78(3), 227–242.

[57] Tew, WP; Fleming, GF. Treatment of ovarian cancer in the older woman. *Gynecol Oncol.*, 2015, 136(1), 136-142.

# INDEX

## #



## A

## B



## C

## D

## E



## F

## I

## J



## K



## L



## M

## N

## Q

## R



## S

## T

## U



## V

## W



## X



## Y



## Z